COCAINE: SCIENTIFIC AND SOCIAL DIMENSIONS

The Ciba Foundation is an international scientific and educational charity. It was established in 1947 by the Swiss chemical and pharmaceutical company of CIBA Limited — now CIBA-GEIGY Limited. The Foundation operates independently in London under English trust law.

The Ciba Foundation exists to promote international cooperation in biological, medical and chemical research. It organizes about eight international multidisciplinary symposia each year on topics that seem ready for discussion by a small group of research workers. The papers and discussions are published in the Ciba Foundation symposium series. The Foundation also holds many shorter meetings (not published), organized by the Foundation itself or by outside scientific organizations. The staff always welcome suggestions for future meetings.

The Foundation's house at 41 Portland Place, London W1N 4BN, provides facilities for meetings of all kinds. Its Media Resource Service supplies information to journalists on all scientific and technological topics. The library, open five days a week to any graduate in science or medicine, also provides information on scientific meetings throughout the world and answers general enquiries on biomedical and chemical subjects. Scientists from any part of the world may stay in the house during working visits to London.

Ciba Foundation Symposium 166

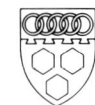

COCAINE: SCIENTIFIC AND SOCIAL DIMENSIONS

A Wiley-Interscience Publication

1992

JOHN WILEY & SONS

Chichester · New York · Brisbane · Toronto · Singapore

©Ciba Foundation 1992

Published in 1992 by John Wiley & Sons Ltd.
Baffins Lane, Chichester
West Sussex PO19 1UD, England

All rights reserved.

No part of this book may be reproduced by any means,
or transmitted, or translated into a machine language
without the written permission of the publisher.

Other Wiley Editorial Offices

John Wiley & Sons, Inc., 605 Third Avenue,
New York, NY 10158-0012, USA

Jacaranda Wiley Ltd, G.P.O. Box 859, Brisbane,
Queensland 4001, Australia

John Wiley & Sons (Canada) Ltd, 22 Worcester Road,
Rexdale, Ontario M9W 1L1, Canada

John Wiley & Sons (SEA) Pte Ltd, 37 Jalan Pemimpin 05-04,
Block B, Union Industrial Building, Singapore 2057

Suggested series entry for library catalogues:
Ciba Foundation Symposia

Ciba Foundation Symposium 166
x + 305 pages, 31 figures, 20 tables

British Library Cataloguing in Publication Data
A catalogue record for this book is
available from the British Library

ISBN 0 471 93179 9

Phototypeset by Dobbie Typesetting Limited, Tavistock, Devon.
Printed and bound in Great Britain by Biddles Ltd., Guildford.

Contents

Symposium on Cocaine: Scientific and Social Dimensions, held at the Ciba Foundation, London, 20–22 July 1991

Editors: Gregory R. Bock (Organizer) and Julie Whelan

Griffith Edwards Cocaine in perspective 1

David F. Musto Cocaine's history, especially the American experience 7
Discussion 14

James C. Anthony Epidemiological research on cocaine use in the USA 20
Discussion 33

Juan Carlos Negrete Cocaine problems in the coca-growing countries of South America 40
Discussion 50

Charles D. Kaplan, Bert Bieleman and **Warren D. TenHouten** Are there 'casual users' of cocaine? 57
Discussion 73

Michael J. Kuhar Molecular pharmacology of cocaine: a dopamine hypothesis and its implications 81
Discussion 89

H. Christian Fibiger, Anthony G. Phillips and **Erin E. Brown** The neurobiology of cocaine-induced reinforcement 96
Discussion 111

Neal L. Benowitz How toxic is cocaine? 125
Discussion 143

William L. Woolverton Determinants of cocaine self-administration by laboratory animals 149
Discussion 161

Marian W. Fischman and **Richard W. Foltin** Self-administration of cocaine by humans: a laboratory perspective 165
Discussion 173

General discussion AIDS and HIV infection in cocaine users (**Don C. Des Jarlais**) 181

Herbert D. Kleber Treatment of cocaine abuse: pharmacotherapy 195
Discussion 200

Charles P. O'Brien, A. Thomas McLellan, Arthur Alterman and **Anna Rose Childress** Psychotherapy for cocaine dependence 207
Discussion 216

Reese T. Jones Alternative strategies 224
Discussion 232

Alan Maynard The economics of drug use and abuse 242
Discussion 251

Harold Kalant Formulating policies on the non-medical use of cocaine 261
Discussion 272

Brenda Almond Drug use and abuse: the ethical issues 277
Discussion 284

Griffith Edwards Summing-up 294

Index of contributors 296

Subject index 298

Participants

Brenda Almond Social Values Research Centre, University of Hull, Hull HU6 7RX, UK

James C. Anthony Department of Mental Hygiene, The Johns Hopkins University School of Hygiene & Public Health, 624 North Broadway, Baltimore, MD 21205, USA

Robert L. Balster Department of Pharmacology & Toxicology, Medical College of Virginia, Virginia Commonwealth University, Box 613, MCV Station, Richmond, VA 23298, USA

Neal L. Benowitz Division of Clinical Pharmacology & Experimental Therapeutics, Department of Medicine, Building 30, 5th Floor, San Francisco General Hospital Medical Center, 1001 Potrero Avenue, San Francisco, CA 94110, USA

Don C. Des Jarlais Beth Israel Medical Center/Narcotic and Drug Research, Inc., 11 Beach Street, New York, NY 10013, USA

Griffith Edwards *(Chairman)* Addiction Research Unit, National Addiction Centre, Addiction Sciences Building, 4 Windsor Walk, London SE5 8AF, UK

H. Christian Fibiger Division of Neurological Sciences, Department of Psychiatry, University of British Columbia, 2255 Westbrook Mall, Vancouver BC, Canada V6T 1Z3

Marian W. Fischman Department of Psychiatry & Behavioral Sciences, The Johns Hopkins University School of Medicine, The Houck Building East-2, 600 N Wolfe Street, Baltimore, MD 21205, USA

Dean R. Gerstein Washington Office, National Opinion Research Center (NORC), University of Chicago, 1350 Connecticut Avenue, Suite 500, Washington, DC 20036, USA

Jerome H. Jaffe Office for Treatment Improvement, Alcohol Drug Abuse & Mental Health Administration, Rockwall II, 10th Floor, 5600 Fishers Lane, Rockville, MD 20857, USA

Reese T. Jones Langley Porter Psychiatric Institute, Department of Psychiatry, University of California, 401 Parnassus Avenue, San Francisco, CA 94143-0984, USA

Harold Kalant Department of Pharmacology, Addiction Research Group, University of Toronto, Medical Sciences Building, Toronto, Ontario, Canada M5S 1A8

Charles D. Kaplan Schepenstraat 87-b, 3039 ND Rotterdam, The Netherlands

Herbert D. Kleber* Office of National Drug Control Policy, Executive Office of the President, Washington, DC 20500, USA

Michael J. Kuhar Neuroscience Branch, Addiction Research Center, PO Box 5180, Baltimore, MD 21224, USA

Alan Maynard Centre for Health Economics, University of York, Heslington, York YO1 5DD, UK

Mark H. Moore John F. Kennedy School of Government, Harvard University, 79 John F. Kennedy Street, Cambridge, MA 02138, USA

David F. Musto Child Study Center (Psychiatry) & History of Medicine, Yale University School of Medicine, 333 Cedar Street, New Haven, CT 06510, USA

Juan Carlos Negrete Department of Psychiatry, McGill University, Montreal General Hospital & Drug Dependence Unit, 1650 Cedar Avenue, Montreal, Quebec, Canada H3G 1A4

Charles P. O'Brien Department of Psychiatry, University of Pennsylvania, Veterans Affairs Medical Center, Philadelphia, PA 19104/6178, USA

**Present address*: Professor Herbert D. Kleber, Department of Psychiatry, Columbia University College of Physicians & Surgeons, 722 W 168th Street, Box 66, New York, NY 10032, USA.

John Strang Drug Dependence Clinical Research & Treatment Unit, The Maudsley Hospital, London SE5 8AZ, UK

Ambros Uchtenhagen Department of Social Psychiatry, Psychiatric University Hospital, Miltärstrasse 8, PO Box 904, CH-8021 Zürich, Switzerland

William L. Woolverton Department of Pharmacological & Physiological Sciences, Drug Abuse Research Center, University of Chicago, 947 E 58th Street, Box 271, Chicago, IL 60637, USA

Cocaine in perspective

Griffith Edwards

Addiction Research Unit, National Addiction Centre, Institute of Psychiatry, London SE5 8AF, UK

> *Abstract.* In a medical text published in 1883, Dr Benjamin Ward Richardson FRS denounced the evils of tea drinking, suggesting that it commonly gave rise to an 'Extremely nervous semi-hysterical condition'. That this distinguished Victorian physician could take such a view invites a sensitivity toward the *perspective* within which any debate on drugs is conducted—the historical, cultural and professional assumptions which will colour views as to what needs to be explained and how explanation is to be accomplished. The reality and significance of 'perspective' is further illustrated by examples drawn from contemporary literature which contrast the laboratory and social science approaches to study of cocaine. No one narrow disciplinary perspective on the cocaine problem will suffice; the challenge is to build bridges.
>
> *1992 Cocaine: scientific and social dimensions. Wiley, Chichester (Ciba Foundation Symposium 166) p 1–6*

In an influential text entitled *Diseases of Modern Life*, published in 1883, Dr Benjamin Ward Richardson, FRS, FRCP, Honorary Member of the American Philosophical Society, and bearer of many other distinctions, alluded to several exotic forms of drug misuse which lie outside the remit of the present symposium. He referred to 'The swallowers of haschisch of Damascus and the East, the amanatine drinkers of Kamschatka; the arsenic eaters of Styria . . . '. But he also dealt with one of the more pervasive stimulants of his and our time, and thus I feel at liberty to quote him a little more fully. He wrote:

'Some functional nervous derangements are excited by fluids commonly consumed with, or as foods. *Tea* taken in excess is one of these disturbing agents. The symptoms . . . are . . . a lowness of spirits amounting to hypochondriacal despondency.

In poverty-stricken districts, amongst the women who take tea at every meal, this extremely nervous semi-hysterical condition from the action of tea is all but universal. In London and other fashionable centres in which the custom of tea-drinking in the afternoon has lately been revived . . . these same nervous symptoms have been developed in the richer classes of society, who, unfortunately, too often seek to counteract the mischief by resorting to alcohol stimulants. Thus one evil breeds another that is worse.'

The perspective from which Richardson developed these ideas can only be understood within the wider context of 19th century medical thinking, with its mixture of moralism and simple faith in science, its campaigns for public health and its fervid belief in the dangers of social degeneration, and its frequently expressed notion that psychologically women were specially vulnerable creatures. Richardson believed in the virtue of cold baths and warned against idleness. In short, he saw the human condition from a Victorian perspective.

The purpose of a chairman's introduction is that of a prologue before the curtains go up on the play. What I want to suggest is that the question of the perspective within which we debate drug problems is important. Let us move from the 19th century argument by moving from Richardson and tea, to a more recent text and the very centre of our present concerns, cocaine. *Cocaine 1980* (Jeri 1980) is a proceedings volume emanating from a meeting held in Lima, in Peru: Marian Fischman (who is taking part in the present symposium), Chris Johanson and Charles Schuster were among the participants. Here is a quotation from a chapter in that book on 'The evaluation of cocaine using an animal model of drug use', written jointly by Schuster and Johanson:

> 'The relevance of data from animal studies to the human problem of drug abuse is based upon the validity of two assumptions: (1) drugs that are reinforcers in infrahuman organisms can serve the same function in humans, and (2) humans and animals are comparable in their sensitivity to the effects, including the toxic ones, of the self administered drug.'

There is nothing in Schuster and Johanson's recently stated scientific position from which any of us is likely to dissent. Let us, though, turn the pages onwards in these same conference proceedings to the chapter by Fernando Cabieses (1980) on 'Ethnological aspects of coca and cocaine':

> 'The author reviews ethnological knowledge about the habit of coca chewing, pointing out the lack of scientific reasons to support repressive and eradiction laws. . . . The act to share coca and chew it, jointly with other people, is an important event which seals the relation of brotherhood and confidence among the participants . . . the factors which have caused condemnation of coca throughout the last four centuries, do not exist and have never existed among the natives. There always have been interests originated in the conflict between the occidental and the Andean culture.'

Here again, we are likely to agree with the author. We agree with Schuster and Johanson and the perspective of the laboratory scientist, and we also agree with, but perhaps feel a little threatened by, Cabieses' hint that the laboratory view—high science, the view from North America—is blind to certain larger realities. Debate on cocaine invites more than one perspective.

If I can group together several different sciences, one highly important viewpoint from which we shall certainly be invited to see these issues over the next few days might, in shorthand, be described as that of the 'laboratory scientist'. Under that heading can be put together behavioural pharmacology, the study of the biological basis of reward mechanisms, the molecular pharmacology of cocaine, and so on. The scientific credentials of such approaches are assured, their funding is relatively generous, and their technical sophistication is enviable. Their unit of analysis extends over a spectrum running from the molecule to the laboratory animal or volunteer experimental subject.

A second perspective might be labelled that of the social scientist, including the historian and the economist. Here the data sets are often dubious, the inferences often outrun the data, and the investigators seek to deal with everything which goes beyond the point where the sensibly cautious laboratory scientist stops. These kinds of investigators do, though, employ a broader-angled lens than their laboratory colleagues. They will see the peasant in the Andean landscape, and surviving in the hard conditions of the *alto plano*, chewing coca and 'establishing brotherhood', rather than focusing down on the synapse or the neurotransmitter.

A third perspective which is going to enter our debates is that of medicine. In some ways, medicine is a bridge between the laboratory and the social science view, if only a rather rickety pontoon construction. Medicine values laboratory science, but is lost (and damned) if it ever forgets the social dimension. As Virchow put it, 'Medicine is a social science in its very marrow'.

In reality this symposium will play host not to just two or three perspectives, but to as many viewpoints as there are individual participants in the room—we each bring to this symposium our own lumber of assumptions. Let me end this prologue by throwing down two modest challenges to the players in the play which is shortly to begin.

(1) Firstly, rather than dismissing Benjamin Ward Richardson as a quaint figure of his distant time, can we, with his views on tea drinking in mind, identify the influences which threaten to dictate and distort our own perceptions of the cocaine issue? What contextual values, given by our wider cultures and the cultures of our professional training, shape our views as to what here has to be explained, how it is to be explained, the likely nature of explanation, and our rights as explainers?

(2) The second challenge relates to the possibility of building bridges between different perspectives. As has already been emphasized, what is both fascinating and difficult about the study of drug problems is that they do not allow retreat to the comfort of any one dominant and assured perspective. It would be all too easy to conduct the symposium in terms of a debate which switched from one alternative perspective to another with polite nods, but no meeting points. The difficulty in finding common ground is not going to be overcome by recourse

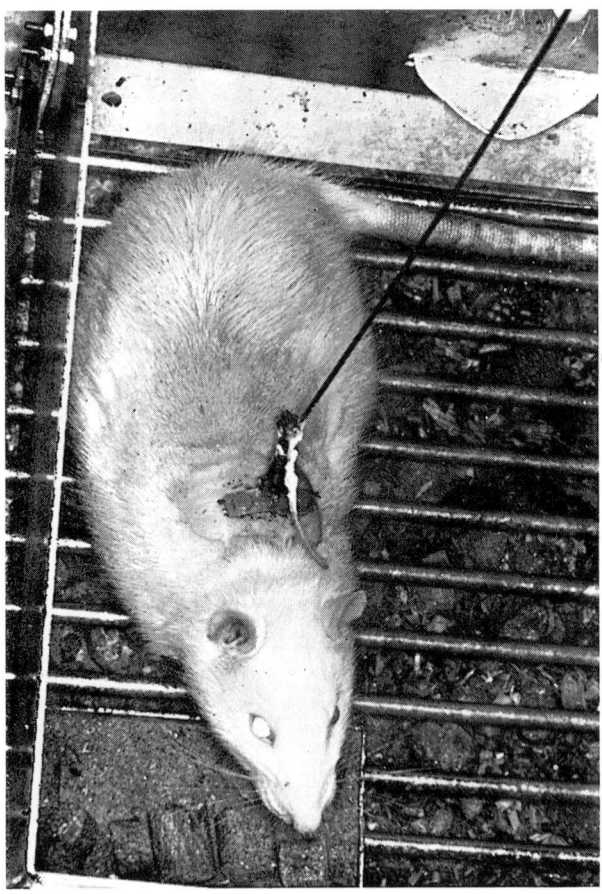

FIG. 1. A chronic preparation permitting intravenous self-administration of drugs by rats. A flexible stainless steel harness is attached to a piece of needle tubing connected to a remote infusion pump. The other end of the needle tubing is cemented to silicone rubber tubing which runs subcutaneously and was inserted into the external jugular vein. (From Thompson & Pickens 1969 with permission of Churchill Livingstone.)

to easy platitudes about the need for multidisciplinary research. Let's, at this point, look at just two images which suggest that a platitudinous approach to bridge-building is unlikely to suffice (Figs. 1 and 2).

How are we, in any honest way, to deal with such disparate images, other than by turning a blind or dismissive intellectual eye to the one or to the other? The challenge to this symposium is that of trying to develop a perspective which can contain both images, and of actively and intentionally seeking connections.

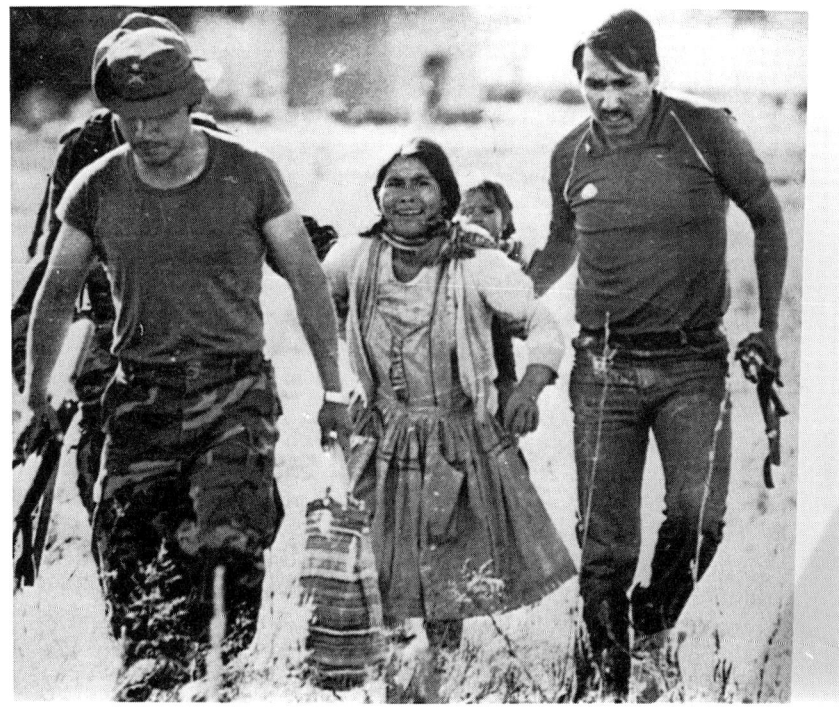

FIG. 2. Peasant woman arrested for involvement in coca paste-making activities in the Upper Cochabamba Valley in Bolivia, in 1985. (From Healy 1986.)

So much for the prologue and its invitations to perspective. The play now begins.

Acknowledgement

I am grateful to Maria Pacan for secretarial assistance.

References

Cabieses F 1980 Ethnological aspects of coca and cocaine. In: Jeri FR (ed) Cocaine 1980. Proceedings of the international seminar on medical and sociological aspects of coca and cocaine. (Pan American Health Office/WHO and the International Narcotics Management, Lima) Pacific Press, Lima, p 246

Healy K 1986 The boom within the crisis: some recent effects of foreign cocaine markets on Bolivian rural society and economy. In: Pacini D, Franquemont C (eds) Coca and cocaine: effects on people and policy in Latin America. Proceedings of the conference: The coca leaf and its derivatives—biology, society and policy. Cultural Survival and Latin American Studies Program, Cornell University, Ithaca, NY, p 101–143

Jeri FR (ed) 1980 Cocaine 1980. Proceedings of the international seminar on medical and sociological aspects of coca and cocaine. (Pan American Health Office /WHO and the International Narcotics Management, Lima) Pacific Press, Lima (pp 264)

Richardson BW 1883 Diseases of modern life. Fowler & Wells, New York

Schuster CR, Johanson CE 1980 The evaluation of cocaine using an animal model of drug abuse. In: Jeri FR (ed) Cocaine 1980. Proceedings of the international seminar on medical and sociological aspects of coca and cocaine. (Pan American Health Office/WHO and the International Narcotics Management, Lima) Pacific Press, Lima, p 29-39

Thompson T, Pickens R 1969 Drug self-administration and conditioning. In: Steinberg H (ed) Scientific basis of drug dependence: a symposium. Churchill, London, p 177-198

Cocaine's history, especially the American experience

David F. Musto

Child Study Center (Psychiatry) and the History of Medicine, Yale University School of Medicine, 333 Cedar Street, New Haven, CT 06511, USA

Abstract. The history of cocaine in America can be traced to the late 19th century. After the discovery of its physiological and psychological effects, cocaine figured in consumables as diverse as hay fever remedies, local anaesthetics and soft drinks. The development of its different usages as well as eventual control of its use through restrictive legislation followed a different pattern in America from that in Europe. In the United States, national laws to control drugs faced constitutional obstacles until the era of World War I. Initially acclaimed as an ideal tonic, within two decades of its introduction in the mid 1880s cocaine was perceived as an extremely dangerous drug. By the 1930s cocaine had declined in use and in the 1960s, when it gradually emerged again, almost no public memory existed of the earlier 'epidemic'. Once again this substance evolved into a threatening and seductive hazard with some similarities to the earlier episode.

1992 Cocaine: scientific and social dimensions. Wiley, Chichester (Ciba Foundation Symposium 166) p 7–19

Cocaine first appeared on the commercial market in the mid 1880s. In earlier decades the appeal of cocaine in the form of extracts from the coca leaf had become increasingly popular. The best-known of these extracts was *Vin Mariani*, a coca wine product that began to be produced in France before 1870. French coca wines, of which Mariani's was the most prominent, developed a European and American following that stimulated the development of other products, one of which evolved to become Coca-Cola, a non-alcoholic coca drink that eclipsed its inspiration in world-wide favour (Helfand 1988, Kahn 1960).

Mariani's wine was advocated for lassitude, poor appetite, melancholy—in short, as a general tonic for the body and mind. In the era of neurasthenia, the preparation became a common remedy and was so recommended by Dr Gilles de la Tourette, among others. Coca extract was not confined to restoring debility, but it was also considered an aid to improve the normal state. Writers, inventors, singers, athletes, painters and sculptors sang praise (Mariani 1901). In the late 19th century an exhibition at Leamington Spa in England not only gave Mariani's wine a gold medal and diploma, but named it the 'wine for athletes'.

In Mariani's own publications its use in athletics is clearly promoted. In 1896 it was reported: 'Professional bicyclists and athletes, after careful trials of our and preparation of others . . . invariably give the preference to our Coca preparations'. It is noteworthy that in this early phase of cocaine's use, the assumption prevailed in Mariani's publications that athletes would naturally seek out the most effective aids to performance. This point of view—in such contrast to our attitude today—is supported by a list of athlete-customers of the 1890s who employed his invigorating wine (Mariani 1896).

The clergy likewise valued the wine. Pope Leo XIII awarded Angelo Mariani a gold medal; Cardinal LaVigerie, Primate of Africa, wrote that 'Vin Mariani gives to my "White Fathers", sons of Europe, the courage and strength to civilize Asia and Africa'. A Capuchin priest gave the wine credit for his ability to preach 512 times in one year. Anyone in a religious vocation or operating an orphanage received a discount on their purchase of the tonic.

In 1892 Thomas Edison sent his photograph to be included in Mariani's compilation of testimonials. Charles Gounod sent Mariani an autograph score of the Soldier's Chorus from *Faust*, but with words praising Vin Mariani. Jules Verne acclaimed it. The Prime Minister of France, Félix Méline, announced he had slightly adjusted his anti-alcohol principles so he could drink the elixir, while his Minister of Justice claimed it made each imbiber a better man and his Minister of the Interior attributed the strength of the Cabinet to the fact that all its members drank Mariani's wine (Mariani 1901).

Mariani's preparations, including a wine, elixir, pastilles and tea, and other less famous concoctions, helped prepare the way for the welcome for pure cocaine in the 1880s. Already in the United States extracts of coca were reported to be a cure for alcoholism and morphine addiction (Huse 1880). This is one of the attributes of cocaine that drew Sigmund Freud's attention to it in 1884: he was seeking a cure for the morphine addiction of his friend Ernst von Fleischl-Marxow. Freud was also interested in the ability of cocaine to increase endurance. Dr Theodor Aschenbrandt had already investigated this characteristic on a battalion of the Bavarian artillery in 1883, using pure cocaine hydrochloride produced by Merck & Company (Aschenbrandt 1883). This energizing feature of coca leaves had been persuasively argued in 1876 by Professor Sir Robert Christison in Britain. Professor Christison, at age 76 and while President of the British Medical Association, found he could walk 15 miles and not become fatigued after chewing a quarter-ounce of coca leaves (Christison 1876). Still, from Freud's perspective, Europe lagged in its use of coca and cocaine. He saw 'some promise of widespread recognition and use of coca preparations in North America, while in Europe doctors scarcely know them by name' (Freud 1885).

One reason for the differing receptions and uses of cocaine can be found by comparing the legal status of the drug and the extent of professional organization in the United States with that in Europe. I am cautious about commenting on

European practices and laws regarding substances like cocaine in the 19th century, for this is an area in which extensive research remains to be done, but I will make some general comments. First, the legal status of cocaine in the United States made it more easily available than in Europe. Aschenbrandt and Freud obtained their cocaine from pharmacists who had been supplied by Merck of Darmstadt. German pharmacy laws were careful to restrict powerful drugs to pharmacies and physicians. In Britain, cocaine apparently fell under the Pharmacy Act of 1868 which limited the availability of certain drugs to pharmacists and physicians. In order to obtain a concentrated or pure form of substances like cocaine, the consumer would be required to be known to a registered pharmacist, to sign a registry and to receive the chemical in a bottle prominently labelled 'poison'. Over-the-counter remedies containing small amounts of cocaine, such as 'medicated wines', could be sold at licensed premises, but these were in forms that did not permit inhalation or injection. The possibility of addiction from these mixtures existed, but the likelihood was small compared to that from pure cocaine salts or injectable solutions. Certainly, after the mid 1880s, cocaine spilled out of professional channels into other hands, but the legal and traditional contexts of availability were the professions of pharmacy and medicine (Musto 1987).

In the United States, however, there existed no national pharmacy or medical laws and the health professions were only in the early stage of organization. Laws controlling the practice of pharmacy and medicine were the responsibility of the several States, according to the contemporary interpretation of the United States Constitution. At the beginning, in 1884, cocaine fell under no law controlling its access in the United States. Furthermore, no law controlled advertising claims for cocaine. The aura of enthusiasm that surrounded cocaine's entry into US commerce, as well as the actual euphoriant effect of the drug, rapidly spread cocaine's use throughout the United States (Musto 1989). As an example of cocaine's entry into everyday life in America, one could note that by 1886 the drug was chosen the official remedy of the United States Hay Fever Association (Hammond 1887b). A former Surgeon General of the Army and a prominent neurologist, Dr William A. Hammond, promoted a coca wine that he boasted had four times more cocaine per ounce than a popular foreign product (Hammond 1887a). Cocaine appealed to Americans and they had far more legal access to it than Europeans.

So far the stimulant properties of cocaine have been emphasized. There were, of course, other specific medical uses which created little controversy. The first of these was described by one of Freud's colleagues, Dr Karl Koller, who demonstrated in 1884 the ability of cocaine to anaesthetize the surface of the eye (Koller 1884). Soon Dr William Stewart Halsted, then a physician in New York, began experimenting on himself and others with injections of cocaine in his attempt to determine the value of cocaine as a local anaesthetic. He and his colleagues were successful in establishing the ability of injections near peripheral nerves to block pain conduction, but the penalty was addiction to cocaine and a profound deterioration of professional ability. Halsted later became Surgeon-in-Chief of the new Johns Hopkins Hospital, but only after a difficult period of treatment that separated him from cocaine. He then started taking morphine, possibly to overcome the desire for cocaine, became addicted to morphine, and remained a morphine user for the remainder of his life (Olch 1975).

Halsted was not the only casualty to cocaine in the early years of its introduction. Compilations of complications appeared in leading medical journals (Brower 1886, Mattison 1887). Yet cocaine continued to be defended by prominent physicians who ridiculed the fear that cocaine had unusual dangers. Dr Hammond has been mentioned. He tried cocaine on himself in large doses and recovered. He assured his readers that the cocaine habit was no more severe than that of coffee or tea, while the unique properties of cocaine were remarkably helpful (Hammond 1887a).

The extravagant claims for cocaine made by professional leaders such as Hammond may have had more impact in the United States, where the public had greater access to the drug, than in Europe, where the medical and pharmacy professions held a closer rein on cocaine's availability. Whatever the reason, it is impressive in retrospect that lurid examples of cocaine's dangers at the very beginning of its availability did not prevent its use from spreading to the extent that 25 years later cocaine would be described by an official government report as the most serious drug problem ever confronted by the United States (Wright 1910).

In the decades after cocaine's introduction, two levels of availability eventually emerged. As laws were being written in reaction to easy access, beginning with local and State legislation and finally in 1914 at the national level, the drug was sold illicitly. Studies of the illicit market in New York City between 1907 and 1914 suggest that the unit sale on the street was commonly one to two grains, or approximately 100 mg. This would be sold as a powder in an envelope for a typical price of 25 cents. This illicit price was roughly equivalent to the hourly wage of an average industrial worker. Curiously, in the second American cocaine epidemic, the price of cocaine on the street in the late 1980s was about the same for the same amount of substance—an hour's wage for 100 mg (Musto 1990).

In the licit market, the arena of French coca wine, Coca-Cola, and some other forms of cocaine such as chocolate cocaine tablets compounded by your local pharmacist, the typical unit dose was much smaller. With regard to Coca-Cola, we know only the amount of cocaine contained in a bottle in 1900, the last year of its presence. It was one four-hundredth per cent, or 2.5 mg per 100 ml (Coca-Cola Bottling Co. of Shreveport v. Coca-Cola: 1983). For a six ounce bottle this would be about 4.5 mg. I am informed by an expert on clinical cocaine use that this amount is at the low end of perception by a person who does not use large amounts of cocaine—that is, an average person. Also, Coca-Cola at that time contained caffeine which added its stimulating effect to the small amount of cocaine. Interestingly, recent animal studies suggest that cocaine's impact is potentiated by caffeine (Schenk et al 1989–1990).

The unnamed foreign coca wine alluded to by Dr Hammond had, he complained, only a half-grain of cocaine to the pint. Taking 1½ ounces as the measure of a wineglass, the amount of cocaine in the recommended dose would be 3 mg. In 1892 a formula appeared in *The Chemist and Druggist* for chocolate cocaine tablets. This called for dividing three grains into 48 tablets, giving each tablet 4 mg of cocaine (The Chemist and Druggist 1892). In Britain a popular 'medicated wine', Hall's Wine, contained one grain of cocaine in 26 ounces, or 4 mg in a 1½ ounce wineglass (House of Commons 1914). One could say that about 4 mg in the unit dose was probably the minimum amount of cocaine in easily available compounds. An analysis of coca wines in 1886 reported a range of 5 to 12 mg of cocaine per ounce (Mariani's wine was recorded as 8 mg per ounce) (The Druggists Circular 1886). The range, then, for popular tonics was from 3 mg to 18 mg in the single dose. In the medicated wines it should be noted the cocaine was in a solution containing about 15% absolute alcohol.

These everyday consumables promoted the positive features of cocaine as an invigorating tonic, but gradually the image of cocaine changed in American society. The alarm caused by cocaine appears to have been linked not to the tonics, but to the inhalation or injection of pure cocaine. From an expensive medicine in the first few years of commercial production, cocaine fell in cost and expanded in distribution (Musto 1990). And yet, in spite of the accumulating record of personal tragedies associated with cocaine use, about 20 years passed before New York State resolved to bring the public's easy access to cocaine under control. Under public pressure, Assemblyman Alfred E. Smith (two decades later the Democratic candidate for the presidency of the United States) introduced a Bill into the New York State legislature that would give physicians and pharmacists control over cocaine. Enacted in 1907, the law did not limit the amount of cocaine the health professionals could provide. The assumption of the law was that the good judgement of the professionals would effectively curb irresponsible use.

As indicated above, an illicit street market was operating after passage of the anti-cocaine law and it appears to have been essentially unaffected by legal access via physicians' prescriptions. For seven years the anti-cocaine laws were strengthened in New York State, and they then were matched by the first federal anti-cocaine law, the Harrison Act of 1914. The Harrison Act also dealt with opiates of which small amounts were allowed in over-the-counter remedies, but for cocaine no amount was permitted without a prescription (Musto 1990).

Cocaine had moved in the 30 years after 1884 from a tonic proclaimed to be without adverse effects to a drug under the most severe restrictions of any substance still permitted for medical purposes. The 1920s were punctuated by cocaine scandals in Hollywood and other dramatic revelations, yet the trend appears to have been downward by the 1930s. The New York City Mayor's Committee on Addiction reported in 1930 that cocaine addiction was no longer a problem, although it had been a serious one 20 years before (Mayor's Committee 1930). The level of cocaine fell so low that by the 1950s it was cited by narcotic law enforcement authorities as an outstanding success of that earlier 'war on drugs' (Harney & Cross 1973).

Cocaine began to reappear in the United States in the late 1960s, as the nation entered another era of drug toleration. Marijuana rapidly increased in use, particularly among youth, and other drugs appeared, including LSD. The similarity in response to cocaine's introduction to the United States 80 years earlier is striking. Cocaine was again seen as a tonic, a harmless, non-addictive lift for everyday life that, for some perverse reason, in 1970 forgotten by almost everyone, was restricted by the most severe penalties. If in the 1880s Dr Hammond calmly compared cocaine use to the tea or coffee habit, one could read a century later that the pattern of cocaine's intranasal use was similar to that of 'peanuts or potato chips' (Van Dyke & Byck 1982)*.

Once again, starting out expensive, cocaine use signified sophistication and the ultimate euphoria. During this time one could locate accounts of cocaine's dangers, but experts and the media commonly adopted a relaxed attitude towards cocaine. In 1980, one prominent psychiatric textbook took cognizance of those who abused cocaine, but assured its readers that use of cocaine two or three times a week was probably safe (Grinspoon & Bakalar 1980). When 'crack', a smokable form of cocaine, appeared in the United States in about 1985, the intense desire for the drug among users and its low cost alarmed the American public. Cocaine laws, which had been softened as a result of widespread use, were now hardened and were included with other anti-drug legislation in two major compendia, the Anti-Drug Abuse Acts of 1986 and 1988.

We have not seen the eclipse of cocaine in the United States and we cannot echo the words of the New York Mayor's Committee of 60 years ago that cocaine addiction used to be a problem, but we have seen enough over the past 25 years to make some preliminary comparisons between the two episodes.

The major similarity is the initial enthusiastic acceptance of cocaine followed many years later by an intense public rejection of the drug in any amount. It is noteworthy that public memory of the earlier epidemic had faded to a degree that optimistic claims for cocaine in the early 1970s were unaffected by past condemnation of the drug. The loss of public memory for the earlier era of disillusionment with cocaine is itself a useful research topic.

A second characteristic is the time required for the transition from tolerance to intolerance of cocaine. About 20 years passed between the introduction of cocaine in the mid 1880s and the Al Smith anti-cocaine law of New York State,

---

*Dr Byck informs me that this phrase was added by an editor, and that it did not appear in the text submitted and does not appear in the authorized reprint of the article.

and 10 more years before the federal government prohibited cocaine except for medical purposes. With regard to the Harrison Act, one should note that a federal law affecting local practitioners was extremely difficult to frame, because of constitutional restrictions on the central government, and delayed action for some years.

About 20 years passed between cocaine's reintroduction in the late 1960s and the recent federal anti-drug abuse acts. These periods are the length of a generation, a rather long period for a drug that is eventually seen as the most fearful of habit-forming substances.

A major difference, however, should be noted between the two episodes. In the first, there were no laws against cocaine at its introduction: increasingly severe laws followed public opinion. In the 1960s the harshest laws were in place when a new generation of Americans welcomed cocaine as an excellent and relatively safe stimulant. The long period of transition to a fear of cocaine and its users led many to believe that the pre-existing laws were built on misconceptions and futile in their efforts. Further, a tolerant attitude toward cocaine while the most severe penalties existed created the opportunity for a lucrative and fairly safe market in illicit cocaine trade over a period of many years. Our perception of the power of the law to affect drug use has been quite different in this era from that in the previous one, when the most severe laws were enacted as the demand for cocaine was apparently in decline.

Finally, the drug problem is commonly thought to be a serious contemporary problem that requires little more study than talking to those now involved with drugs. There is, however, a past that is relevant to our current problem and the way we conceptualize and approach it. Through this essay I have attempted to demonstrate that both the European and the American experiences with cocaine are worthwhile fields for historical investigation.

Acknowledgement

I wish to thank Jennifer Spiegel for assistance in the preparation of this paper.

References

Aschenbrandt T 1883 Dtsch Med Wochenschr No. 50:730–732
Brower DR 1886 The effects of cocaine on the central nervous system. JAMA (J Am Med Assoc) 6:59–62
The Chemist and Druggist 1892 Vol 36, p 299
Christison R 1876 Observations on the effects of the leaves of Erythroxylon Coca. Br Med J p 527–531
Coca-Cola Bottling Co. of Shreveport v. Coca-Cola, 563 F. Suppl. 1222 (1983) at 1131
The Druggists Circular and Chemical Gazette 1886 Vol 30, p 32
Freud S 1885 Ueber Coca [On Coca]. Zentralbl Ges Ther 2:289–314. English translation: Byck R (ed) 1974 Cocaine papers by Sigmund Freud. Stonehill Publishing, New York, p 48–73

Grinspoon L, Bakalar JB 1980 Drug dependence: non-narcotic agents. In: Kaplan HI, Freedman AM, Sadock BJ (eds) Comprehensive textbook of psychiatry, 3rd edn. Williams & Wilkins, Baltimore, p 1621-1622

Hammond WA 1887a Coca—its preparations and their therapeutical qualities, with some remarks on the so-called cocaine habit. Va Med Mon p 598-610

Hammond WA 1887b Coca: its preparations and their therapeutical qualities. Trans Med Soc Va p 212-226

Harney ML, Cross JC 1973 The narcotic officer's notebook, 2nd edn. Charles C Thomas, Springfield, IL

Helfand WH 1988 Mariani et le vin de coca. Psychotropes 4 (no. 3):13-18

House of Commons 1914 Report from the Select Committee on Patent Medicines, p 456

Huse EC 1880 Coca Erythroxylon: a new cure for the opium habit. Therapeutic Gazette, NS 1:256-257

Kahn EJ, Jr 1960 The big drink: the story of Coca-Cola. Random House, New York, p 56

Koller C 1884 On the use of cocaine for producing anaesthesia on the eye. Lancet 2 p 990-992

Mariani A (ed) 1901 Contemporary celebrities from the album of Mariani. Mariani & Co, New York

Mariani A 1896 Coca and its therapeutic application, 3rd edn. JN Jaros, New York

Mattison JB 1887 Cocaine dosage and cocaine addiction. Lancet 1:1024-1026

Mayor's Committee on Drug Addiction 1930 Report of the Mayor's Committee on Drug Addiction to the Hon. Richard C. Patterson, Jr., Commissioner of Correction, New York City. Am J Psychiatry 10:453

Musto DF 1987 The history of legislative control over opium, cocaine and their derivatives. In: Hamowy R (ed) Dealing with drugs. Lexington Books, Lexington, MA

Musto DF 1989 America's first cocaine epidemic. Wilson Quarterly 13 (no. 3):59-64

Musto DF 1990 Illicit price of cocaine in two eras: 1908-1914 and 1982-1989. Conn Med 54:321-326

Olch PD 1975 William S. Halsted and local anesthesia: contributions and complications. Anesthesiology 42 (no. 4):479-486

Schenk S, Horger BA, Snow S 1989-1990 Caffeine exposure sensitizes rats to the motor activating effects of cocaine. Behav Pharmacol 1:447-451

Van Dyke C, Byck R 1982 Cocaine. Sci Am 246 (3):108-119 (p 128-134, US edn)

Wright H 1910 Report on the International Opium Commission and on the opium problem as seen within the United States and its possessions. Opium Problems: Message from the President of the United States Senate Doc. no. 377, 61st Cong., 2nd Sess., 21 Feb 1910, p 47

DISCUSSION

Kleber: During that period early in this century when the street price of cocaine in New York was roughly the same as the hourly wage of an industrial worker (25 cents for 100 mg), what was the price paid if it was obtained by medical prescription?

Musto: It has proved remarkably difficult to answer that. Of course, the prescription price varied from one pharmacist to another, but even the American Institute of the History of Pharmacy lacks information on that interesting question. We know that the wholesale cost when cocaine was purchased in kilogram and larger lots on the international market was about 25 cents a gram, and we are reasonably certain that the illicit street price in New York City from 1907 to 1914 was ten times that minimum. I assume the prescription price would be less than that multiple. One must keep in mind that in the United States in the period I am discussing, about 1900 to 1914, the average industrial hourly wage was between 20 and 25 cents. Interestingly, the cost, in real terms, of street cocaine was about the same then as it was in the 1980s (Musto 1990).

Kleber: You said that by the end of the first era, in the 1930s, the laws had become very strict against cocaine possession or sale, and therefore when cocaine use increased again (in the late 1970s), the laws were already in place. What do you feel was the role of those laws in diminishing cocaine use in the *earlier* period? I am unclear whether the laws came in as the decline in cocaine use was already beginning, earlier this century, or whether they helped to cause that decline.

Musto: The laws represented a powerful shift in attitude toward cocaine that peaked in the period shortly before World War I. The Harrison Act of 1914 eliminated any legal availability of cocaine without a physician's prescription—the first drug to be so severely restricted. I believe the laws helped speed the decline of cocaine use over the next 20 years or so, although the chief reason was the changed public attitude. Still, history doesn't allow control groups. But I don't believe that anyone could have persuaded a large number of Americans in that era to forego legal sanctions against cocaine. Americans demanded laws against the easy availability of cocaine and the drug proved to be the most successfully prohibited of any previously widely used psychotropics.

As for the timing of the laws in relation to the peak of use, I cannot yet say anything confidently regarding cocaine, but the anti-opiate laws generally came after the peak of consumption in the mid 1890s. That isn't surprising, however, because the fall in demand had to gain momentum for a consensus that strict controls were necessary. I suspect the same for cocaine, but cocaine's rise and fall were swifter than those of the opiates.

Finally, the experience regarding law enforcement of those who have lived through our current cocaine episode and that of our great-grandparents is quite different. We have, I believe, more questions about the efficacy of law enforcement, at least of legal statutes, than our ancestors had. They saw the imposition of legal restrictions as demand declined and popular attitudes hardened against cocaine. Our experience has been that the most severe legal restrictions did not prevent a resurgence of cocaine and that law enforcement is weak against popular enthusiasm for cocaine. We have had perhaps two decades of law enforcement trying to curb the use of cocaine with less than satisfactory results. So although both epidemics may eventually have a similar 'shape', we are less sanguine about the unique ability of severe laws to curb use.

Uchtenhagen: I wonder how much is known about the characteristics of people taking cocaine in the two US epidemics, and in different phases of the epidemics?

Musto: Cocaine in the 1880s was initially quite expensive. Freud complained about this in his first essay *Ueber Coca* (1885). Its first distribution in America appears to have been to the middle and upper classes as a new and sophisticated treatment for hay fever, sinus problems and melancholia, and as a tonic for what were then called 'brain workers'—professionals in medicine, law and religion. Soon the cost became lower and it was more commonly available in patent medicines for asthma, toothache and hay fever and in common drinks. The non-medical use also spread and seemed worrisomely popular among criminals, prostitutes and in the South among African-Americans. These negative perceptions helped fuel the drive for legal control, but there is reason to believe that use by Blacks in the South was not greater than that by Whites (Green 1914).

There is, then, a pattern similar to what we have experienced in the 1970s and 1980s: cocaine is used at first by the affluent and later undergoes a mass distribution, the effect of which is to create great concern among the public about the behaviour of 'lower classes' using or seeking cocaine. Commission of crimes to get money to buy cocaine was a common complaint when cocaine was unrestricted, as well as now. Cocaine has not been cheap, if the user developed an addiction, in either era.

Kalant: When Hans Maier wrote his book on cocaine in 1926, his historical review showed very clearly the evolution of use that you described; but, by that time, his patients consisted either of physicians who had access to cocaine professionally, or of people who may have been gainfully employed in 'respectable' fields, but became acquainted with cocaine through the *demimonde* of prostitution or petty crime. Cocaine had obviously already fallen into disrepute, and was seen as a drug that was unacceptable to the majority of society. This would certainly fit with the downturn in use and its virtual disappearance during the middle part of this century, at least in Europe and North America. The relation between the change in public attitude and the enactment of drug control laws fits well with the argument that laws are really a codification of public opinion rather than a determinant of that opinion; they are passed when the public demands the laws, and are disregarded when the public no longer believes in what the laws represent.

One question: how exactly did cocaine first appear as an illicit commodity in the United States?

Musto: My view is that as there became greater concern over cocaine, in the 1890s, physicians and pharmacists became more hesitant in providing it, and it was then easily available only from a minority of pharmacists or some physicians, or from other sources in which the price was somewhat higher. The reason we know about the illicit price in New York City after the 'Al Smith' anti-cocaine law of 1907 is that detailed reports of people arrested for violation of that act then appeared. We found from those reports that there was a steady price for illicit cocaine of about 25 cents for a packet containing approximately

100 mg. I don't know when that street market began, but there are reasons to believe that it may have started late in the 19th century or early in this century.

Kalant: Even before the laws were enacted, then?

Musto: In New York City, I believe there was a street market before the 'Al Smith' Act of 1907, although I am not sure I can call it 'illicit'. I believe this to be likely because the growing fear of cocaine was leading health professionals to be more and more circumspect in providing the drug, and a street market would make it available with no questions asked, at any time and for a price that, although not cheap, was affordable.

Kuhar: In the earlier cocaine epidemic in the US, what was the distribution system? Was it like the one that exists now, with cocaine being smuggled from South America, and so on?

Musto: Smuggling may have occurred, but there were no serious restrictions, such as very high tariffs on cocaine and coca leaves. It's hard at this date to estimate smuggling. The most typical distribution system would start with coca leaves imported from South America. US drug companies would extract cocaine from these, or import cocaine itself, often from Germany. Cocaine would then be distributed by syndicates in New York City and sold on the streets by dealers ranging from newsboys to full-time gang members. Unlike the last two decades, there was no enormous overproduction by illicit producers to compensate for interdiction. After the Harrison Act (1914), evidence of smuggling appeared and there were diversions from licit supplies, but by this time the growing disenchantment with cocaine, coupled with legal penalties, gradually reduced demand in the United States, so that by the 1930s cocaine had become a minor problem in New York City.

Negrete: I feel rather uncomfortable with the comparison between the current cocaine epidemics and the one occurring in the first decade of the century. I am not sure they are the same thing. We have no idea, of course, of the prevalence of cocaine use then; I think there were no population surveys. But I suspect that there were not the same patterns of use. Is there any precedent for smoked cocaine before the recent episode, for example?

We all smile when we hear the praises given to, say, Vin Mariani, but they were not off the mark; that is exactly what it did! I am sure that if we had such preparations of cocaine now, we would have the benefits of it. The energy that is given, *without* the immediate central nervous system perception of stimulation, is a very important difference from what you see in cocaine abuse. Mariani in fact copied from the Incas, who knew about the energizing properties of the drug. They measured distances for their couriers by cocadas. A *cocada* was a pouch full of coca leaves; so the number of *cocadas* you need to chew in order to get to your destination is a way of telling you how far you have to go!

Musto: There were coca cigarettes and coca cheroots produced by the Parke-Davis company within one year of cocaine's introduction into the United States, in 1884, and by other companies, but whether coca paste was smoked or not, then, I am not sure. There was complete availability of hypodermic syringes and cocaine in the late 1880s and 1890s, so a user could either sniff it, use an atomizer to inhale it, which was also provided in the 'cocaine kits', or inject it. There was no limit to what you could take. But I don't know of any smoking apart from the cigarettes and cheroots composed of coca leaves.

Edwards: Dr Musto, you are suggesting, very persuasively, that an epidemic may reach its peak and start to decline because of social resistance—when people turn against it—rather than because of the law; then the change in the law follows and may reinforce the decline. But are you sure that you are right? Do epidemics of drugs 'burn themselves out'? What about an alternative explanation in terms of changes in economic or market determinants? Or some other drug moving in to substitute for cocaine? And, in terms of your theory, who 'turns against'? Do the media turn against cocaine, or does some emergent social movement? You are making such an important assertion, but how firm do you think the evidence is?

Musto: First, my observations are based chiefly on a study of the American experience, in which a rapidly expanding legal consumption of cocaine elicited a strong opposition to the drug and strong support for the enactment of the most severe legal restrictions applied to any drug still available for medical purposes. I believe the reduction in cocaine use during the 1920s and 1930s was facilitated by the criminal justice system. I can't establish this by re-running the experiment without anti-cocaine laws, but I think it is reasonable to assume that a widely shared conviction of cocaine's dangers would lead to narrowing those niches in society in which cocaine continued to be used and that legal sanctions would further discourage use—in that context of public disapproval.

Second, the change in attitude toward cocaine and the opiates was part of a much broader movement in the United States against risk-taking behaviour that flourished from about 1890 to 1920. This concern was not confined to the prohibition of alcohol (1920–1933) but extended to national laws affecting pure food and drugs, meat inspection, clean streams, preservation of the forests and natural resources, and so on. We are now in another era similar that of nearly a century ago.

With regard to drugs like cocaine, public opinion moved from seeing them as useful if well-understood and used in moderation, to seeing them as bad in any amount, unless required for medical purposes like analgesia.

When this change took place, research and treatment were both adversely affected. When drugs were seen so negatively, the solution to the drug problem appeared to be a simple one—separate the drug from the user. Research interest fell, and earlier optimism about treatment by medical means almost disappeared in the United States. Law enforcement became the public's focus, as it is becoming now in the USA. So the change in attitude toward drug use carried with it many related consequences and was part of a larger movement aiming at risk reduction in the things we take into our body and in hazards in the environment.

Gerstein: On this point of what effects the law has, we should pay attention to the distinction between use by the elite and by the *demi-monde*, although in the USA it is perhaps more important to take the rather different dimensions of use by Whites and use by Blacks, because I think the drug laws in the USA have been used most aggressively and extensively against Blacks.

The spread of cocaine use, particularly in the middle class and among wealthier people, White or Black, during the period of the present cocaine epidemic in the USA, could be viewed as an instance in which, no matter how harsh the laws on the books, they were never applied with force to the White elite but were prosecuted much more vigorously among the poor, and the Black poor particularly. This might explain why, despite the apparent difference in the status of the law between the early and later periods of cocaine use, we see in both cases an epidemic occurring among White users who are well-off and otherwise respectable, and a strong backlash of prosecution and police action when cocaine use becomes strongly identified with Blacks.

References

Freud S 1885 Ueber Coca [On Coca]. Zentralbl Ges Ther 2:289–314. English translation: Byck R (ed) 1974 Cocaine papers by Sigmund Freud. Stonehill Publishing, New York, p 48–73 (see p 58)

Green EM 1914 Psychoses among negroes: a comparative study. J Nerv Ment Dis 41:697–708

Maier HW 1926 Der Kokainismus. Georg Thieme, Berlin. English translation: Kalant OJ 1987 Maier's Cocaine addiction (Der Kokainismus). Addiction Research Foundation, Toronto

Musto DF 1990 Illicit price of cocaine in two eras: 1908–1914 and 1982–1989. Conn Med 54:321–326

Epidemiological research on cocaine use in the USA

James C. Anthony

Department of Mental Hygiene, The Johns Hopkins University School of Hygiene and Public Health, Baltimore, MD 21205, USA

> *Abstract.* In the study of cocaine, epidemiology offers a way to reckon the experience of human populations, from time to time, from region to region, from community to community, and from group to group. Continuing surveillance of cocaine experiences in diverse segments of the United States population has allowed us to plot the course of our most recent cocaine epidemic in more detail than in the past. Still, much remains to be learned about the dynamics of the cocaine epidemic before public health agencies or anyone else should ride to glory on the descending limb of this epidemic curve. Beyond basic surveillance, epidemiology has the capacity to teach us about the conditions under which human cocaine use starts, is maintained, and stops, including the array of perceived and actual consequences of cocaine use that may determine specific patterns of use. In this respect, there is some value in making a chronicle of cocaine users' life experiences, with a comparison to the life experiences of others. However, the perceptions of cocaine users do not always map onto observations made under controlled conditions of laboratory research. Finally, it is not essential for epidemiology to rely solely upon what individuals perceive and report as causal linkages between cocaine use and their other life experiences. One effective alternative is to use the epidemiological case–control method and related strategies to probe suspected causal linkages involving cocaine. As demonstrated in recent research, these strategies have a resolving power that goes beyond that of standard epidemiological survey reports. Of course, the resulting epidemiological evidence does not stand alone. Rather, it complements laboratory and clinical research, giving a more complete view of cocaine's impact on human health.
>
> *1992 Cocaine: scientific and social dimensions. Wiley, Chichester (Ciba Foundation Symposium 166) p 20–39*

In this paper I intend to touch on three epidemiological topics that concern cocaine use in the United States. The first topic is our most recent cocaine epidemic. A time series of prevalence estimates, shown in Fig. 1, may suggest that the epidemic has recently ended or subsided.

For those who lead public health agencies or government, there is temptation for an exhilarating ride to glory on the descending limb of an epidemic curve such as this one. The ride is a moment of pleasure mixed with apprehension.

Epidemiology of cocaine use in the USA

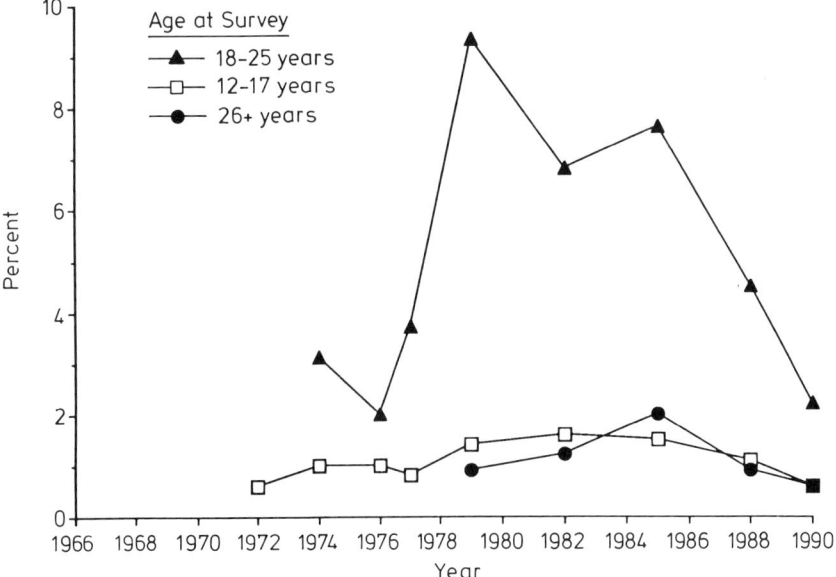

FIG. 1. Estimated prevalence (%) of active cocaine use by year of survey and age of respondent (any cocaine use in the 30 days prior to interview). Data from the National Household Surveys on Drug Abuse sponsored by the National Institute on Drug Abuse, 1972-1990.

Age stratum in year of survey	Years of each household survey								
	1972	1974	1976	1977	1979	1982	1985	1988	1990
12-17	0.6	1.0	1.0	0.8	1.4	1.6	1.5	1.1	0.6
18-25	—	3.1	2.0	3.7	9.3	6.8	7.6	4.5	2.2
26+	—	*	*	*	0.9	1.2	2.0	0.9	0.6

These trend data were provided by Mr Joseph Gfroerer, Division of Epidemiology and Prevention Research, National Institute on Drug Abuse, June 1991.

Pleasure is from knowing that one's efforts might make a difference, and might be appreciated. Apprehension is from knowing that public health work is ruled by 'out of sight, out of mind'. Soon there will be budget cuts. These cuts will harm our capacities to learn from the epidemic experience, and to prevent, delay, or curtail the next epidemic.

It is my belief that no one should ride to glory as this cocaine epidemic subsides. We know too little about the dynamics of this epidemic. By posing several unanswered questions, I shall try to show how little we know.

My second topic relates to the epidemiological study of conditions under which human cocaine use starts, is maintained, and stops. I shall make specific note of perceived consequences of cocaine use that are thought to determine specific patterns of use. As we will see, we cannot expect cocaine users always to perceive and report cocaine effects that map directly onto observations from more controlled laboratory studies of cocaine.

My third and final topic concerns the major challenges that have engaged a small cocaine epidemiology research group at Johns Hopkins, put together with support from the National Institute on Drug Abuse (USA). I asked the group to focus on a set of related questions about suspected hazards of using cocaine, namely, a suspected impact on the mental life and behaviour that generally occurs too infrequently for study in controlled environments of the laboratory (Anthony & Petronis 1991).

By way of illustration, we now appreciate that clinicians, especially psychiatrists, see many cocaine users with a disturbed mental life (e.g. Gawin 1991). For example, clinicians have told us that cocaine use causes or precipitates panic attacks or panic disorder. Others have described cocaine-induced suicide attempts. Because these clinical hypotheses have some basis in observations on the neurobiological actions of cocaine, our own work has included a test of whether cocaine use might signal an increased risk of having a panic attack or of making a suicide attempt, while controlling for suspected confounding variables.

These are troublesome issues, because we might well expect psychiatrists to see an excess of cocaine users with mental disturbances. Further, major mental disturbances such as panic attacks and suicide attempts are events that pharmacologists have not yet brought down on their subjects in the bio-behavioural laboratory, for a variety of reasons.

Our alternative has been to probe the linkage of cocaine use with panic attacks, suicide attempt, and other psychiatric disturbances in the epidemiological context, using samples of community residents rather than help-seeking cocaine users or cocaine-using volunteers in the biobehavioural laboratory. Furthermore, in our epidemiological work, we use stratification and matching, as well as multiple regression modelling, in order to hold constant suspected confounding variables.

The other psychiatric conditions we have studied in this fashion have ranged from sustained episodes of mood disturbances to possibly more severe psychotic experiences, each of which has some plausibility as an effect of cocaine use, not only in the clinical observations, but also in the pharmacological and neurobiological evidence. In our most recent work, we have investigated a suspected association between cocaine use and the occurrence of obsessive–compulsive disorder, a linkage that might well be mediated through the serotonergic activity of cocaine or its metabolites. My hope is that our discussion will centre on these studies of cocaine use and subsequent psychiatric disturbances, since this work offers more challenges than basic descriptive epidemiology.

The cocaine epidemic

Returning to the topic of the US cocaine epidemic, I must point out that the data in Fig. 1 concern the *prevalence* of active cocaine use—that is, the proportion using cocaine in some defined period of time, such as the 30 days prior to interview. Also, please note that the prevalence values are given for broad bands of age—not for the surviving members of individual birth cohorts. This is important, because the observed relationships between age and cocaine use have often been strong and sometimes non-linear (Abelson & Miller 1985, Kandel et al 1985, Anthony et al 1986, Trinkoff et al 1990).

To illustrate, in the broad band from age 12 to 17 years, active cocaine use is concentrated among individuals age 15–17 years and is found much less frequently among 12–14-year-olds. Given these facts, simple algebra can be used to show that today's overall number of active cocaine users age 12–17 years will be influenced heavily by the size of individual cohorts born some 12–17 years ago and surviving to the present. During an era of constant age-specific prevalence rates, a dramatic baby boom can produce a drop, followed by an increase in the prevalence of active cocaine use. These changes occur in sequence, as the baby boomers pass through puberty, and then through later adolescence.

Dr Morton Kramer (unpublished work 1991) has used these basic principles of epidemiology and demography to forecast future trends in the number of adult male Americans with active drug abuse-dependence syndromes. Assuming no change in prevalence rates, and applying US Census projections for changes in the age structure of the population between 1990 and 2010, he found that there should be increases in the number of Hispanic males with drug abuse-dependence, increases in the number of Blacks with drug abuse-dependence, and decreases in the number of non-Hispanic Whites with drug abuse-dependence. A similar forecast was obtained for adult women.

Having noted that trends in summarized prevalence values for broad age bands can be influenced by population demographics, we can turn to a more fundamental set of interdependent relationships between prevalence of active cocaine use, the average duration of cocaine use, and the incidence of cocaine use, where 'incidence' refers to the occurrence rate at which individuals become users for the first time.

When we hold constant the demographic factors, prevalence of active cocaine use can be expressed as a dynamic function of incidence × average duration. That is, a prevalence value is an estimate that mixes the forces determining the incidence of (first-time) use, and combines them together with the forces determining the duration of use among users. For this reason, epidemiologists typically plot epidemic curves as time series of *incidence* estimates, not as time series of *prevalence* estimates. The forces determining duration are allowed to influence the epidemic, but these forces typically deserve separate consideration.

To my knowledge, there are no recent published estimates or technical reports that give us estimates for the incidence of (first-time) cocaine use in the United States population, or for the average duration of cocaine use. As a result, apart from Dr Richard Clayton's report of preliminary data from the late 1970s and early 1980s (Clayton 1985), we have no clear view of the year or years in which the epidemic reached peak incidence. We do not know the extent to which current prevalence of cocaine use is being sustained by continuing accrual of new users, or alternatively, by lengthened average duration of use, or by both of these determining influences.

A more complete view of progress along the cocaine epidemic curve might also be provided if we were to allow for varying degrees of susceptibility in the population. For example, we can expect changing characteristics of incident (first-time) users and sustained (continuing) users as any epidemic progresses, in part as a reflection of changes in susceptibility or exposure.

In epidemiology and public health generally, the concept of variation in susceptibility has proved to be very useful. There is a long history of epidemics that have ended because the pool of susceptibles effectively was used up: the epidemic stopped because there were no more susceptibles to be affected. Further, public health strategies designed to control epidemics have been based on the principle of reducing 'exposure opportunities' for susceptible individuals. In the case of smallpox, one strategy was to surround infected persons with non-susceptibles. In the case of rubella, there have been successful efforts to break the chain of transmission from susceptible to susceptible. The utility of these infectious disease models for drug abuse epidemics is no longer subject to debate, in view of the pioneering work by de Alarcon and others (e.g., de Alarcon 1969, Brill & Hirose 1969, Ellinwood 1974).

As we retrospectively plot the course of the recent cocaine epidemic in the USA, and plan for the control of future epidemics, it would be useful to illuminate a distinctly individual variation in susceptibility. Changing tides in the epidemic might be discovered by studying the relative balance of different groups among the incident users and among the sustained users. Given what we know about the age-specific prevalence of cocaine use, one might find evidence that this cocaine epidemic started to decline once incident users began to be drawn more heavily from the ranks of 12–15-year-olds ('virgin' susceptibles), and less heavily from the ranks of persons born in the post-World War II baby boom (a residual pool of 'mature' susceptibles).

Before turning to my second topic, I offer a summary by way of a series of unanswered questions about the dynamics of the recent cocaine epidemic:

1. The downward trend in the prevalence of cocaine use and other illicit drug use in the USA has run parallel with demographic shifts in the age structure of the population. In the US population generally, the number of younger people

has declined while the number of older adults has increased. This shift implies declining overall prevalence.

The decline in prevalence surely has taken place not only because fewer individuals are in the ages of highest prevalence, but also because of changes in social mixing within- and across-age strata (D. B. Kandel, unpublished work 1991). The result implies variations in the conditional probability of being offered an opportunity to use cocaine. That is, there is plausible evidence that boyfriends, girlfriends, and other social intimates are key elements in the diffusion of cocaine (e.g. Boyd & Mieczkowski 1990). To the extent that cocaine use is concentrated differentially in the age stratum from 18 to 25 years, it is more risky to be intimately acquainted with 18–25-year-olds. As the number of 18 to 25-year-olds in the population has declined, the conditional probability of being offered an opportunity to use cocaine quite likely has declined.

Because diffusion of cocaine use depends in this fashion upon demographic shifts in the population, it is reasonable to ask whether a fairly simple model of demographic shift might account for the observed peak and decline in the overall prevalence of cocaine use in the general population.

2. In a similar vein, we might make projections for broad age strata (12–17 years, 18–25 years, and older adults), using the methods described by M. Kramer (unpublished work 1991), and substituting values for age-specific prevalence of cocaine use in the middle 1970s. If these projections were made, it would be useful to know how closely the projected values for the late 1970s and the 1980s compare with observed values in the general population and in subgroups defined by sex and race-ethnicity. We might ask: after what interval do the projected values begin to decline?

3. The functional relationships between prevalence, incidence, and average duration lead to several speculations that have some additional basis in recent ethnographic and clinical observations. In particular, one might speculate that (i) the year or years of peak incidence of (first-time) cocaine use have occurred at least 1–2 years prior to the year of peak prevalence, and (ii) the values on the descending limb of the prevalence curve reflect in part an increase in the average duration of cocaine use.

Here, we must ask whether evidence from the available epidemiological surveys rings true with this speculation. If so, there are clear implications for the assessment of public policy and for planning current and future public health initiatives, especially for treatment of continuing cocaine users.

4. Is there evidence that this cocaine epidemic began to decline once incident users were drawn more heavily from the ranks of 'virgin' susceptibles and less heavily from a residual pool of 'mature' susceptibles characterized by use of marijuana or psychedelic drugs in the 1970s? At the current stage in the cocaine epidemic, is there any basis for characterizing the older adult incident (first-time) users as less cosmopolitan and less socially integrated than at earlier stages? This would be an implication drawn from theory and observations on the social diffusion of technological innovations.

5. As the epidemic has progressed, have the continuing users been drawn more heavily from disadvantaged sectors of the population, where there is a limited array of alternative reinforcers to compete with cocaine use?

6. Finally, considering that the cocaine supply in the USA is relatively abundant, particularly in the inner cities, can we be certain that the epidemic of cocaine use has subsided in all areas and segments of the population? Should we be confident that the epidemic has ended?

These are a few of the epidemiological questions about our recent cocaine epidemic that remain unanswered. Aside from preliminary reports (e.g. Clayton 1985), we have no evidence that the already-gathered field survey data have been analysed to answer these basic questions, and we must infer that these analyses have not been done. An alternative kinder and gentler perspective is that attempts have been made, but the available data are not adequate to answer the questions posed in this paper. Whatever the explanation, it would seem that much remains to be learned about the dynamics of the cocaine epidemic before anyone should ride to glory on its descending curve.

Determinants of progression in cocaine use

My second topic relates to epidemiological study of conditions under which human cocaine use starts, is maintained, and stops. Several research groups are addressing these issues, but in this brief paper I can only sketch an outline of what my colleague Chris Ritter and I found in analyses of data from the National Institute on Mental Health Epidemiologic Catchment Area Program. For these analyses, we concentrated on prospectively gathered data from interviews with adults sampled from community populations in three American metropolitan areas: Baltimore (Maryland), the Raleigh-Durham-Piedmont area (North Carolina), and Los Angeles (California). In this study, we used fairly conventional epidemiological strategies to sharpen the focus on personal and behavioural attributes that might be associated with the initiation or progression of cocaine use, while holding constant so-called 'macrosocial' influences such as cocaine availability and cost in local neighbourhoods, poverty levels, and poor access to health services (Ritter & Anthony 1991).

Drawing from a much larger community sample with thousands of subjects, we matched 78 cocaine users with 131 controls, holding constant their age and neighbourhood. Using conditional multiple logistic regression models, we found that initiation or progression of cocaine use at that time was associated with conditions designated in Table 1: a recent history of illicit use of marijuana and/or other federally controlled drugs; having recently gained a job after a period of no employment; and level of personal income. There was an inverse association with being married at the time of interview (Ritter & Anthony 1991).

Through separate analyses, we found that a prior history of major depression did not predict initiation or progression in cocaine use. However, there was

TABLE 1 Conditions associated with initiation or progression of cocaine use. Prospective study data from the Epidemiologic Catchment Area surveys conducted with community samples in Baltimore City (Maryland), Raleigh-Durham-Piedmont (North Carolina) and Los Angeles (California), 1981–1985

Conditions that signalled increased risk of initiation or progression of cocaine use
Recent illicit use of marijuana and/or other controlled drugs (besides cocaine)
Having recently gained a job after a period of no employment for pay
Personal income in the previous year

Conditions that signalled lower risk of initiation or progression of cocaine use
Being married

Conditions found to have no strong association with initiation or progression of cocaine use
Being male
Being Black or Hispanic
Being employed continuously during the observation interval
Educational achievement (years of schooling)
Previous history of major depression
Occupational prestige rank

Source: Ritter & Anthony 1991.

some evidence that syndromes of depression developed concomitantly, possibly in response to cocaine use (Ritter & Anthony 1991), a topic to which we shall return.

Other characteristics found to have no strong association with initiating or progressing in cocaine use included sex (being male), race-ethnicity (being Black, being Hispanic), being employed continuously during the entire observation interval, educational achievement, and the prestige associated with one's occupation.

Subsequent analyses have demonstrated that the neighbourhood matching did not lead us to underestimate associations involving social class, as indicated by educational achievement or job prestige. There were no important associations with education or job prestige in either matched or unmatched analyses of the study data (C. J. Ritter & J. C. Anthony, in preparation).

Some observers, in offering a critique of epidemiological findings of this type, have argued that these analyses neglect the potential importance of perceived drug effects as determinants of cocaine use. Our studies have not included measurement of the full array of perceived beneficial or detrimental consequences of cocaine use. None the less, what we have observed prompts us to urge caution when interpreting what users of cocaine and other drugs might perceive and report about the consequences of their drug use.

For example, according to evidence from controlled studies in the biobehavioural laboratory, the reinforcement potential of cocaine use exceeds that of heroin. Notwithstanding these results, upon studying cocaine users and heroin users identified by probability sample surveys in four metropolitan areas

(Baltimore, Raleigh-Durham, Los Angeles and St Louis, Missouri), our research group has found that fewer cocaine users report having become dependent, having failed to cut down on their drug use, and other indicators of drug dependence, than heroin users. This was true even under reported conditions of daily cocaine use for two weeks or more, as shown in Table 2 (Anthony & Petronis 1989). Thus, it seems that the perceptions of cocaine users do not always map onto observations made under controlled conditions of laboratory research.

For reasons such as these, members of my research group, among others, have been reluctant to rely solely upon what cocaine users perceive and report as causal linkages between cocaine use and their other life experiences. While reports of perceived cocaine effects bear information of great value to ethnographers and social psychologists, members of this symposium are well aware that the reporting of drug effects is determined in part by culture, personality and setting, perhaps more than by the chemical structure of a drug and its activity at receptor sites.

Cocaine's suspected impact on health, especially mental health

In order to gain a more complete view of cocaine's potential impact on human health, we have turned to the epidemiological case–control method and related strategies (e.g. Anthony 1988). Within this framework for epidemiological research, we have not been obliged to ask cocaine users, or anyone else, what they might perceive about the consequences of cocaine use. Instead, this strategy

TABLE 2 Prevalence of self-reported dependence indicators among 69 sustained daily users of cocaine (but not heroin), and 57 sustained daily users of heroin

	Among 69 daily cocaine users		Among 57 daily heroin users	
Self-report	Number reporting this symptom	Percentage reporting this symptom	Number reporting this symptom	Percentage reporting this symptom
Ever felt dependent on drug	15	22.1	44	78.6
Ever unable to cut down on amount used	8	11.6	23	40.4
Ever felt tolerance to drug's effects	29	42.0	39	68.4
Ever experienced withdrawal	9	13.0	43	75.4

Estimates based on Diagnostic Interview Schedule data from Epidemiologic Catchment Area household and institutional probability samples in Baltimore, St Louis, Durham-Piedmont and Los Angeles, 1980–1984. Percentages in row 1 are based on 68 cocaine users and 56 heroin users.
Source: Anthony & Petronis 1989.

requires an inquiry about cocaine exposure, either by asking questions or by using laboratory bioassays. There also is a need to define and measure the suspected health consequences in an independent manner that controls for spurious artifacts due to our unwarranted beliefs or biases about cocaine toxicity.

It was this type of careful work that has led the medical community to be confident that tobacco smoking signals an increased risk of dying from lung cancer, and that this risk might be reduced by not smoking. Several of the original studies of suspected causal linkages between tobacco smoking and lung cancer were of the case-control variety, with the relative risk of lung cancer estimated by asking cases and non-diseased controls whether they had been tobacco smokers. Later studies have been prospective or longitudinal, following individuals over time to see whether tobacco smoking was associated with increased risk of lung cancer.

Of course, there are necessarily limited opportunities to conduct controlled human experiments with randomized tobacco or cocaine exposure followed by observation to detect toxic consequences such as lung cancer. This means that we must use stratification, matching, and data analysis strategies to hold constant or adjust for extraneous conditions that might be confounded with drug effects.

Because we cannot be sure that our observational studies have achieved total experimental control of error, we hesitate to regard the results of any single study as definitive. Instead, we look for a consistency of replicated findings across these studies. Further, we depend heavily on whether the results are coherent within the context of findings from clinical observations and more controlled laboratory studies of related phenomena.

A study of suicide attempts serves to illustrate an application of the case-control strategy in epidemiological research on cocaine. There is a long history of clinical observation relating to episodes of mood disturbances and suicide attempts among cocaine users, and there is at least circumstantial evidence to link suicide, serotonergic or dopaminergic systems, and cocaine.

Against this backdrop, we have used the epidemiological case-control strategy to probe for evidence that recent cocaine use might signal an increased risk of suicide attempt in the population. We have done so in a manner that has allowed us to hold constant many of the other suspected causes of suicide attempt that otherwise might confound relationships involving cocaine use.

Specifically, we sought to estimate the risk of making a suicide attempt during a 1-2 year observation interval in the early 1980s by studying 13 673 adults who were sampled and who completed baseline and follow-up interviews for the National Institute of Mental Health Epidemiologic Catchment Area multi-site collaborative study, in this study drawing from all five sites of the multi-site study.

A total of 40 adults in the sample reported making suicide attempts during the observation interval; these were our suicide attempt 'cases'. One to 17 non-cases were grouped with each case by Census tract of household residence and by age (4+/−years). The grouping by Census tract of residence effectively matched for, and held constant, suspected macrosocial influences on suicidal behaviour, some of which have figured prominently in the sociological literature on suicide. As described in relation to the study of cocaine use, this strategy allowed us to sharpen our focus on personal and behavioural attributes suspected of influencing the risk of making a suicide attempt, including recent use of cocaine (Petronis et al 1990).

As shown in Table 3, recent use of cocaine signalled a moderately increased risk of making a suicide attempt, with a relative risk estimate of 4.45 ($P=0.076$) against a null relative risk value of unity (1.0). Additional multiple logistic regression analyses offered an opportunity to hold constant other suspected risk factors, such as a history of major depression, and alcohol abuse–dependence syndromes, being separated or divorced, and social class.

In these analyses, we found evidence of a more substantial degree of association between recent use of cocaine and risk of making a suicide attempt. The corresponding relative risk estimate was 61.9 ($P=0.012$), a substantial departure from 1.0, the null value. A relative risk of 61.9 is a remarkably high value considering the circumstances, a value not likely to be explained away by an appeal to uncontrolled confounding variables.

There are a number of limitations in this work on suicide attempts, and it would certainly be premature to draw firm conclusions from a single epidemiological study. None the less, it is important to recognize that these findings complement careful observations made by clinicians who care for cocaine-using patients. Additional plausibility rests on associations observed

TABLE 3 Cocaine use signalled an increased risk of making a suicide attempt

Risk of suicide attempt for cocaine users versus non-users: initial model

Type of psychiatric disturbance	No. of incident cases in risk sets	Remaining candidates in risk sets	Estimated relative risk	P value
Suicide attempt	40	160	4.45*	0.076

Risk of suicide attempt for cocaine users versus non-users, holding constant neighbourhood, age, marital status, education, history of alcohol disorder, history of major depression

Type of psychiatric disturbance	No. of incident cases in risk sets	Remaining candidates in risk sets	Estimated relative risk	P value
Suicide attempt	40	160	61.9*	0.012

Estimates from conditional multiple logistic regression modelling of prospective study data gathered from Epidemiologic Catchment Area household probability samples in New Haven, Baltimore, St Louis, Durham-Piedmont and Los Angeles, 1980–1984.
*95% confidence interval for relative risk estimate: (2.5, 1527.8).
Source: Petronis et al 1990.

TABLE 4 **Estimated relative risk of specific psychiatric disturbances in relation to cocaine use**

Type of psychiatric disturbance	No. of incident cases in risk sets	Remaining candidates in risk sets	Estimated relative risk	P value
Panic attack	122	387	3.6	0.003
DSM Panic disorder	18	59	3.2	0.133
DSM Major depression	192	621	1.7	0.148
Depression syndrome	259	776	2.0	0.017
Simple depression	232	591	1.8	0.121
DSM Manic episode	24	104	11.8	0.031
Mania syndrome	42	164	5.5	0.006
Delusion/hallucination	477	1818	1.6	0.047
Suicide attempt	40	160	4.4	0.076
DSM Obsessive–compulsive disorder	105	514	2.6	0.055

Estimates from conditional logistic regression analyses of epidemiological data from Epidemiologic Catchment Area household probability samples in New Haven, Baltimore, St Louis, Durham-Piedmont and Los Angeles, 1980–1984.
DSM, Diagnostic and Statistical Manual of Mental Disorders, third edition.
Sources: Anthony & Petronis 1991; R. C. Crum & J. C. Anthony, under review.

by the research groups of Asberg, Mann and others that involve suicide and serotonin (e.g. Mann et al 1986), and, separately, cocaine's involvement with serotonergic systems (Balster 1988, Lakoski & Cunningham 1988).

Table 4 summarizes other work by our research group in which we have tested for the potential impact of cocaine use on other health hazards in the form of specific psychiatric disturbances. As shown, we have found that cocaine use signals reliably increased risk for panic attack, a syndrome of sustained depression, syndromes of mania, and experiences resembling delusion and hallucinations. There is reason to pursue these findings in future research, given the involvement of cocaine in multiple neurobiological systems, as well as accumulated clinical observations about cocaine and these psychiatric disturbances (e.g. Gawin 1991). The future studies can go beyond a mere search for replication of these observed epidemiological associations, strengthening the research design through better and more comprehensive measurements of cocaine use, the psychiatric disturbances under study, and other characteristics that might create a spurious appearance of cocaine's involvement (Anthony et al 1989, Petronis et al 1990, Tien & Anthony 1990, Anthony & Petronis 1991). It is also important to test for possible differences involving different methods of ingesting cocaine (e.g., crack smoking), which were not common in the samples we drew in the early 1980s.

Before closing, I should mention that ours is not the only epidemiology research group that is applying the epidemiological case–control method and other population research strategies to the study of cocaine's potential health impact. Recent publications reflect progress made by other epidemiologists in the study of cocaine and primary infertility (Mueller et al 1990), cocaine and seizure (Ng et al 1990), cocaine and stroke (Kaku & Lowenstein 1990), and other suspected health hazards.

In summary, epidemiological research on cocaine use in the United States reflects a growth beyond a mere description of progress in the cocaine epidemic and the consequences of cocaine use as perceived and reported by active cocaine users. We are in a period during which the cocaine epidemic has subsided for the time being, and in this period there has emerged a more complete picture of the potential impact of cocaine use on the public health. We have entered a period during which our attention is focused more securely on hypothesized models for cocaine's impact on human health. An important challenge for future epidemiological research on cocaine is to determine whether these impressions of important public health impact can be sustained through systematic replications and more rigorous inquiry.

Acknowledgement

This research was supported by a grant from the National Institute on Drug Abuse (DA03992).

References

Abelson HI, Miller JD 1985 A decade of trends in cocaine use in the household population. In: Kozel NJ, Adams EH (eds) Cocaine use in America: epidemiologic and clinical perspectives. (National Institute on Drug Abuse Research Monograph 61) US Government Printing Office, Washington, DC, p 35–75

Anthony JC 1988 The epidemiological case–control strategy, with applications in psychiatric research. In: Henderson AS, Burrows GD (eds) Handbook of social psychiatry. Elsevier Science Publishers, Amsterdam, p 157–172

Anthony JC, Petronis KR 1989 Cocaine and heroin dependence compared: evidence from an epidemiologic field survey. Am J Public Health 79:1409–1410

Anthony JC, Petronis KR 1991 Epidemiologic evidence on suspected associations between cocaine use and psychiatric disturbances. In: Schober S, Schade C (eds) The epidemiology of cocaine use and abuse. (National Institute on Drug Abuse Research Monograph 110) US Government Printing Office, Washington, DC, p 71–94

Anthony JC, Tien AY, Petronis KR 1989 Epidemiologic evidence on cocaine use and panic attacks. Am J Epidemiol 129:543–549

Anthony JC, Ritter CJ, Von Korff MR, Chee EM, Kramer M 1986 Descriptive epidemiology of adult cocaine use in four U.S. communities. In: Harris LS (ed) Problems of drug dependence, 1986. (National Institute on Drug Abuse Research Monograph 76) US Government Printing Office, Washington, DC, p 283–289

Balster RL 1988 Pharmacological effects of cocaine relevant to its abuse. In: Clouet DH, Asghar K, Brown RM (eds) Mechanisms of cocaine abuse and toxicity. (National Institute on Drug Abuse Research Monograph 88) US Government Printing Office, Washington, DC, p 1–13

Boyd CJ, Mieczkowski T 1990 Drug use, health, family and social support in 'crack' cocaine users. Addict Behav 15:481–485

Brill H, Hirose T 1969 The rise and fall of a methamphetamine epidemic: Japan 1945-1955. Semin Psychiatry 1:179–194

Clayton RR 1985 Cocaine use in the United States: In a blizzard or just being snowed? In: Kozel NJ, Adams EH (eds) Cocaine use in America: epidemiologic and clinical perspectives. (National Institute on Drug Abuse Research Monograph 61) US Government Printing Office, Washington, DC, p 8–34

de Alarcon R 1969 The spread of heroin abuse in a community. Bull Narc 21:17–22

Ellinwood E 1974 The epidemiology of stimulant abuse. In: Josephson E, Carroll E (eds) Drug use—epidemiological and sociological approaches. Hemisphere Publishing Company. Washington, DC, p 303–329

Gawin FH 1991 Cocaine addiction: psychology and neurophysiology. Science (Wash DC) 251:1580–1586

Kaku DA, Lowenstein DH 1990 Emergence of recreational drug use as a major risk factor for stroke in young adults. Ann Intern Med 113:821–827

Kandel DB, Murphy D, Karus D 1985 Cocaine use in young adulthood: patterns of use and psychosocial correlates. In: Kozel NJ, Adams EH (eds) Cocaine use in America: epidemiologic and clinical perspectives. (National Institute on Drug Abuse Research Monograph 61) US Government Printing Office, Washington, DC, p 76–110

Lakoski JM, Cunningham KA 1988 The interaction of cocaine with central serotonergic neuronal systems: cellular electrophysiologic approaches. In: Clouet DH, Asghar K, Brown RM (eds) Mechanisms of cocaine abuse and toxicity. (National Institute on Drug Abuse Research Monograph 88) US Government Printing Office, Washington DC, p 55–77

Mann JJ, Stanley M, McBride PA et al 1986 Increased serotonin, and β-adrenergic receptor binding in the frontal cortices of suicide victims. Arch Gen Psychiatry 43:954–959

Mueller BA, Daling JR, Weiss NS, Moore DE 1990 Recreational drug use and the risk of primary infertility. Epidemiology 1:195–200

Ng SKC, Brust JCM, Hauser WA, Susser M 1990 Illicit drug use and the risk of new-onset seizures. Am J Epidemiol 132:47–57

Petronis KR, Samuels J, Moscicki E, Anthony JC 1990 An epidemiologic investigation of potential risk factors for suicide attempts. Soc Psychiatry Psychiatr Epidemiol 25:193–199

Ritter C, Anthony JC 1991 Factors influencing initiation of cocaine use among adults: findings from the Epidemiologic Catchment Area Program. In: Schober S, Schade C (eds) The epidemiology of cocaine use and abuse. (National Institute on Drug Abuse Research Monograph 110) US Government Printing Office, Washington, DC, p 189–210

Tien AY, Anthony JC 1990 Epidemiological analysis of alcohol and drug use as risk factors for psychotic experiences. J Nerv Ment Dis 178:473–480

Trinkoff AM, Ritter C, Anthony JC 1990 The prevalence and self-reported consequences of cocaine use: an exploratory and descriptive analysis. Drug Alcohol Depend 26:217–225

DISCUSSION

Jaffe: Are your questionnaires designed so that they can give you data on people who use cocaine exclusively and not heroin, and also heroin exclusively but not cocaine? Because of considerable overlap in use, often when we ask people whether they experience withdrawal symptoms, we have to depend on them to tell us which drug it is withdrawal from—and they may not know. This may be of some interest when we try to understand the factors that lead to continued use of cocaine, the duration of the cocaine withdrawal syndrome, and other factors. How did you do the analyses on tolerance and withdrawal?

Anthony: We shared your concern about the co-occurrence of daily heroin use and daily cocaine use. For this reason, we studied 69 daily cocaine users who reported essentially no experience with heroin, certainly no pattern of daily heroin use (see Table 2, p 28). These 'heroin-free' daily cocaine users were drawn from a much larger pool of cocaine users found in our epidemiological samples, as we deliberately tried to restrict our attention to people who would be informative about daily cocaine use and not heroin use.

Kleber: Something we began to learn in the early 1980s was that the cocaine addict was more likely to have a pattern of use consisting of 'binges' (1–3 days of heavy use followed by a few days of non-use) than to be a daily user of cocaine, and that the daily user was more likely in fact to be a 'self-medicator'. So, if you are equating the daily heroin user and the daily cocaine user, this may not be an appropriate comparison.

Anthony: Please understand the context of this particular comparison of daily cocaine users and daily heroin users. Our point of departure was a published study of *treated* drug users, from which it was claimed that daily cocaine users were dependent on cocaine just as frequently as heroin users were dependent on heroin. Our goal was to see whether epidemiological samples of cocaine users and heroin users, selected by probability sample survey methods, would lead us to the same conclusions, otherwise using the same standardized research methods. It is possible to over-generalize from clinical experience and clinical samples. The broad population experience with cocaine will sometimes be quite different from the experience of cocaine users who enter treatment facilities.

Kleber: Secondly, is there the possibility of circular thinking in your data relating to the idea that cocaine use might increase suicide risk? If I were already depressed, and at risk of suicide, I might use cocaine to deal with my depression. In other words, is there an implication of a chicken-and-egg causal process, from your results?

Anthony: In this instance, we would not have chosen to study suicide attempts in relation to cocaine use had there not been repeated clinical observations that cocaine users were at increased risk of suicide attempt. Further, there was some evidence of cocaine's involvement in neurobiological systems that also might be related to making suicide attempts, as Asberg and others have found. These two elements together provided a theoretical basis for examining this question with epidemiological data. If it were true that cocaine use signals an increased risk of making a suicide attempt, then we should see this in the epidemiological data. This was indeed what we saw.

You also asked whether this association might be confounded by a history of depression. We had three separate measures of depression. One was a diagnosis of major depression, which we also found to be strongly related with making a suicide attempt. A second measure involved a less specific syndrome of depression, which did not make much difference, once we took into account the lifetime history of major depression. The third measure was simply a self-report to identify those persons who had had a period of two weeks in their lives when they had felt sad or blue, or had lost all interest in their usual activities. Holding constant any or all of these three measures of depression did not change the relationship between cocaine use and occurrence of suicide attempt, except to make the association more potent. This evidence suggests that 'confounding' by pre-existing depression is not the explanation of the link we found between cocaine use and making a suicide attempt.

Now, we admit that there are other ways to measure a history of depression, and there are other risk factors that we did not hold constant in this study. A family history of affective disorder, for example, might put a person at increased risk of making a suicide attempt. We did not control this type of risk factor because it was not measured in our multi-site collaborative study in any uniform way. One direction for future studies of the association between cocaine use and suicide attempt is in relation to suspected confounding variables like family history. We need better measurement and control of such variables.

Edwards: Does anyone want to take further this important issue of causality?

Des Jarlais: Yes, and specifically on Herb Kleber's question. In one of our studies of heroin addicts (Des Jarlais et al 1992) we asked about suicide attempts in the period when the use of crack was still uncommon among heroin addicts in New York City. We found that attempted suicide in 1985 predicted persistent crack use in 1987–1989. In this case, because the crack epidemic came after these people had attempted suicide, the causal relation was clearly *from* a previous suicide attempt *to* persistent crack use in a later period. So I would be cautious about saying that all of the causation goes *from* cocaine use *to* suicide attempts. Here clearly the suicide attempt was occurring before a particularly dangerous form of cocaine use.

Anthony: I agree that we need to be cautious in drawing the inference of causality, but we have to direct our attention toward systematic replications and more rigorous inquiries. To allow our scepticism to deter others from attempting to replicate would be wrong.

Moore: What happened to the suicide attempt rates in the heroin users when the crack epidemic occurred?

Des Jarlais: There were no real changes in rates over the time of crack use.

Kleber: Dr Anthony, one of your more interesting results relates to panic attacks. We know from clinical experience that persons with such attacks are less likely to use cocaine because it can make the attacks worse. The fact that panic attacks showed an increased relative risk supports the suggestion of direct causality, namely that these people didn't *previously* have panic attacks, but took cocaine and then developed them.

Fibiger: I am still a little confused, Dr Anthony. Do your data allow you to say, with respect to depression, for example, that cocaine use eventually resulted in depression, or did it exist before the cocaine use?

Anthony: Our study indicated that cocaine use signalled an increased risk of panic attack, and also an increased risk of depression, as well as other disturbances listed in Table 4 of my paper (p 31). Let me take panic attack as an illustration. At baseline in our surveys we used a systematic interview to identify persons who reported ever having had a panic attack at any time prior to the baseline assessment. Those individuals were then excluded from the analysis, in order to exclude the possibility that the panic attack had preceded the cocaine use. Then, after a follow-up interval of one year, we studied this 'at-risk' set of individuals with no prior history of panic attack, and we estimated whether cocaine users were more likely to develop panic attack than non-users. We produced these estimates in a manner that allowed us to hold constant potentially confounding variables such as a history of alcoholism or other psychiatric disorders, unemployment status, being divorced or separated, and so on. The panic attack estimate in Table 4 shows that cocaine use signalled increased risk of panic attack. A result based on the same type of standard prospective research strategy was obtained for the syndrome of depression, and for other psychiatric disturbances. Thus, the historical influence of prior panic attack or major depression and the like has been eliminated, as far as we can manage it.

I have to admit that if an interviewee has a liability for depression that has not yet fully expressed itself in the way we measured depression, then such a person deserves attention in future studies, provided this liability can be measured. The liability for depression might lead them to cocaine use, and then the two factors together perhaps, or the liability for depression by itself, might lead them on to a suicide attempt. This remains an issue for future enquiry.

Almond: I wonder if there is an important distinction in your work between attempted suicide and suicide? I notice that you talked only about attempts, and usually it is thought that the psychological factors and type of people involved are quite different in the two cases.

Anthony: Yes. There's a very clear distinction between suicide and suicide attempt. We studied suicide attempt. In our epidemiological samples, we have evidence that there might have been one successful suicide, but no more than a few successful suicides, as you might expect for 18 000 American adults over a one-year span of time.

Negrete: I am interested in the epidemiological evidence of psychiatric disturbance and cocaine use. I think we are much too ready to assume that a suicide intention, or a suicide attempt, is a reflection of a psychopathological state which is independent of cocaine use. In clinical experience, most of the severely addicted cocaine users, during the 'crash' (which they experience even if they are daily users), feel very bad about themselves and think of suicide. Some patients take some action, but the majority just feel they could or should die, and are worthless. These feelings subside rather quickly, if these people remain abstinent. I would not necessarily say that it was pre-existing depression that led them to use cocaine. The experience of suicidal intention is not necessarily a reflection of a co-existing depressive disorder; it is a short-lived, morbid way of thinking, linked to cocaine toxicity.

Finally, were there any gender differences in this question of suicidal intent, or attempt, among cocaine users?

Anthony: There were no gender differences in the degree to which cocaine use signalled an increased risk of attempted suicide. As to the survey measurements, we measured making a suicide attempt, rather than a stated intention to do so.

O'Brien: My experience with cocaine users who are applying for treatment is very similar to Dr Negrete's, but I also think that there are great numbers of cocaine users out there in the population who never come to clinicians such as Dr Negrete and me, and whose experience may be very different. My patients are mostly 'bingers' who have lost control and have a high frequency of psychosis, suicide attempts and other problems, but they may not be representative of the broader population of cocaine users.

Benowitz: I want to ask about the duration of cocaine use. Jim Anthony's data showing much higher use rates in 18–25-year-olds compared to people 26 years or older (Fig. 1, p 21) suggest that the duration of cocaine use for an individual is relatively brief. Do you have specific data on this, or does anyone have data on duration of use?

Anthony: The data on duration of cocaine use exist but have not been analysed or published; members of my research group hope to secure the national survey data needed to make these estimates. Your point brings us back to the dynamics of the cocaine epidemic and allows me to tie my paper in with David Musto's paper.

I wonder whether the public's *tolerance* of cocaine use is the dynamic factor behind the current cocaine epidemic? I can think of at least two other dynamically changing factors that might be explanatory. These might resonate with the experience of the first cocaine epidemic that Dr Musto described.

One dynamically changing factor might be variation in the number of persons who are susceptible to trying cocaine use, but then stop using it. Illicit use of marijuana or other controlled substances (besides cocaine) might be important here.

It seems plausible that the use of marijuana or some other illegal drug use might be a signal of a different susceptibility to try cocaine, at least in the USA where the probability of becoming a cocaine user has been exceedingly small for those who never tried marijuana or engaged in other illicit drug use.

Almost all of our cocaine users have been drawn from the pool of individuals who have used marijuana at some time or another (see Clayton 1985, Ritter & Anthony 1991). I have wondered whether the present epidemic might be an expression of our having created in the 1960s and early 1970s a large pool of susceptibles for cocaine use at a time when the availability of cocaine was relatively low.

Then, as air traffic increased between North and South America, and as South America became an increasingly common travel option for young American citizens, the traffic channels increased the opportunities to use cocaine in a previously 'primed' and more susceptible population. So, we had an intermixing of a more susceptible population at a time of low cocaine supply, and then cocaine becoming more available during a later period when that population was still in early adulthood, taking on new life experiences, and not yet settled into the pattern of alcohol consumption that is more normative for fully middle aged adults in the USA.

Now, consider that the size of this pool of susceptibles is determined by the number of young adults in the population (in recent years, largely dominated by survivors of the post-war baby boom), and also by the proportion who have been 'primed' for cocaine use by virtue of the prior experience of taking marijuana or some other drug illegally. The bulk of this pool of susceptibles (a carry-over from the post-war baby boom and the marijuana epidemic in the late 1960s and early 1970s), given an increase in cocaine supply, could have been 'burned out' by 1980, certainly by 1985—long enough for these susceptibles to have had an opportunity to try cocaine or to complete the passage into early middle age.

This is the other dynamically changing factor: a pool of more susceptible persons eventually is burned out, unless the number starting cocaine use is replaced by an equivalent number of new susceptibles, such as persons age 18–22. In the United States, the number of persons aged 18–22 has been declining in parallel with the reported decline in the cocaine epidemic, so perhaps the pool of susceptibles is being depleted. Once a pool of susceptible individuals has been depleted (in this case, by having tried cocaine and moved on, or simply by becoming middle-aged), then the epidemic should decline.

Kalant: On this speculation of a role of marijuana as a primer setting the stage for cocaine use, the Ontario and US school data indicate that alcohol use precedes or is associated with marijuana use, and that there are no people who are specifically primed for cocaine by marijuana who have not already used alcohol (Erickson et al 1987). I would suggest that the broad waves of drug use, both in the original period of cocaine use and in the second phase, were preceded by 20–30 years of increasing alcohol use. I also suggest that there is a general level of public acceptance of drug use that is first expressed with respect to alcohol, for the obvious reason that it is licit, easily available, and poses no great problems of social deviance; but then the acceptance of alcohol sets the stage for the increased acceptance of not only cocaine but a variety of other drugs.

Musto: With regard to susceptibility to cocaine after marijuana use, I am reminded of Freud's response to the accusation that he had unloosed in Europe a cocaine epidemic. He retorted that cocaine addiction only occurred in those who had previously used morphine to excess. In Freud's words, 'Cocaine has claimed no other, no victim on its own' (Freud 1887). Dr Anthony's hypothesis is a most interesting one—and I am certain Freud would be inclined to agree!

Anthony: I was of course referring to the illicit use of marijuana and other controlled substances (i.e., to illicit drug-using behaviour congeneric with illicit cocaine-taking), and not to the more normative use of alcohol or tobacco.

Edwards: To me, the question remains, after Jim Anthony's paper, of what the epidemiologists are really doing. When are epidemiologists in this particular arena going to stop being blind empiricists, and to start measuring things which will explain and generalize?

Anthony: I take your point, but it is worth mentioning that many practising epidemiologists date the modern origins of our discipline to 1850 or so, when John Snow worked right here in London. Snow tested his theory of cholera, versus the miasma theory, using data on the cholera epidemic. Snow's work stands as a model for theory-driven epidemiology. In this context, I wonder if it is fair to allege that epidemiology represents blind empiricism. For the most part, practising epidemiologists work from a biologically plausible hypothesis, arising either through the careful observations of clinicians, or from laboratory evidence, or from a brilliant deduction—perhaps the result of sitting under apple trees and waiting for apples to fall! With time, we shall learn whether the right hypotheses have been selected, and whether we have measured what matters. Meantime, some of us will continue being blind empiricists and some of us will not.

References

Clayton RR 1985 Cocaine use in the United States: in a blizzard or just being snowed? In: Kozel NJ, Adams EH (eds) Cocaine use in America: epidemiologic and clinical perspectives. (National Institute on Drug Abuse Research Monograph 61) US Government Printing Office, Washington, DC, p 8–34

Des Jarlais DC, Wenston J, Sotheran JL, Maslansky R, Marmor M 1992 Crack cocaine use in a cohort of methadone maintenance patients. J Subst Abuse Treat, in press

Erickson PG, Adlaf EM, Murray GF, Smart RG 1987 The steel drug: cocaine in perspective. Lexington Books, Lexington, MA

Freud S 1887 Beitrage ueber Anwendung des Cocain. Wiener Med Wochensch No. 28: p 929–932. English translation: Byck R (ed) 1974 Cocaine papers by Sigmund Freud. Stonehill Publishing, New York, p 170–176 (see p 173)

Ritter C, Anthony JC 1991 Factors influencing initiation of cocaine use among adults: findings from the Epidemiologic Catchment Area Program. In: Schober S, Schade C (eds) The epidemiology of cocaine use and abuse. (National Institute on Drug Abuse Research Monograph 110) US Government Printing Office, Washington, DC, p 189–210

Cocaine problems in the coca-growing countries of South America

J. C. Negrete

Department of Psychiatry, McGill University, and Alcohol & Drug Dependence Unit, Montreal General Hospital, Montreal, Canada H3G 1A4

Abstract. The problems of cocaine present a rather particular profile in the Central Andes region from which this drug originates. On the one hand there is a relatively harmless pattern of use (coca leaf chewing) in the countries concerned which minimizes the drug's most hazardous properties. On the other hand the region suffers from some of the most severe cocaine-related problems to be observed anywhere: (a) easy access to the newer, highly toxic preparations of the drug (such as coca paste) and a rapid growth in the number of new users; (b) the abandonment of certain traditional and essential agricultural activities in favour of the more profitable coca leaf production; (c) the severe ecological damage being caused in the coca growing areas; and (d) the establishment of a powerful coca trade economy which is subverting the very fabric of society and is creating corruption, lawless violence and political anarchy.

1992 Cocaine: scientific and social dimensions. Wiley, Chichester (Ciba Foundation Symposium 166) p 40–56

Coca growing and cocaine production

There are at present two major species of cocaine-yielding shrubs: *Erythroxylum coca* and *Erythroxylum novagranatense*. Each of these has two varieties, thus accounting for the four types currently in commercial cultivation. *Erythroxylum coca* var. *coca* is by far the most frequently used variety; its habitat is the moist forest conditions which prevail on the eastern slopes of the Andes mountains, in Peru and Bolivia. A second variety (*E. coca* var. *ipandu*) has been developed in recent years for growth in the rain forest lowlands of the upper Amazon basin (Colombia, Brazil and Ecuador). This new variety, of course, is almost exclusively destined for the illicit drug market. A third variety (*E. novagranatense* var. *truxillense*) has been adapted to the drier conditions of the northwest of Peru, in the semi-desert area around the city of Trujillo. The fourth variety— *E. novagranatense* var. *novagranatense*—has long been farmed in the northernmost regions of the Andes mountain range, where it supplies the needs of some isolated native groups with coca leaf chewing traditions (e.g. the Kogi of the Sierra Nevada de Santa Marta).

Peru and Bolivia are still the largest producers, and the only countries to operate a legal, government-controlled coca leaf market. Authorized growers supply the international demand for coca-flavoured products (such as cola drinks) and for the cocaine intended for pharmaceutical use. More significantly, they cover the demand generated by several million coca leaf chewers; in Peru alone they consume each year the yield of some 12 000 hectares of intensive coca farming (Lerner 1991, p 25, 26).

As a traditional habit of significant cultural impact that is difficult to eradicate, coca leaf chewing is one of the few drug-taking practices which qualified for deferral of the immediate ban laid down by the 1961 International Convention on Narcotic Drugs. Such practices, it was agreed at that Convention, were to be progressively eliminated, within 25 years of the date on which the international agreement became effective (1964). This goal has of course not been attained; in 1989, coca growing was still a major economic activity in the traditional producer societies (Peru and Bolivia) and it had been newly introduced into countries such as Colombia and Brazil where there was practically none in the 1960s. The annual yield of coca leaf in Peru increased from 11 068 tonnes in 1959 to an estimated 250 000 tonnes in 1987 (Leon & Castro de la Mata 1989, p 213, 264). Official records show that the production authorized by the Peruvian government grew almost seven-fold between 1967 and 1987. But it is the non-registered, illegal cultivation, which has developed since the mid 1970s, that is the most important source of coca leaf supply at the present moment (see Fig. 1).

Total cultivated area and annual yield figures can nowadays only be estimated, for aerial surveys have found that illegal coca farming accounts for as much

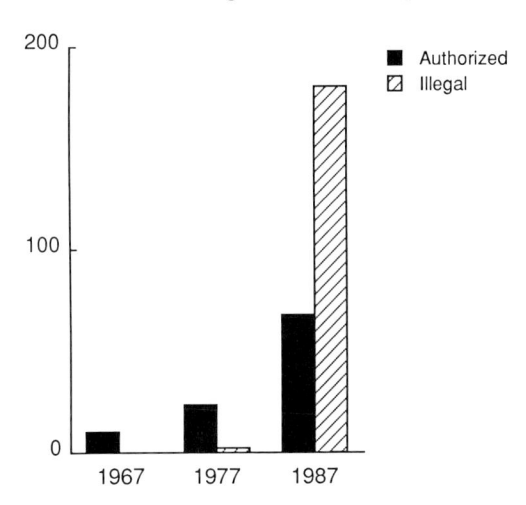

FIG. 1. Coca leaf production in Peru, in rounded annual figures, expressed in thousand tonnes. (Adapted from data of Jeri & Perez 1990 and Leon & Castro de la Mata 1989.)

as 80% of the current production (Leon & Castro de la Mata 1989, p 264). Unauthorized coca farming in Peru takes place in a myriad of smallish plots of land, frequently hidden in dense forest and scattered across an extensive territory on the eastern slopes of the Andes (Leon & Castro de la Mata 1989, p 264). The same occurs in Bolivia, where coca growing has expanded well beyond the traditional farming area in the Yungas highlands, down into the tropical region of Chapare and the Beni, where many growers operate without government authorization (Jeri 1980, p 154–158). Coca growing has indeed undergone major changes over the last 20 years. From the centuries-old, orderly and socially stable farming activity it was until the 1960s, it has become a rather ruthless, expedient and profit-oriented industry, which shares none of the traditions of the trade and is largely practised by transient farmers who avoid official controls, must hide from law-enforcing repression, and are only interested in producing for the illicit drug market.

A number of growers, whose production from duly registered farms is cleared for trade in the legal coca leaf market, have been selling part of the crop in the parallel illicit market. They trade the leaves as such or—quite frequently—their yield of coca paste, which many of these farmers are capable of preparing on their own premises (see below).

In the Bolivian regions of the Chapare, a substantial volume of leaves is offered for sale each week in the market place. Much of this large supply, however, is not being bought by coca chewers for their own use, but rather by individuals who intend to divert it into the production of coca paste (Knox 1991). Thus, the illicit cocaine market is not only supplied by an underground farming system, but it absorbs a sizeable amount of the legal coca leaf crop as well.

Coca farms in Peru must sell their produce to a State monopoly (ENACO), which has exclusive control over pricing and distribution. The price paid by this agency for the coca leaf has been consistently lower than the one offered by middlemen of the underground trade. In fact, for several years, ENACO has been paying only about one-sixth of the illegal rates (Table 1). Not suprisingly, many growers sell at least part of their crop in the parallel market.

TABLE 1 Potential revenue from coca growing in Peru for the period 1985–1987[a]

Average yield per 1 Ha coca field	Local market value ($)	
	Legal	Underground
1000 kg coca leaf	600	3600
10 kg 'raw' coca paste	N/A	5000
4.5 kg 'cleansed' coca paste	N/A	5500
3.15 kg cocaine HCl	N/A	94 500

[a]Adapted from data published by Morales (1989) and by Leon & Castro de la Mata (1989), p 265–268.

Moreover, a sizeable number of them—both registered and underground—rather than selling the leaves, are producing coca paste *in situ*; this not only fetches a higher price, but is considerably easier to transport and to trade on. Dealers would much rather buy coca paste than the equivalent in leaves which is a hundred times the weight and much bulkier.

The making of coca paste is a relatively simple chemical procedure which can be carried out under rather primitive technical conditions. Most of the illegal farming units, and some of the registered growers, have ready access to the necessary facilities. Many have developed their own individual 'laboratories', and others make use of collective coca paste plants operating in the community. A major hindrance is the local unavailability of the large volumes of sulphuric acid, sodium carbonate (or other alkaline substances) and organic solvents (kerosene or gasoline) which are needed in the process. These chemicals must be brought over long distances to the rural areas where coca paste is produced. Coca-paste makers are none the less able to obtain their supplies by securing the cooperation of law enforcement agents, who are paid to overlook the telltale cargoes, or from deliveries made by underground dealers, who fly the chemicals into clandestine airstrips in the area.

The paste is the first byproduct of coca leaf, an essential step in the manufacturing of the salt, cocaine hydrochloride (HCl). Its content in alkaloids varies from about 60% of the total weight in the 'crude' preparations, to nearly 80% in the more refined ones (*pasta lavada* or 'cleansed' paste). In South America, this product is called *pasta basica* (cocaine base paste), in reference to the fact that much of the alkaloid contained in it is in the form of cocaine free base, rather than as the salt. The Colombian slang term *basuca* evokes both the chemical nature (cocaine base) and the potency of the psychotropic effects (i.e. as powerful as a bazooka gun).

In the preparation of cocaine HCl powder, the crude coca paste is first 'cleansed' through the use of an oxidizing agent (potassium permanganate) and a more refined solvent (ether), and then precipitated once more by the addition of hydrochloric acid. The drug is usually manufactured in large clandestine laboratories around the area where coca growing has been recently introduced, but more often this is done in remote locations in the Colombian hinterland (Morales 1989). The latter activity has been curtailed recently by more effective policing in Colombia, and considerably larger amounts of coca paste are now being sold within the local market in Bolivia and Peru (Lerner 1991).

Local patterns of cocaine use

Coca leaf chewing

Coca leaf chewing is still the most prevalent form of cocaine use in the Central Andes region. It involves millions of people, mostly highland Quechua peasants, who make it part of their daily habits—much the same as coffee drinking or tobacco smoking are elsewhere (Heath 1990). This traditional drug practice has changed little over the centuries; it consists in keeping a wad of leaves in the mouth, between cheek and gums, and sucking the juices from it steadily during two or three hours at a time ('chewing' is a misnomer). Small quantities of an alkaline powder (such as sodium bicarbonate, or wood ashes) are deposited on the wad every so often, with the purpose of increasing salivation and facilitating the release of the alkaloids. There can be no doubt that this method effectively extracts cocaine and results in its absorption into the blood stream. Chewers do experience the local anaesthetic effects of the drug, and blood level readings show detectable amounts only minutes after the leaves are put into the mouth (Paly et al 1980a). Cocaine blood concentrations rise steadily during the chewing session and peak shortly after the used leaves are discarded. Experienced users, taking moderate amounts of leaves (12–15 g), attain a peak blood concentration of about 100 ng/ml. When larger amounts (50 g) are chewed during the same period, the peak concentration levels can be much higher (800 ng/ml). Such blood cocaine levels, of course, are pharmacologically significant.

Ferrando (1990) found that one-third of the population at risk (aged 12–50) in towns of the mountain region in Peru report having chewed coca leaves at some time in their lives. The figure would most likely be higher had the rural population been included in the sample. The habit is less frequent in the coastal centres, where Quechua Indians form only a minority of the population, and in the riverside towns of the eastern jungle region, where coca chewing is culturally alien (see Table 2). Coca chewing, traditionally identified with the lifestyle of impoverished highland peasants, carries a social stigma and is shunned by those sectors of Peruvian society who wish to assert a higher standing—such as *mestizos* (people of mixed European and Indian race) and Whites, urban dwellers, the better educated, and white collar workers. The size of the population involved is therefore expected to diminish as more opportunities for upward social mobility become available. Indeed, overall rates of coca chewing have been decreasing over the years (Caravedo & Almeida 1972, Lerner 1991). But another likely explanation for this decline is the significant increase in the retail price of coca leaf, caused by competition from the illegal drug market (Heath 1990). While the number of chewers may be falling in the highlands, the rates in Lima and the Amazon region remain stable, or are even slightly higher than before. This is quite probably due to the accelerated influx of highland migrants, who have been moving into the urban centres in search of better opportunities.

Lerner (1991) reports that coca leaf chewing shows the youngest average age of onset (17.7 years) among all forms of cocaine use in Peru. This can be explained in part by the association this habit has with heavy manual labour, which also starts early in life around the farming and mining communities of the Andes. Coca chewing appears to be the most persistent form of use as well,

TABLE 2 Rates of cocaine use (lifetime) per 100 respondents in different regions of Peru[a]

	Lima	Highlands	Amazonia
Coca leaf	13.4	30.5	5.3
Coca paste	3.6	0.6	2.5
Cocaine HCl	1.8	0.2	0.6

[a]Urban population aged 12–50. Adapted from data published by Ferrando (1990) and Lerner (1991).

for Ferrando (1990) has found that only 28% of chewers have ever tried to quit the habit, while six out of 10 users of coca paste or cocaine powder assert that they did make such attempts.

Coca paste smoking

Coca paste, practically unknown in South America before the 1970s, is now widely available and quite frequently used in the coca-growing countries of the region. The modal pattern of intake is by smoking; pyrolysis is easily effected by burning the paste in pipes of different types, or by adding it to tobacco or cannabis cigarettes. Solid cocaine turns liquid at relatively low temperatures (98 °C); at higher temperatures it may sublimate—that is, pass directly from the solid to the gaseous state (Budavari et al 1989). The volatile nature of the drug facilitates inhalation and accounts for the high blood levels attained through coca paste smoking (Paly et al 1980b). In fact, smoking is the most effective method of making cocaine bioavailable. No other form of intake delivers comparable amounts to the brain in as short a time. The psychoactive reward effects are both immediate and intense, and the well-known reinforcing properties of the drug are more fully exerted with this mode of use. Coca paste smokers purposely seek the mind-altering effects of cocaine—something coca chewers rarely do, for absorption through the digestive tract is much slower and seldom leads to the required blood levels.

Paste smoking is a deviant practice, culturally not legitimized and still largely attracting the marginal sectors of society: mainly the emotionally unstable, the social misfits and the idle; the street youth and the homeless; the criminal underworld; and those involved in the cocaine trade. Consequently, a higher prevalence is found in larger urban centres than in the more socially stable and traditional communities. In Peru and Bolivia, for instance, there is an apparent negative correlation between frequency figures for coca chewing and those for cocaine smoking or snorting. In areas where the former are higher the latter are lower, and vice versa (Table 2).

As is the case with most deviant habits, the prevalence of coca paste smoking among South American women is only a fraction of the prevalence among men.

TABLE 3   Male and female rates of cocaine use (lifetime) per 1000 respondents, established through household surveys[a]

	Colombia (1987) M	Colombia (1987) F	Peru (1988) M	Peru (1988) F	Mexico (1988) M	Mexico (1988) F	Canada (1989) M	Canada (1989) F
Cocaine HCl	4	1	25	1	4	0.1	45	27
Coca paste	10	3	57	1	—	—	—	—

[a]Adapted from data published by Organizacion Panamerican dela Salud (1990), Ferrando (1990) and Eliany (1989). Samples in Colombia: urban, aged 12–64; in Peru: urban, aged 12–50; in Mexico: countrywide, aged 12–65; in Canada: countrywide, aged 15+.

But the latter has reached an alarming magnitude: more than one in 20 Peruvian males in the age range 12–50 years (Table 3). These data derive from self-reports in interviews in household surveys, and the figures can be assumed to underestimate the actual prevalence, for respondents would be naturally wary of inquiries dealing with this issue at a time of increased law-enforcing activity. Moreover, since these surveys systematically exclude potential respondents who do not live in single-family dwellings, the high risk groups previously mentioned are unlikely to be represented in the samples. The size of the transient and homeless population in the cities involved is significant indeed; and—as demonstrated by Masur et al (1990) in Sao Paulo—rates of cocaine use among South American street dwellers can be many times higher than those in the community at large.

Cocaine HCl

The use of this preparation is relatively infrequent in South America, for most drug users opt for the less expensive and more readily available coca paste. Prevalence figures have nevertheless increased steadily over the years, and comparably obtained rates are much higher now (Ferrando 1990) than they were in 1979 (Carbajal et al 1980) or even in 1986 (Jutkowitz et al 1987). It is also apparent that cocaine powder users are to be found mainly within the better-educated older and higher income groups in the urban population. The current prevalence rate in Lima, for instance, is nine times that in the highlands and threefold the rate in the Amazon region (Table 2).

Most cocaine powder users in South America just snort the drug; 'free-basing' or 'crack' smoking is practically unknown in the region. There may well be differences in social perception between snorting, a pattern which attracts people from the upper classes as well, and coca paste smoking, which is more typical of the less desirable groups in society. Social attitudes notwithstanding, eight out of ten cocaine HCl users admit to having smoked coca paste some time in their lives—which points to the possible existence of a process of upward mobility in drug choices.

Cocaine-related problems

The public belief in coca-producing countries was for years that there was no such thing as a local cocaine problem. Those naive attitudes reflect both a social unease about the coca-growing issue, and the shortsighted assumption that illegal cocaine production will continue to be 'for export' only. Actually, as shown in Table 3, cocaine use in those countries is now reaching the same high levels as those observed in major 'consumer' societies (e.g. Canada), and the rates are lower in Latin American countries where there is no cocaine production (e.g. Mexico). Producer countries are indeed experiencing serious consequences; the following is a brief summary.

Health problems

Coca chewing is not known to cause behavioural or mental disturbances of clinical significance, particularly in the early stages of the habit. However, it does induce a nicotine-like dependence and is associated with an impoverishment of mental function—as well as general neglect—in the more advanced phases. Gutierrez Noriega & Zapata Ortiz (1947) had published relevant clinical observations already some 50 years ago, and controlled field studies (Negrete & Murphy 1967, Murphy et al 1969) later confirmed the existence of a mild but significant deficit in cognitive functions, which increases with years of chewing (Fig. 2). Such impairment could certainly help to perpetuate the conditions of social backwardness in which most coca chewers live.

Coca paste smoking, of course, is associated with the most severe consequences of any form of cocaine addiction. The first clinical cases were reported in Lima in the mid 1970s and incidence figures are still increasing. This habit is currently responsible for the largest number of hospital admissions among all drug practices in the region (Jeri & Perez 1990, Luna 1984), and has been identified as the top cause of drug casualties by the RENAD—a 1990 registry of the drug abuse cases in hospital emergency rooms in Lima (Instituto Nacional de Salud Mental [Peru] 1991).

Social, economic and ecological problems

Apart from the well-known state of violent anarchy and public corruption into which the cocaine-producing countries have fallen, the vertiginous growth of this major activity is causing social–environmental harm of incalculable consequences. A sizeable sector of the population is now involved in the deviant activities related to the trade. Large numbers of people are flocking to the newly developed coca-growing areas in the hope of sharing in the bounty. There they live, in social anomie, an unsettled existence, full of danger and unpredictability. Rural dwellers in their majority, they are lost to the traditional agricultural

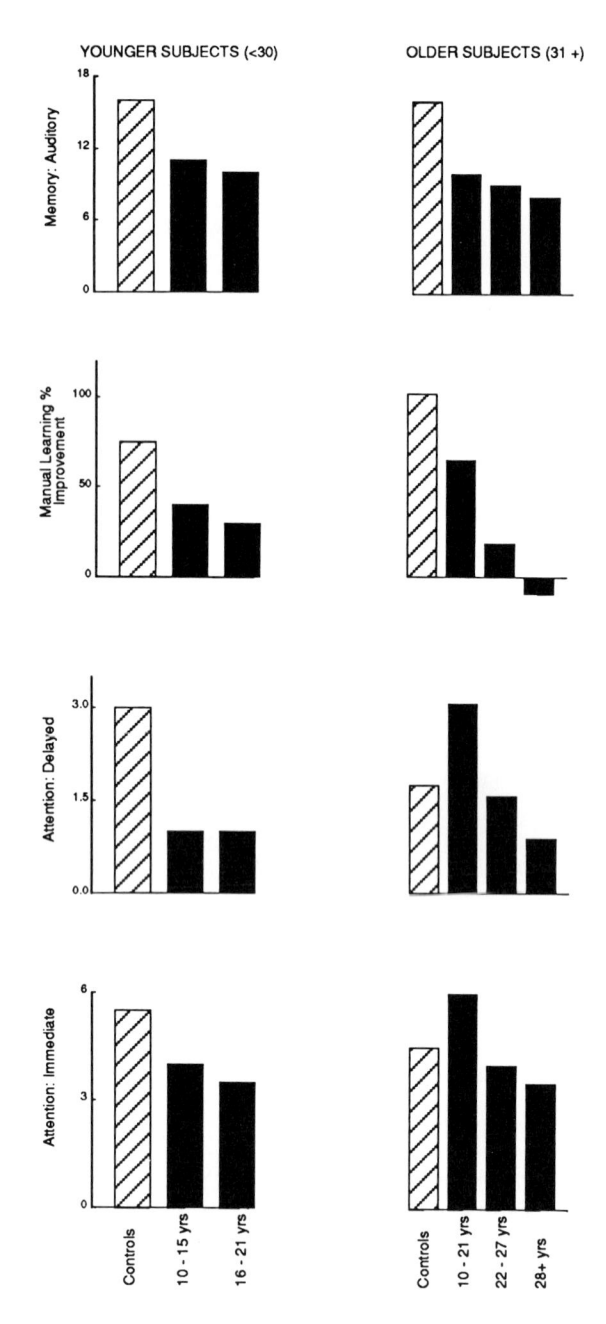

FIG. 2. Cognitive test scores in chronic coca chewers and control subjects, for two age groups (up to 30 years and 31 years or over). Horizontal axis shows the length of time for which cocaine has been used. (Adapted from data of Negrete & Murphy 1967.)

activities which occupied their elders. Squatters in a land that they don't plan to settle, they destroy and mistreat it, clearing patch after patch of precious forest in pursuit of the high yields of which the rapidly eroding terrain is capable for only two or three growing seasons. Tonnes of chemical waste from the coca paste plants are being spilled on the ground or drained into neighbouring rivers; large areas have already been affected by this highly toxic pollution (Leon & Castro de la Mata 1989, 281-299).

Thus, the coca-growing countries of South America are suffering considerable public health, sociocultural and ecological damage. The adverse consequences of the current cocaine upheaval are likely to be long lasting in those societies. Some, indeed, may even be irreversible.

Acknowledgements

The author gratefully acknowledges the helpful comments and useful information provided by Drs R. Jeri, A. Perales and R. Lerner (Peru); E. Velasquez and J. Luna (Colombia); and E. Madrigal (Pan American Health Organization/World Health Organization, Washington, DC).

References

Budavari S, O'Neil MJ, Smith A, Heckelman PE (eds) 1989 The Merck index, 11th edn. Merck & Co, Rahway, NJ
Carbajal C, Jeri R, Sanchez C, Bravo C, Valdivia L 1980 Estudio epidemiologico sobre uso de drogas en Lima. Rev Sanidad Fuerzas Policiales 41:1-38
Caravedo B, Almeida M 1972 Alcoholismo y toxicomanias; un informe actual sobre los problemas de alcohol, el coquismo las drogas en el Peru. Ministerio de Salud, Lima (pp 62)
Eliany M (ed) 1989 Licit and illicit drugs in Canada. Health & Welfare Canada, Ottawa
Ferrando D 1990 Uso de drogas en las ciudades del Peru. Monografia de investigacion 5, CEDRO, Lima (pp 172)
Gutierrez Noriega C, Zapata Ortiz V 1947 Estudios sobre la coca y la cocaina en el Peru. Ministerio de Salud, Lima (pp 144)
Heath DB 1990 Coca in the Andes: traditions, functions and problems. Rhode Island Med J 73:237-241
Instituto Nacional de Salud Mental (Peru) 1991 Sistema de Registro del Uso y Abuso del Alcohol y Drogas (RENAD), INSM, Lima (pp 91)
Jeri FR (ed) 1980 Cocaine 1980. Proceedings of the international seminar on medical and sociological aspects of coca and cocaine. (Pan American Health Office/WHO and the International Narcotics Management, Lima) Pacific Press, Lima (pp 264)
Jeri FR, Perez JC 1990 Dependencia a la cocaina en el Peru. Monografia de investigacion 4, CEDRO, Lima (pp 73)
Jutkowitz JM, Arellano R, Castro de la Mata R et al 1987 Uso y abuso de drogas en el Peru. Monografia de investigacion 1, CEDRO, Lima
Knox P 1991 The economics of coca leaves. The Globe & Mail (Toronto), April 20 1991, p B18

Leon F, Castro de la Mata R (eds) 1989 Pasta basica de cocaina. CEDRO, Lima (pp 428)

Lerner R 1991 Drugs in Peru: reality and representation. Drukkerij Quickprint BV, Nijmegen (pp 200)

Luna JA 1984 Aspectos generales de la cocaina y sus derivados en Colombia. In: Seminario internacional sobre la coca y sus derivados. Ministerio de Salud, Bogota, p 29–32

Masur J 1990 Cited in Abuso de drogas. Publicacion cientifica 522. PAHO/WHO, Washington, DC, p 164

Morales E 1989 Cocaine: white gold rush in Peru. University of Arizona Press, Tucson (pp 267)

Murphy HBM, Rios O, Negrete JC 1969 The effects of abstinence and re-training on the chewer of coca-leaf. Bull Narcotics 21(2):41–47

Negrete JC, Murphy HBM 1967 Psychological deficit in chewers of coca leaf. Bull Narcotics 19(4):11–18

Organizacion Panamericana de la Salud 1990 Abuso de drogas. Publicacion cientifica 522. PAHO/WHO, Washington, DC (pp 217)

Paly O, Jatlow P, Van Dyke C, Cabieses F, Byck R 1980a Plasma levels of cocaine in native Peruvian coca chewers. In: Jeri FR (ed) Cocaine 1980. Proceedings of the international seminar on medical and sociological aspects of coca and cocaine. (Pan American Health Office/WHO and the International Narcotics Management, Lima) Pacific Press, Lima, p 86–89

Paly D, Van Dyke C, Jatlow P, Jeri FR, Byck R 1980b Cocaine: plasma levels after cocaine paste smoking. In: Jeri FR (ed) Cocaine 1980. Proceedings of the international seminar on medical and sociological aspects of coca and cocaine. (Pan American Health Office/WHO and the International Narcotics Management, Lima) Pacific Press, Lima, p 106–110

DISCUSSION

Musto: How much cocaine is absorbed from the average wad of coca leaves that is chewed? I recall that I was told in Bogota that it is only about 4–5 mg per wad.

Negrete: No. The average coca leaf chewer uses some 20 g of leaves in a wad; the maximum would be 40–50 g. The leaves contain about 1–2% by weight of cocaine, so 20 g would yield 200 mg of cocaine—considerably more than was told to you.

Musto: So it is *not* 4 mg per wad? I had been interested in this figure, because it appeared to match the 4 mg of cocaine formerly in a bottle of Coca Cola, and in the typical chocolate tablet of cocaine, and also in Hall's medicated wine, which had 4 mg in the dose. Yet a number of people who work with individual users, and give them cocaine, tell me that 4 mg turns out to be too small a dose to provide any effect.

Jones: The 'wad' described by Dr Negrete would contain an oral dose of cocaine adequate to give a predictable pharmacological effect, namely 200–400 mg.

Fischman: My laboratory uses, as a 100 mg placebo intranasal cocaine dose, 4 mg cocaine mixed with 96 mg lactose. This dose has no cardiovascular or subjective effects that we can measure, other than a momentary numbing (or 'freezing') of the nasal mucosa (e.g. Javaid et al 1978, Foltin et al 1988). Four mg of cocaine taken by the oral route of administration, where absorption is less efficient and slower than via the intranasal route (Fischman 1988), is unlikely to have any discriminable effect at all.

Negrete: You are referring to subjective effects, of course. The coca chewer does not in any case seek to feel 'high' or to have a mood-altering effect; he just wants to feel well. In fact his pulse rate, blood glucose level and metabolic rate are all elevated; and he has more muscular endurance. These effects are also cocaine effects (Gutierrez Noriega & Zapata Ortiz 1947).

Fischman: It is likely that the coca leaf chewer is getting a discriminable dose of oral cocaine, because a 'wad' of coca can provide 200-300 mg cocaine. The person who drinks a beverage containing 4–5 mg cocaine, however, does not receive a discriminable dose of cocaine.

It is important that we do not confuse the coca chewer, and the traditional use of coca in South America, with the illicit cocaine user. There is a sociocultural history associated with coca chewing which is interwoven with many of the traditional aspects of everyday life. This is distinct from the drug use culture in which cocaine is taken.

Negrete: I agree, and I tried to distinguish these distinct practices in my paper.

Strang: Dr Negrete, how much information do we have about the years in which the smoking of coca paste came in, in South America? The 1980 book edited by Dr Jeri already had reports of this practice (Jeri 1980). Do we know the link between coca paste smoking and the development of the use of free base, and later with crack, in North America?

A related question concerns your impressions of the different smoking routes. Should we just regard smoking of *pasta* and *basuca* as slightly dirtier versions of crack but pharmacodynamically the same?

Negrete: The first cases of coca paste smoking to come to the attention of physicians in Lima were in the mid 1970s. I would say that there probably wasn't a very long time gap between the onset of the practice in the community and the occurrence of the first cases seen by the health services, because what we are talking about here is a tremendously heavy use of cocaine, which I think is unparalleled in North America. For example, Dr Jeri has accumulated 616 cases of coca paste smokers who have been treated in hospitals in Lima for cocaine-related symptoms (Jeri & Perez 1990). Of these, a great majority, more than 90%, were smoking daily, or 2–4 times a week. They used cigarettes of coca paste, either alone, or with tobacco or with cannabis; the cocaine is in the *pasta basica* (cocaine base paste) form, which contains as much as 60–80% cocaine free base. They were smoking between 11 and 30 times per day, in the majority of cases, according to Jeri's data. I haven't seen anyone in my clinic in Montreal who reports such a high quantity/frequency rate of use. It may be that some crack smokers do so for two or three days, but these Lima patients have been doing this for a month: the data are a frequency-quantity record over one month. It is essentially free-basing, and is therefore the same as crack, which you asked about.

Kalant: These data were obtained from a clinical population. Does the fact that they include very few occasional users mean that the data can't be representative of the general population of coca users in Lima?

Negrete: That is so; these are cases in treatment, not in the community at large. But even among cases in treatment in North America, we don't see that rate of consumption.

Benowitz: What are the health consequences of cocaine abuse in this population, compared to crack users in the USA?

Negrete: There are a lot of CNS complications—seizures and cerebral vascular accidents, according to Dr Jeri. There are also frequent cardiovascular accidents, as you would imagine, and, it would seem, more admissions to mental hospitals than in North America. Of course, psychiatric admission is the customary way of treating these patients there.

Jones: Jeri presented data on patterns of coca paste smoking in 1980 (Jeri 1980). Has there been any shift in the pattern of coca paste use since then, or is it decreasing in Lima, as it seems to be in the United States?

Negrete: In fact coca paste smoking is still increasing in Lima. Comparable population surveys indicate that the rate of consumption had gone up between 1986 and 1989.

Kleber: Roberto Lerner from CEDRO in Lima has said that they are estimating in Lima a rate of growth of *pasta* use of 20% per year, and similar kinds of growth in Bolivia and in Colombia (unpublished communication; CEDRO Conference, Lima, Peru, 24 October 1990).

Fischman: With reference to the health consequences, we have to be careful not to relate those to the cocaine, necessarily; *pasta basica* is full of solvents and other chemicals that will certainly have substantial health consequences of their own.

Negrete: That is true. This has been one argument, because gasoline and kerosene are used in the preparation of coca paste. The crude paste is however 'cleansed' afterwards, as I described.

As to the symptoms shown, it is hard to differentiate; some may even be due to lead poisoning.

Kleber: One point should be emphasized which may have major implications for the public health of the Andean countries in relation to the new growth of cocaine. As Dr Negrete said, this new growth of cocaine is a different variety, and of higher potency than *Erythroxylum coca* var. *coca*, which makes it too irritating to the mouth for it to be chewed. So the only uses of this new, high potency coca leaf are as *pasta* and as the hydrochloride; if the US market dries up, and other markets do not take up the slack, these countries are left with a big growth of coca leaf which can only be used for the more destructive forms of the drug. That may be one of the reasons why *pasta* use is increasing so fast in Lima and other places.

Kalant: I am puzzled by some of the figures, Dr Negrete. Dr Jeri's clinical data, which you have referred to, indicate that among *pasta* smokers the modal value was high, 15–20 *ketes* (doses) per day, whereas among the users of cocaine HCl, the modal value was 1–2 g per week, which is a much lower dosage range. I wonder how the figures fit together. Also the statement that the use of *pasta* is increasing now, *after* the market for sale to Colombian middlemen has been substantially inhibited, doesn't fit with the correlation found between use and production for other drugs in other parts of the world.

Negrete: There has been a larger supply of *pasta* in recent years, but the use of cocaine HCl is very rare in Peru and Colombia. As I mentioned, there seems to be a social perception of a hierarchy there; cocaine hydrochloride is mostly for upper-class people. If such people want to use cocaine, they will not smoke *pasta* any more, because they find it too common and too toxic. They consider the snorting of cocaine HCl to be preferable (there is no injection, practically, of cocaine HCl in Peru and Colombia). So those who prefer to snort cocaine are fewer and tend to be more moderate users. *Pasta* smokers however are not only found in the marginal social groups; middle-class youngsters and university students also smoke *pasta*. So there is a wide range of *pasta* users, but as you get richer and have more social standing, you would tend to prefer cocaine HCl. The data (Lerner 1991) show that most cocaine hydrochloride users have used *pasta* previously. These are the people who can pay the higher price and can move on to the higher status pattern.

Kalant: But they are apparently using less (lower doses)?

Negrete: Yes, they use cocaine HCl in relatively small quantities, but we don't have information about the amounts they used to take when they were smoking coca paste.

Kaplan: Usually when we talk about traditional coca use in South America we are speaking about the Indians, but what is known about the current casual use of cocaine in Latin America? I know from ethnohistorical accounts that in Colombia a popular way of getting up in the morning, among some circles, is with a *blanco y negro*, which is a varying amount of cocaine and a very small cup of black coffee (*tinto*). A vivid description of this so-called 'Santa Marta breakfast' has been published in the account of Charles Nicholl's (1985, p 198) trip through the international cocaine underworld. This is almost like the potentiation found in the old Coca-Cola. Likewise, the Afro-Cuban jazz and dance musicians of Havana, New York and Miami for many years took small amounts of cocaine before performing and dancing after midnight in the clubs (Winick 1950). Does this sort of use ever come up in the current epidemiology?

Negrete: I am sure there has always been some use of cocaine HCl in the South American continent, and perhaps in the milieux that you just mentioned, it is much the same as in North America, among musicians and other Bohemian types. But this is nothing like the extent of coca chewing among the Indians, which is the traditional pattern. Of course, there is coca chewing outside the Indian population as well; some non-native people pass coca leaves around after dinner as a digestive! But by and large the use of cocaine HCl powder is a new phenomenon in South America.

Moore: In the second part of your paper, Dr Negrete, you were trying to estimate the *consequences* of cocaine use for users in South America, using epidemiological data to help make those estimates. This is a move away from the epidemiology which simply tells you whether levels of drug use are going up or down with some reasonable degree of precision and accuracy, that is so helpful to policy makers. Now, epidemiology is moving into the attribution and prediction of *consequences*; not just estimates of levels of use. That may be hazardous for historians, and for policy-making, because we might then lose valuable information about simple trends. So I am concerned to know what is going on in epidemiology now: are we using epidemiological data to get better estimates of consequences of drug use; or are we still doing some of the 'blind empiricism' of which Griffith Edwards spoke (p 39), but which turns out to be very valuable?

Another comment that occurs to me is that we now have three quite different pictures of the determinants of the aggregate demand for drugs in general. One picture could be thought of as the *epidemiological* model, which begins with a population of susceptible subjects, and then sees drug use moving through that population at a particular rate.

The second model is that drugs are *substitutes* for one another in economic terms; if we have an increase in cocaine use, we shall have a decrease in heroin use; if there is an increase in marijuana use there will be a decrease in any of the other drugs.

The third picture is that, in economic terms again, these drugs *complement* one another. If we have an increase in alcohol use, then later we shall see an increase in marijuana use, and then, subsequently, an increase in cocaine use.

Those are three quite different pictures of the current determinants of the aggregate demand for drugs. For the proper development of public policy, it is important that we develop a sense of which of those we think is true. So far as I can tell, there is very little understanding of how we might use empirical evidence to allow us to distinguish which among those hypotheses is the correct view of what is happening in the aggregate demand for drug use.

Balster: Taking up the question of the role of epidemiological research raised by Mark Moore, I wonder about a possible role in looking at natural experiments, in which large-scale interventions are made, laws are passed, advertising campaigns are mounted, etc. Can epidemiological research be used to answer questions about whether or not these large-scale social 'experiments' have an impact on drug use?

Gerstein: The term 'epidemiological' is being used here in a rather broader meaning than usual. For example, the matched case–control method, which is a standard procedure in clinical epidemiology and has been applied in this field, is not something that one can use readily to look at the effect of policy changes. It is a method of 'micro' analysis, which creates the equivalent of an experimental protocol in biomedical science. That is, it selects carefully and narrowly within the general population. But the notion of using population-wide surveys outside a clinical context, to examine the effect of policy changes and the like, is now common in many fields.

One particular point is pertinent to Professor Edwards' description of 'blind empiricism', although the phrase Samuel Stouffer coined, of 'dust-bowl empiricism', may be more appropriate. In the large-scale survey of 18 500 or 20 000 subjects (or 32 000, to which the National Household Survey on Drug Abuse in the US is now growing), the design is not produced by someone in a single laboratory who collects a set of data and then publishes the method and results, which others in similar laboratories can try to replicate and expand on. There is frustration that the large survey data in the USA are not necessarily accessible to qualified researchers. We collect huge and very expensive amounts of data, which give the impression of epidemiologists knocking on every door in every city, but then the extent of analysis performed is not commensurate. The ratio of mind applied to data available is far too low, in my view.

Anthony: In the USA we spend more than $14 million a year in the gathering of drug surveillance data, but there is a meagre investment in the analysis of these data, or in the prior design of the data-gathering so that it could answer pertinent questions—perhaps $1 million per year, if that. This disparity between the annual USA budget for drug data-gathering, and that for preparation and analysis, is worrying. One effect is our inability to test questions of the type that Bob Balster just mentioned—questions about relationships between policy change and patterns of drug use. Under proper circumstances, these might be tested using an interrupted time series design to take careful measurements for lengthy periods before and after the implementation of a specific policy, or with some other quasi-experimental research design. However, the experience in this arena has not been altogether satisfactory (e.g. Anthony 1979).

It should be added that the Epidemiologic Catchment Area data are available as public-use data tapes, and can be purchased for the cost of the tape.

Kleber: The tapes of the High School Senior Survey done yearly by Lloyd Johnson at the University of Michigan under a grant from the National Institute on Drug Abuse are available to university-based scholars for, I believe, about $500 per tape. However, I agree that there is far too little secondary analysis done.

Gerstein: The tapes are available in principle, but in practice it takes a call from the White House to shake loose a copy.

Maynard: It is ironical to hear the American participants lamenting how much information they have and how little they analyse it! All things are relative; in the UK we have a tradition of not confusing policy-making with facts at all. What few data are available are certainly not analysed enough.

On another relativity point, which refers back to Jim Anthony's paper, it was interesting to see all the measures of damage done by drugs, but one inevitably asks the question: relative to what? He showed that if I use cocaine I have a greater risk of attempting suicide and having psychiatric disturbance, but that's life, isn't it? Life is a risky activity! How should we compare the results coming out of his cocaine user population with those from other populations? What should be the norm? Is cocaine use worse than alcohol use?

Anthony: That is a good question, but not sufficiently precise to be answered with our epidemiological data. We can't answer the question of whether alcohol use or cocaine use is 'worse' without getting into issues of how much cocaine use, how frequently, by what route of administration, and under what conditions. And there are corresponding questions for alcohol: how much alcohol? Under what conditions? And so on.

References

Anthony JC 1979 The effect of federal drug law on the incidence of drug abuse. J Health Polit Policy Law 4:87–108

Fischman MW 1988 Behavioral pharmacology of cocaine. J Clin Psychiatry 49(2)(suppl):7–10

Foltin RW, Fischman MW, Pedroso JJ, Pearlson GD 1988 Repeated intranasal cocaine administration: lack of tolerance to pressor effects. Drug Alcohol Depend 22:169–177

Gutierrez Noriega C, Zapata Ortiz V 1947 Estudios sobre la coca y la cocaina en el Peru. Ministerio de Salud, Lima (pp 144)

Javaid JJ, Fischman MW, Schuster CR, Dekirmenjian H, Davis JM 1978 Cocaine plasma concentration: relationship to physiological and subjective effects in humans after intranasal administration. Science (Wash DC) 202:227–228

Jeri R (ed) 1980 Cocaine 1980. Proceedings of the international seminar on medical and sociological aspects of coca and cocaine. (Pan American Health Office/WHO and the International Narcotics Management, Lima) Pacific Press, Lima (pp 264)

Jeri R, Perez JC 1990 Dependencia a la cocaina en el Peru. Monografia de investigacion 4, CEDRO, Lima (pp 73)

Lerner R 1991 Drugs in Peru: reality and representation. Drukkerij Quickprint BV, Nijmegen (pp 200)

Nicholl C 1985 The fruit palace. St Martin's Press, New York

Winick C 1950 The use of drugs by jazz musicians. Social problems 7:240–253

Are there 'casual users' of cocaine?

C. D. Kaplan, B. Bieleman and W. D. TenHouten

INTRAVAL, 's-Gravendijkwal 1A, 3021 EA Rotterdam, The Netherlands

Abstract. Medical and public opinion about cocaine use have shifted dramatically over the past decade. New research methodologies and definitions to evaluate the impact of cocaine are needed. This paper presents a theoretical definition and empirical analysis of the 'casual user' of cocaine. Data have been drawn from a subsample of 58 cocaine users and their cocaine-using contacts in Rotterdam. The methodology of the study presents a novel approach to patterns of cocaine use involving the integration of social network variables with 'snowball' sampling data collection techniques. The theoretical definition is systematically related to two social context variables: (1) the scope of settings where contacts use cocaine; (2) the degree of involvement in social network relations of actual cocaine use. Scope of settings has been defined in terms of the number of cocaine-using social circuits contacts are drawn from: i.e. 'narrow' setting where all contacts originate from one circuit while a 'wide' setting indicates contacts come from two or more circuits. Involvement has been defined in terms of the percentage of contacts where the relation with study participants is characterized by cocaine use most or all of the time. Additional social network variables measuring the mean duration (in years) of contacts' cocaine use and the use of cocaine with contacts in the last six months are subsequently related to the scope and involvement variables. The implications of the analysis for a new cross-classification of cocaine use patterns are discussed with special reference to public health policy issues.

1992 Cocaine: scientific and social dimensions. Wiley, Chichester (Ciba Foundation Symposium 166) p 57–80

Within the past decade, public and medical opinion on the use patterns and consequences of cocaine have shifted dramatically. This shift has been nowhere more striking than in the United States. A decade ago, cocaine had been perceived by medical opinion as a non-addictive substance that could have some negative psychological consequences. Public opinion had also reflected this view. By 1984 a shift had started to occur. The Director of the National Institute on Drug Abuse warned the American public that cocaine use had become 'the drug of greatest national concern from a public health point of view' (Pollin 1984, p vii). The latest American epidemiological results estimate a lifetime prevalence of cocaine use in the general population at 11% and a current prevalence of cocaine use of 1%, after reaching a high point in 1985 of more than 2% (National Institute on Drug Abuse 1990, Rouse 1991). Comparable data on national epidemiological trends do not exist in Europe, but differences between countries in the extent of the cocaine problem can be inferred. For example, a general population survey conducted in Amsterdam (hardly representative of the typical European city with respect to drugs) indicated a lifetime prevalence of 'only' 5.6% and a current prevalence of less than 1% (Sandwijk et al 1988). Public and medical opinion in Europe reflect these relatively lower prevalence levels of cocaine use. In Europe an attitude of watchful concern rather than of a public health emergency prevails on the issue of cocaine.

In order both to monitor the situation and to better link scientific research to practical health policy requirements, we now need new field research methodologies, just as we need the methods and models that have been recently called for in laboratory and clinical research on cocaine (Gawin 1991). New methodologies are necessary for answering the most basic of questions, such as, 'are there casual users of cocaine?' For example, numerous animal cocaine self-administration studies have demonstrated in the laboratory that cocaine is an extremely potent pharmacological reinforcer and therefore must be considered a drug of high human abuse potential (Johanson 1984, Siegel 1989). Yet, the epidemiological evidence shows that millions of Americans have used cocaine without encountering serious clinical problems. This suggests that subtle patterns such as 'casual use' exist and are also rather prevalent.

Studies of clinical populations are not particularly suitable in defining use patterns that do not present a clinical dependency syndrome. Intensive, targeted community-based field investigations are needed to identify a wider range of patterns relevant for prevention. Yet only a handful of such surveys have been published (van Meter 1990a, Cohen, 1989, Erickson & Murray 1989, Chitwood 1985). In this paper the preliminary results of an on-going community research project among cocaine users in Rotterdam are presented with special reference to the question of casual use. Rotterdam has been designated as the pilot research development site of a coordinated multi-city investigation of the nature and extent of cocaine use in the European Community. This project has been designed with the results and limitations of previous community-based surveys in mind. The study is focused upon the questions of the nature and extent of use of cocaine in a modern city and is characterized by a novel methodological and theoretical approach.

Defining casual use

Previous community-based studies of cocaine use have offered little help toward the definition of subtle patterns such as 'casual use'. They do provide evidence supporting the results of general population surveys which suggest that cocaine dependency, like clinical alcoholism, is a rather exceptional case. Yet, carrying further the similarity with alcohol, the relatively low prevalence of clinical cocaine dependency in the general population may be partly a function of time.

A relatively long period may elapse in the person (and in society) from the onset of use to the appearance of dependence symptoms. This may especially be the case when cocaine (as with alcohol) is used in less potent forms. Given this possibility, the issue of 'casual use' has become a priority in recent American drug abuse policy pronouncements. The rationale of these is preventive: by pursuing and punishing the 'casual user' of cocaine the 'pipeline' going from casual to addictive use can be shut down (H. D. Kleber, paper on illicit drugs presented at an international conference on Drugs, alcohol and tobacco: making the science and policy connections, University of London, 16–19 July 1991; Office of National Drug Control Policy 1989, Ostrow 1990). From a policy point of view, casual users seem to exist, but can scientific research provide any clarification of this vague social construct?

Community-based surveys of cocaine use conducted in Miami and Amsterdam have constructed definitions of cocaine use patterns based upon an implicit behavioural science perspective. Both studies have employed Morningstar & Chitwood's (1983, 1984; see also Chitwood 1985, Cohen 1989, p 41–58) 13-point composite index of level of cocaine use. This index gives equal weight to three factors: self-reported route of ingestion, frequency of use, and quantity of use. A low-medium-high measure of level of use has been reported in these studies. Taken in the perspective of variations in use across time, this measure profiled six distinct developmental patterns of cocaine use in both Amsterdam and Miami: (1) much cocaine use at first, then slowly decreasing use; (2) a slow and steady increase in cocaine use; (3) a stable level from first to current use; (4) 'up-top-down', i.e. a relatively low cocaine use at first that rises to a peak and then drops to the early levels; (5) intermittent use at the same level, but with significant breaks in time; and (6) varying cocaine use with peaks and troughs in an irregular trajectory. None of these patterns corresponds precisely to a definition of casual use.

In the Amsterdam study the most prevalent patterns were Pattern 4 (39% 'up-top-down') and Pattern 6 (33% irregular trajectory). Only 3% of the sample presented Pattern 2 (slow and steady increase), the developmental profile that would characterize classical opiate dependence (Cohen 1989, p 57). The Miami study reported that approximately one-half (48%) of the sample were using cocaine at a level higher than in the first year, one-fifth remained low-level users, and nearly as many (18%) progressed from low-level use during their first year to higher levels in subsequent years (Chitwood 1985, p 118–120). The Miami and Amsterdam results are similar: cocaine use presents a wide variation of patterns. Both studies also found that only a minority of users progressed in a way that was similar to the course of opiate dependency.

In addition to these community-based surveys, an eleven-year follow-up of a 'friendship network' of 27 San Francisco cocaine users has been published (Murphy et al 1989). This unique study presents complementary data on the long-term patterns of cocaine use. Unlike the community surveys, however, the

San Francisco study provided a definition of casual use. Murphy and her co-workers used the term 'casual use' to refer to their subjects when they were first interviewed in 1974–1975. The great majority of these subjects did not use cocaine daily and did not believe cocaine to be addictive. They had experienced only a few negative effects from the use of the drug. At follow-up eleven years later, Murphy and her co-workers found four specific patterns of variation over time (with their frequency in the sample): continuous controlled use (33%); progression from controlled to heavy to controlled use (33%); progression from controlled to heavy use to abstinence (24%); and progression from controlled use to abstinence (10%). They also reported 'the exception'— the one person who continued heavy use, i.e. the classical opiate dependency pattern.

In adopting the terms 'controlled' and 'heavy' use, Murphy et al (1989) showed their commitment to an ethnographic approach. In ethnography the definitions and meanings of members of a specific subculture are given considerable weight (Sacks 1972, Adler & Adler 1987). 'Controlled use' is a term by which members of the drug subculture refer to non-addictive or non-dependent patterns. Murphy and her co-workers also employed the term 'casual' use to describe the patterns of use encountered at the first interview. This application makes good ethnographic sense. The term 'casual' was widespread in California in the 1970s and was used by members of newly emerging lifestyles to characterize their relationships. Thus, in one ethnographic study of new sexual lifestyles in California, 'casual sex' was defined as sex 'consented to . . . it is here and now, situated, not everywhere and forever . . . You have it for now when it is here. . . . Do it for pleasure' (Douglas et al 1977, p 146). The casual use of cocaine conveys the same localized meaning. However, 'casual use' was not retained by Murphy et al (1989) in their classification of long-term non-addictive patterns. This change in terminology seems to be related to changes in use patterns that occurred over time. As Murphy and her co-workers write: 'From our current perspective we realize that our description would have been less sanguine had we studied the group longer. We now know, for example, that several subsequently had physical and psychological problems when they began to use more cocaine over a longer period' (p 428).

Both the community surveys and the ethnographic follow-up study of cocaine use defined patterns of cocaine use in terms of intrinsic, individualistic behavioural categories. In contrast, this paper takes a novel approach to the definition of use pattern. Our beginning point is to introduce social context variables in which the individual behaviours take place. This novel approach is consistent with the recent trend in cross-cultural psychiatry (de Vries 1987, Littlewood 1990). Further confidence in this approach is obtained from the results of a Toronto community-based cocaine survey. In comparing those respondents who intended to continue to use cocaine with those who intended to quit, Erickson & Murray (1989, p 146) found that a variable measuring the proportion of friends who used cocaine was associated with the greatest differences. Of those who intended to continue using cocaine, 61% reported that at least half of their friends also used cocaine, compared to only 33% of those who intended to quit. These results indicate that social context variables can have a particular significance in constructing definitions of subtle cocaine use patterns.

In defining casual use in terms of social context variables we do not mean to eliminate individual behavioural variables. Rather, we propose that social relations can be specific indicators of use patterns in their own right, by reason of their well-documented role in the social definition of drug-related problems. In our image of casual use, any basic definition should be integrally related to 'secondary' social relational properties, not necessarily related to the psychopharmacological properties of the drug. To illustrate, Littlewood's (1990, p 322) cross-cultural psychiatric conjecture 'Does the biomedical notion of "dependence" in substance use correlate with a limited variety of social institutions which employ the substance in a central experience?' represents an approach to psychiatric definition that would have notions such as 'casual use' integrally tied to specific social structural contexts.

In operationalizing our theoretical definition of 'casual use', we considered many social context variables. In this paper, a limited and preliminary selection has been made from the total array of social network variables. We have hypothesized that two social context variables should be specifically relevant to the definition of casual use: (1) the scope of settings where the study participants' contacts use cocaine; and (2) the degree of social network involvement between study participants and their contacts in mutual cocaine use. In the analysis to be presented here, the scope of settings has been defined in terms of a study participant's contacts being drawn from a 'narrow' setting (e.g. one social circuit alone, such as an intimate friendship circuit) or a 'wide' setting (e.g. two or more social circuits, such as intimate friendship plus work circuits). Involvement has been defined in terms of the percentage of contacts where the relation with the study participant is characterized by the use of cocaine most or all of the time. Both the scope of settings and the social involvement variables have been initially defined at the ordinal level of measurement. The scope of settings ranged from 1 to 4 with a median value of 2 in the study sample. This median value has been used to distinguish the 'narrow' participants with contacts from only one setting from the 'wide' participants who drew their cocaine contacts from two or more settings. The qualitative social circuits which were set equivalent to 'settings' included: entertainment, work, intimate friends, sport, and the hard-drug scene. The involvement variable ranged from ranks of 9% or less to 90% or more of the study participants who used cocaine with this percentage of their contacts most or all of the time. The median value for the study sample was the rank of 20%. As with the scope of settings variable, the median value has been used to distinguish 'low involvement participants'.

A 'low involvement participant' has been defined as using cocaine most or all of the time with less than or equal to 29% of his or her contacts (i.e. the rank was computed from values ranging from 20% to 29%), while a 'high involvement participant' used most or all of the time with 30% or more of his or her contacts.

These variables are well grounded theoretically. Thus, our positing of a 'scope of settings' variable as integral to a definition of 'casual use' corresponds to Littlewood's conjecture that a limited variety of social institutions (i.e. 'narrow' scope of settings) which accept cocaine use would correlate with a higher presentation of biomedical drug dependency symptoms. By definition, then 'casual' users should have a relatively wider scope of settings from which their cocaine contacts are drawn. A relatively wider variety of social contexts should be related to a greater likelihood of non-dependent use patterns. This theory is predicated on the assumption that secondary social definitions play a determining role in the probability of the presentation of pathological symptoms. Therefore, that a casual user has contacts from a wider scope of settings indicates that he or she has adopted a pattern of use and self-definition that 'fits' to the expectations of other users drawn from multiple social circuits. This pattern, in turn, seems likely to present a 'normal' common denominator of cocaine-related behaviour acceptable to a wide range of different kinds of people.

Similarly, the selection of the 'social involvement' variable is based on the specific finding of Erickson & Murray (1989) that the intention to continue to use cocaine was highly associated with the percentage of friends using the drug. Given that 'intention' is a critical theoretical construct when one is defining individual human behaviour, its relationship with social network variables as found by Erickson & Murray should be seen as important. Carrying this result further, the concept of 'social network density', defined as 'the ratio of the number of social relations that actually exist in a system to the number of possible relations', can be applied to a network of cocaine contacts (Kadhushin 1982, p 147). Our 'social involvement' variable corresponds to the 'cocaine use density' of the network of contacts. The variable can be interpreted as a measure of the relationship between possible cocaine use relations and actual use relations. As Kadhushin has demonstrated, the relationship between high social density of the interpersonal environment and lowered stress reaction exists for young men in moderately sized urban areas. However, as Kadhushin himself concludes: 'The larger social context may well affect the relationship between density and mental health. . . . Some urban circles may be knowledgeable and supportive with respect to mental health issues but others may not be' (p 155). Interaction effects between density and the particular mental health stressor are therefore quite likely in specific situations. By defining 'casual users' as those who display a relatively low percentage of frequent use with their possible cocaine relations, we have posited that there is an interaction between the 'cocaine stressor' and the 'cocaine use density'. 'Casual users' seem to be involved in cocaine-using networks where 'intentions' other than frequent cocaine use carry more weight.

In this specific case, the interaction is one of a low cocaine use density with a 'good' mental health outcome. In that 'casual users' are not relating to their contacts through cocaine use, they are obviously defining these relations in ways other than drug use. Implicit to this interaction is that 'casual users' are keeping their cocaine use in social circles who are 'knowledgeable and supportive with respect to mental health issues' related to cocaine.

Methodology

The majority of the published community surveys of cocaine use have employed, for the most part, a 'snowball' sampling methodology for acquiring respondents (van Meter 1990b, Cohen 1989, Erickson & Murray 1989, Chitwood 1985). In this methodology, sample selection begins by making contact with members of a specific population that may be characterized as 'rare', 'elusive' or 'hidden' (see Kaplan et al 1987, Sudman et al 1988, Watters & Biernacki 1989, Biernacki & Waldorf 1981). The knowledge accrued in this initial fieldwork (a simple or stratified random sample may also be used) is used to find the 'starters', composing the 'zero stage' of a snowball sample. These starters, in turn, 'nominate' other members of the population. Interviews with the starters and nominees are routinely conducted. The snowball procedure 'ascends' through these chains of referrals into more general levels of the population. Snowball sampling provides a practical technique in research situations where probability samples are not feasible. This practical advantage is usually offset by the disadvantage of the uncertain generalizability of the sample. If it is not known how representative the sample is, valid results may be difficult to obtain. There is, however, promising work being done aimed at overcoming some of these methodological disadvantages (van Meter 1990a, Frank 1979).

The data presented here have been collected in Rotterdam using a design employing snowball sampling in different settings of cocaine use (Intraval 1990). Fieldwork began at the end of 1990. Key informants were contacted and a social map of the organizations and institutions important for the study was drawn. A large number of locations and events (cafes, bars, discos, parties, and so on) were visited by the research fieldworkers. Informal conversations explained the aim of the study and built trust in the community of cocaine users. Study participants were recruited in these contexts and appointments were made for an interview. Participants were also recruited by means of advertisements placed in national and regional newspapers and in prison.

The recruited participants completed a focused interview of one to four hours. The interview consisted of two parts. A qualitative part elicited narrative data on the following topics: social background; present lifestyle; first drug and alcohol experience; the when, where and why of first cocaine use; cocaine career; functions, effects and consequences of cocaine use; setting and estimations of present use; income; criminal behaviour; and social assistance. The second part consisted of a 'closed ended' schedule with fixed response categories. This part provided the basis for a network analysis. The participant estimated the number of cocaine users he or she was aware of in each of the following social circuits: entertainment; work; intimate friends; sports and the hard-drug scene. From each of these social circuits the participant was asked to nominate a maximum of 10 persons. Information was provided by the participant for each nominee on their sex, age, whether their primary contact involved cocaine, the nominee's knowledge of the participant's cocaine use and their profession or occupation. From each setting, two of the nominees were selected using a random number table. The participant was then asked to provide information on the relations with the nominee including: the length of the relationship; presence at nominee's first cocaine use; knowledge of whether the nominee was still using cocaine or when the nominee had stopped using cocaine; where the nominee uses cocaine; contact with the nominee in the last six months; where the contact took place; and did the current contact have anything to do with cocaine? The two nominees with the lowest random number assignment were then selected for the next stage of the snowball sample. If the participant said that he or she would or could not reach the selected nominees, then he or she was asked if any of the other nominees named could be reached. If the participant said that none of the nominees could be contacted, then he or she was asked if there was another way, or other persons who could be considered. The inclusion criteria for participants and nominees were the same: an estimated lifetime prevalence of 25 times or more of cocaine use and/or a current prevalence of five times or more of use in the past six months.

A total of 110 participants were interviewed for the study. In turn, these participants named over 1000 nominees and additionally provided social network data on between 400 and 500 of them. A subsample consisting of the first 58 participants was selected for the purposes of this paper. The participants nominated a mean of 4.3 contacts (standard deviation = 2.5). Within the subsamples, 14 'within' references occurred; i.e. a participant was nominated by another participant. Three participants were named twice and eight participants once. Seven participants refused some information on nominees.

The unit of analysis was the participant. A cross-classification analysis of the scope of settings and the social involvement variables was done in order to tighten the connection between our theoretical definition of 'casual' use and our hypothetical, empirical indicators. This produced a 2×2 cross-classification table representing the association between the two variables. This table presented a four-fold classification of patterns of cocaine use, based upon two independent social context indicators. Since this cross-classification employed ordinal level variables, a Gamma statistic was computed evaluating the association between the two indicators. This statistic provides a summary of the strength and direction of the association between the variables.

TABLE 1 Cross-classification of Scope of Setting by Social Involvement variables: percentages of total N (58) and (n)

		Scope of setting	
		Narrow	Wide
Involvement	Low	29% (17)	29% (17)
	High	14% (8)	28% (16)

Subsequent two-way analyses of variance were used to systematically refer the indicator variables to other social network variables. Two social network variables were selected as dependent variables. We hypothesized that they would be predicted or differentiated by our definitional variables. These dependent social network variables were (1) the percentage of participants within a defined subgroup who had used cocaine with nominees in the past six months; and (2) the mean duration in years of cocaine use by the participants' nominees. The percentage of participants who had used with a nominee was computed by adding the number of participants who had used with a nominee within each specific subgroup defined by the cross-classification variables and dividing by the total in that subgroup. The mean duration was calculated by averaging the number of years of cocaine use reported by the participant of his or her total number of nominees. The percentage of participants who had used cocaine in the past six months with a contact was taken as a good measure of the current prevalence of cocaine use within a specific subgroup. The mean duration of use by contacts was seen to be a useful measure of the incidence of cocaine use in a specific subgroup. Therefore, both dependent variables can be seen as social network equivalents of the standard epidemiological indicators that are routinely measured at the individual self-report level.

Results

Table 1 presents the results of the cross-classification of the scope of setting by social involvement variables. A Gamma value of 0.33 was obtained for the table. This value showed a moderate degree of association between the two social context indicator variables. The positive direction of the orders of the variables gave us confidence that the connection of our theoretical definitions and their ordered indicators was sufficiently tight. The Gamma value gave us a theoretically satisfying result; i.e. for most of the pairs of participants the same order was predicted. Thus, most of the participants who were either narrow or wide in their scope of settings were also correspondingly low or high in their cocaine use involvement with these same contacts. The cell percentages in the table are illustrative and have been computed on the base of a total subsample of 58. A relatively even distribution was found among the narrow-low 17 (29%),

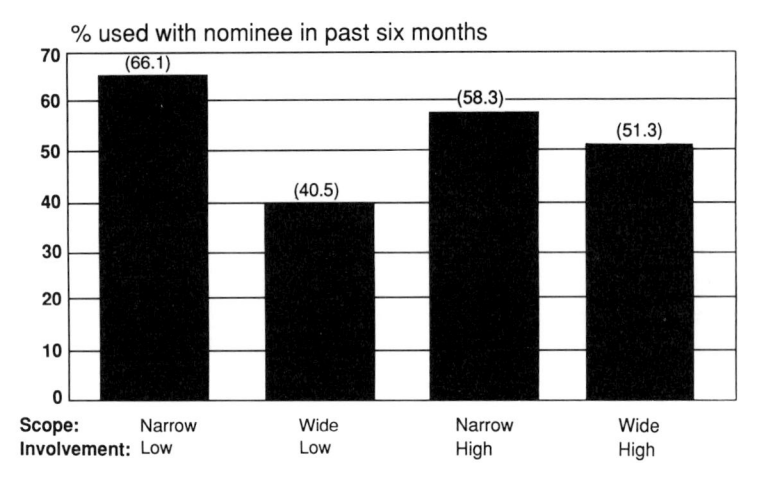

FIG. 1. The percentage of study participants using cocaine with the nominee in the past six months, by scope of setting and network involvement in cocaine use.

wide-low 17 (29%) and wide-high 16 (28%) cells. The narrow-high cell had an exceptionally low frequency 8 (14%).

Figure 1 displays the results of the two-way analysis of variance demonstrating that the indicator variable 'scope of setting' is indeed predictive of the dependent variable, percentage of participants using cocaine with nominees in the past six months. The scope of setting variable had a significant main effect ($F = 3.59$, $df = 52$, $P = 0.03$). The figure shows clearly that those participants distributed in the 'wide-low' cell (40.5%) (i.e. our 'casual' users, by definition) have the

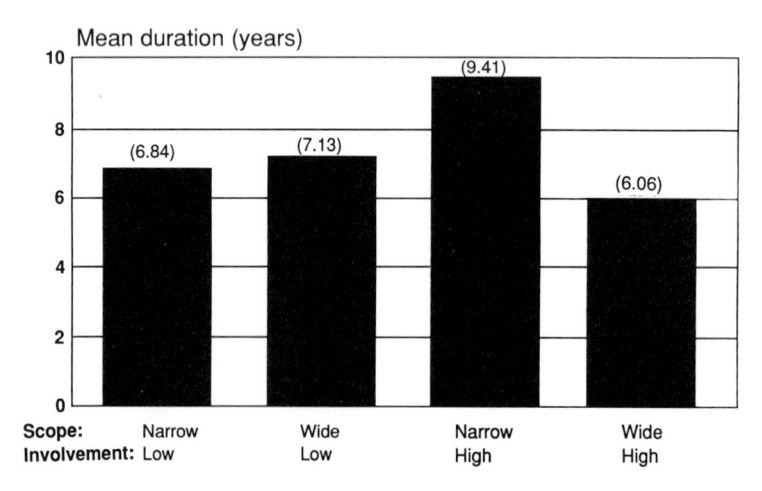

FIG. 2. The duration of the nominees' cocaine use, by scope of setting and network involvement in cocaine use (in years).

lowest levels of 'using with nominee' relations. The 'wide-high' participants are higher in their percentage levels (51.3%), but are lower than those participants who were characterized by a narrow scope of settings (narrow-low, 66.1%; narrow-high, 58.3%).

Figure 2 presents the results of the two-way analysis of variance of the 'scope of setting' and 'network involvement' variables on the dependent variable, mean duration of cocaine use by nominees, in years. A significant interaction effect between the two social context variables on the dependent variable was found ($F = 5.84$, $df = 48$, $P = 0.019$). Figure 2 shows that 'mean duration of use' can also differentiate between participants; that is to say, both narrow scope-high involvement (9.41) and wide scope-low involvement (7.13) participants know nominees who have used longer than the participants who are characterized as narrow scope-low involvement (6.84) or wide scope-high involvement (6.06).

Discussion

The results of the analysis indicate that an analytical strategy of including social context variables in the definitions of cocaine use patterns can be useful, especially for subtle variations and under conditions in which self-reports of personal use might be unreliable. Our theoretical definition of 'casual use' related statistically to the social contextual indicators of a wide scope of settings of contacts' use and a low involvement in social relations with those where frequent use of the drug occurs. These variables taken together suggest a typology of subtle cocaine patterns of use that may escape individual behavioural typologies such as 'high-medium-low', or ethnographic ones such as 'controlled' and 'heavy' use. However, a future typology of subtle cocaine use patterns is unlikely to be composed of only two variables. It is indeed necessary that future research be oriented toward specifying other variables (including behavioural, ethnographic and contextual ones) suitable for a classification system of subtle use patterns.

Nevertheless, on the basis of the two social context variables used (scope of setting and social network involvement), an empirically grounded cross-classification of cocaine use patterns did emerge. Therefore, on the basis of our analysis an affirmative (if also preliminary) answer to the research question, 'are there "casual users" of cocaine?' can be given. The 'casual user' can be identified with those whose social context of use consists of cocaine contacts from a wide scope of settings and whose social network involvements with other cocaine users cannot be characterized by cocaine use most of the time. This definition becomes more satisfying when contrasted with its logically opposite type: the cocaine user who can be designated as 'compulsive'. The 'compulsive' user exists in a social network where there is a high involvement of use with other cocaine contacts. Most or all of the time compulsive users will take cocaine with their cocaine contacts.

This identification of 'compulsive' cocaine use with a high social network involvement fits well with the World Health Organization's redefinition of drug dependency (Edwards et al 1982). In this redefinition, the leading common factor across all kinds of drug dependency is the subjective awareness of the drug user of a craving to take the drug. This craving is brought on by internal and external cues. Thus, the interaction between compulsive users and their cocaine contacts reflects a cueing situation leading to use most or all of the time. This interaction, in turn, is likely to correspond to a subjective awareness of compulsion. In addition, following Littlewood's conjecture, since our society has severely limited the institutional variety of the cocaine experience, we should expect 'compulsive' users to reflect this narrowing of options, by also limiting the scope of settings from which they draw their cocaine contacts. This 'coping style' by 'compulsive' users would be a functional adaptation to the prevailing social conditions of socially undesirable definitions and repression. The 'compulsive' user can be expected to have internalized this negative social complex to such an extent that he or she restricts the scope of his or her own cocaine experience.

Following through our cross-classification, a redefinition of a 'controlled' use can also be made. Like the casual user, the controlled user is someone who has a low involvement of cocaine use in his or her cocaine network. But, like the compulsive user, they are adapting themselves to a narrow scope of settings, probably for many of the same coping reasons. However, unlike the compulsive users, they may have learned that their own personal use can 'escalate' into negative consequences if the pleasure of the 'social euphoria' (i.e. sharing the cocaine experience with friends) develops a momentum of its own (Reinarman 1979, p 244-246). In this regard, the 'controlled' user minimizes, as a rule, exposure to social contexts where the risk of 'social euphoria' is high.

In contrast to the 'controlled' user, the class of user characterized by a wide scope of settings with a high network involvement can be introduced. Again drawing on Edwards et al (1982), this pattern can be termed 'salient' use insofar as drug-seeking behaviour is given a high priority over other considerations. The 'salient' user spends a large part of the day in cocaine-related activities and other activities and relations become less significant. This is indicated by a social context that includes taking cocaine with one's contacts most of the time and drawing these contacts from a relatively wide scope of settings. If this interpretation is plausible, then it can be expected that the 'salient' users are more likely to be users who are still in the beginning phases of their cocaine careers and have not yet experienced enough negative social consequences to narrow their scope of settings.

The frequency distributions shown in Table 1 across the 'casual' (wide-low; 29%), 'controlled' (narrow-low; 29%), and 'salient' (wide-high; 28%) classes are rather even; 86% of the sample was characterized by these specific contexts. As has been documented in both the community-based surveys and the long-term follow-up, as discussed earlier, 'compulsive' use characteristic of the opiates is 'an exception' when considering cocaine. These findings are supported by our results. By our social context definition of 'compulsive' ('narrow-high') use, only 14% of the sample fell into that class. Looking specifically at our class definitive of 'casual' use, the frequency distribution of 29% compares favourably with the results of the community-based surveys and the long-term follow-up, reviewed earlier. While casual use was not specifically an interest in those surveys, a rough equivalent type for our purposes might be the continuous low level user; that is, the user who started at low level use, whose period of heaviest use was also at a low level, and whose current use was also low. Although the definitions were somewhat different in the Amsterdam and Miami surveys, making comparisons difficult, the relative percentage of the continuous low level use type was 34.8% of the sample in Amsterdam and 21% in Miami. Our results at 29% fall into this range. While Murphy and co-workers did not retain casual use as a term in reporting their follow-up results (Murphy et al 1989), their 'continuous controlled user' at 33% is close to both our 'casual' and 'controlled' user frequencies. This convergence of prevalences of 'casual use' equivalents in multiple samples using multiple methods in multiple sites and times suggests that our definition based upon social context variables alone represents a robust contribution to drug use and abuse classification.

The results of our analyses of variance provide supporting evidence for the plausibility of our definition of casual use and other subtle use patterns. Thus, Fig. 1 shows that the definitional variable, 'scope of settings', effectively predicted the dependent variable percentage of respondents who had used cocaine with their contacts in the past six months. Interestingly, both the 'controlled user' (66.1%) and the 'compulsive user' (58.3%) have been using cocaine more often with some of their contacts than either the casual or salient users. In addition, a subtle difference between the compulsive and controlled user can be seen. Both are using the drug relatively frequently with their contacts, but the controlled user is selective about whom she or he uses with. Unlike the compulsive user, he or she is not using with many of them most of the time. But, with those fewer contacts, the controlled user is taking cocaine more often. In contrast, and consistent with our definition, the casual user has the lowest percentage of use with cocaine contacts in the past six months (40.5%).

Our analysis presented in Fig. 2 demonstrates that an interaction of our two social context variables can differentiate the relative 'age' of the cocaine network of a participant. This result has several important implications. First, the data show that the 'salient' user has the shortest duration of use among his or her contacts (6.06 years). Like their contacts, therefore, these users may be relatively less experienced with cocaine and therefore give it a higher consideration than the casual and controlled users who have cocaine contacts who have been using longer. In contrast, the compulsive user has contacts who have been using far longer (9.41 years). The 'salient' users seem to be at the middling phases of their career, while the compulsive user may well be toward the end. Second, the results in Fig. 2 seem to contradict the remark by Murphy and her co-workers (1989) that casual use is an unstable pattern that appears at the beginning of a cocaine career and breaks down later into 'controlled' or 'heavy' use. As can be seen in Fig. 2, casual users know others who have a relatively long duration of use (7.13 years). Only the compulsive users tend to know others who have used cocaine longer. This suggests that both casual and compulsive use can be the long-term ends of the cocaine career.

The research reported here should be seen as preliminary. The correlation between social context variables and the psychobehavioural variables that are well-documented in the literature will need to be explored before fixing any final redefinition of cocaine use patterns. Nevertheless, despite the limitations of our preliminary analysis, several important health policy issues relating to cocaine have been clarified by our approach. Our results now join the numerous other studies suggesting that the pattern of 'compulsive' use of cocaine is not comparable to the use patterns of opiates. Furthermore, casual and controlled use patterns may be assumed to characterize the majority of the cocaine-using population at any given point in time. This 'social fact' has probably provided the real basis for the popular myth that cocaine is not an addictive drug. From the viewpoint of prevention policy, it is necessary to balance this myth with the possibility that the introduction of rapid delivery forms of cocaine in wider availability (e.g. 'crack') can change the prevalence profile in a given subpopulation. The likelihood of cocaine addiction is strongly influenced by the route of administration of the drug. Crack cocaine is marketed to smoke rather than to sniff. Thus, shifts in the prevalent route of administration of cocaine from intranasal to smoking or injection should also produce a higher prevalence of compulsive use. Thus, the Miami study discussed in this paper included a subsample selected from the drug treatment population who tended to smoke or inject cocaine. Therefore, it is not surprising that a higher prevalence of compulsive use was also observed. A similar finding has been reported in a field study of cocaine use in the Rotterdam heroin addict population where smoking and injecting cocaine are the prevalent routes of administration (Grund et al 1991).

Our research suggests that the 'pipeline' image of a singular flow of cocaine users from entry to compulsive use at the exit may be a useful metaphor in some respects, but is wrong on the issue of casual use. The pipeline metaphor implies that casual use is equivalent to 'beginning' use and, therefore, by 'targeting' the casual user, we shall prevent later compulsive use. Making casual use a policy priority would seem to do little to close down the cocaine pipeline. Even if relatively 'older' casual users would be eliminated, the controlled and salient user would still exist in high numbers to feed the pipeline toward compulsive use. In times of scarce resources, our analysis could be used to support the recommendation that casual users are a relatively older and stable group that should remain a low prevention priority. In our view, a higher priority should be given to the salient and controlled users. Especially, the salient users should be receiving attention. These younger users have been vividly portrayed in a New York ethnographical study by Williams (1989). For these 'cocaine kids' prevention is challenged to provide a viable alternative to a cocaine-centred lifestyle that has become socially functional in their group. In any case, 'secondary' prevention efforts are called for, specifically directed toward salient and controlled users (Jekel 1987). A bold corollary of such a policy would be to try to redirect these salient and controlled users toward the 'casual' end of the pipeline. This could mean prevention strategies that do not focus on the goal of complete abstinence from cocaine, but cleverly try to stimulate cocaine users to become involved in health promotion within their own cocaine networks. Such a strategy would encourage non-dependent cocaine users to be aware of the relationship between the prevention of addiction and their own subtle use patterns. New opportunities for involvement with those of their cocaine contacts who do not require the use of cocaine most of the time need to be specified and promoted. For this strategy to be consistent, social definitions of cocaine should also be subtly changed, to allow for a slight widening of the scope of current cocaine settings. Abstinence is indeed a real possibility for many cocaine users, but we should also be prepared to contemplate the possibility that casual use may also be a relevant goal of 'secondary' prevention.

Acknowledgements

The research presented in this paper has been supported by grants from the City of Rotterdam and the Commission of the European Communities Health and Safety Directorate. Valuable criticisms, comments and advice have been given by Professor Tom Snijders, Edgar de Bie and Marinus Spreen. Careful attention and persistent editorial stimulation have been provided by Julie Whelan and the editorial staff of the Ciba Foundation. The views presented in this paper are the sole responsibility of the authors and do not reflect the policies of the funding agencies or our scientific advisers.

References

Adler PA, Adler P 1987 Membership roles in field research. Sage Publications, London
Biernacki P, Waldorf D 1981 Snowball sampling: problems and techniques of chain-referral sampling. Sociological Methods & Research 10:141–163
Chitwood DD 1985 Patterns and consequences of cocaine use. In: Kozel NJ, Adams EH (eds) Cocaine use in America: epidemiologic and clinical perspectives. (National Institute on Drug Abuse Research Monograph 61) US Government Printing Office, Washington, DC, p 111–129
Cohen P 1989 Cocaine use in Amsterdam in non-deviant subcultures. (Onderzoek-Programma Drug Beleid Gemeente Amsterdam 10) Universiteit van Amsterdam, Amsterdam
de Vries MW 1987 Introduction. Investigating mental disorders in their natural setting. J Nerv Ment Dis 175:509–513

Douglas JD, Rasmussen PK, Flanagan CA 1977 The nude beach. Sage Publications, London

Edwards G, Arif A, Hodgson R 1982 Nomenclature and classification of drug- and alcohol-related problems: a shortened version of the WHO memorandum. Br J Addict 77:3-20

Erickson PG, Murray GF 1989 The undeterred cocaine user: intention to quit and its relationship to perceived legal and health threats. Contemp Drug Problems 16:141-156

Frank O 1979 Estimation of population totals by use of snowball samples. In: Holland PW, Leinhardt SL (eds) Perspectives on social network research. Academic Press, New York, p 319-347

Gawin FH 1991 Cocaine addiction: psychology and neurophysiology. Science (Wash DC) 251:1580-1586

Grund JPC, Adriaans NFP, Kaplan CD 1991 Changing cocaine smoking rituals in the Dutch heroin addict population. Br J Addict 86:439-448

Intraval 1990 Cocaine use in Rotterdam. A preliminary study. Intraval, Groningen & Rotterdam

Jekel JF 1987 Public health approaches to the cocaine problem: lessons from the Bahamas. In: Allen D (ed) The cocaine crisis. Plenum Press, London, p 107-116

Johanson CE 1984 Assessment of the dependence potential of cocaine in animals. In: Grabowski J (ed) Cocaine: pharmacology, effects, and treatment of abuse. (National Institute on Drug Abuse Research Monograph 50) US Government Printing Office, Washington, DC, p 54-71

Kaplan CD, Korf D, Sterk C 1987 Temporal and social contexts of heroin-using populations. An illustration of the snowball sampling technique. J Nerv Ment Dis 175:566-574

Kadhushin C 1982 Social density and mental health. In: Marsden PV, Lin N (eds) Social structure and network analysis. Sage Publications, London, p 147-158

Littlewood R 1990 From categories to contexts: a decade of 'new cross-cultural psychiatry'. Br J Psychiatry 156:308-327

Morningstar PC, Chitwood DD 1983 The patterns of cocaine use: an interdisciplinary study. Final report No. R01 DA03106. (National Institute on Drug Abuse, Rockville, MD) US Government Printing Office, Washington, DC

Morningstar PC, Chitwood DD 1984 Cocaine users view of themselves. Implicit behavior theory in context. Human Organization 43:307-318

Murphy SB, Reinarman C, Waldorf D 1989 An 11-year follow-up of a network of cocaine users. Br J Addict 84:427-436

National Institute on Drug Abuse 1990 Population estimates of lifetime and current drug use, 1990. NIDA Capsules. (National Institute on Drug Abuse, Rockville, MD) US Government Printing Office, Washington, DC

Office of National Drug Control Policy 1989 First, get the casual user. US Government Printing Office, Washington, DC

Ostrow R 1990 Casual drug users should be shot, Gates says. Los Angeles Times (Thursday 6 September) A1:19

Pollin W 1984 Foreword. In: Grabowski J (ed) Cocaine: pharmacology, effects, and treatment of abuse. (National Institute on Drug Abuse Research Monograph 50) US Government Printing Office, Washington, DC, p vii-viii

Reinarman C 1979 Moral entrepreneurs and political economy: historical and ethnographic notes on the construction of the cocaine menace. Contemp Crises 3:225-254

Rouse BA 1991 Trends in cocaine use in the general population. In: Schober S, Schade C (eds) The epidemiology of cocaine use and abuse. (National Institute on Drug Abuse Research Monograph 110) US Government Printing Office, Washington, DC, p 5-18

Sacks H 1972 An initial investigation of the usability of conversational data for doing sociology. In: Sudnow D (ed) Studies in social interaction. The Free Press, New York, p 31–74

Sandwijk JP, Westerterp I, Musterd S 1988 Het Gebruik van legale en illegal drugs in Amsterdam: verslag van een prevalentie-onderzoek onder de bevolking van 12 jaar en ouder. (Onderzoek-Programma Drug Beleid Gemeente Amsterdam 9) Universiteit van Amsterdam, Amsterdam

Siegel RK 1989 Intoxication: life in pursuit of artificial paradise. EP Dutton, New York

Sudman S, Sirken MG, Cowan CD 1988 Sampling rare and elusive populations. Science (Wash DC) 240:991–996

van Meter KM 1990a Methodological and design issues: techniques for assessing the representatives of snowball samples. In: Lambert EY (ed) The collection and interpretation of data from hidden populations. (National Institute on Drug Abuse Research Monograph 98) US Government Printing Office, Washington, DC, p 31–43

van Meter KM 1990b Sampling and cross-classification analysis in international social research. In: Øyen E (ed) Comparative methodology: theory and practice in international social research. Sage Publications, London, p 172–186

Watters, JK, Biernacki P 1989 Targeted sampling: options for the study of hidden populations. Social Problems 36:416–430

Williams T 1989 The cocaine kids: the inside story of a teenage drug ring. Addison-Wesley, New York

DISCUSSION

Moore: I would have expected that the concept of controlled drug use would have something to do with the *quantity* of drug consumed, as well as the *settings* in which people use particular drugs. Controlled drug use would then mean keeping use below the intoxicating or disruptive level, or that when a person uses it at such a level, he or she makes sure of using it in a setting where that level is 'safe'. The key idea of controlled drug use, I think, is that a controlled drug user can keep him or herself out of danger with drug use. With that definition, what you are offering is explanatory variables about what might prove to be predictive of, or determinative of, whether a person is able to maintain a controlled drug use. Your explanation focuses on how much of his or her social environment consists of drug users. The implicit assumption is that other drug users are either elevating that person's consumption, or extending it over time, or pushing it into contexts where things become more dangerous. To me, trying to define a pattern of drug use by variables that describe how many different settings you use it in, and how many people you know who have also used drugs, is a slightly odd procedure.

Kaplan: Most studies of 'controlled' use have used variations of Morningstar & Chitwood's (1984) index, which I reviewed in my paper and which fit your expectation. We have these data, but we wanted to try to define patterns of use (including controlled use) purely by social context variables for the purposes of this paper. The concept of 'controlled' use comes from the users; they say they are in control, and we believe them, as we have to do as ethnographers. We have to take their point of view. 'Controlled' use is, at its origin, a social construct, a users' category. So we chose to start our analysis with data from another level—the social relations level. In a more comprehensive, later analysis we want to see where the two levels come together. Our implicit assumption is indeed that social relations—for example, the frequency and kind of people you use drugs together with—are good indicators of the settings component that you yourself recognize as intrinsic to a concept of use pattern. Thus, the 'scope' variable is what you say it is—a variable related to the settings of the social relations of use. From an ethnographic point of view, the controlled user is seeking out a specific setting where he or she feels in control, and an intrinsic part of the setting is its social relations. This type of user starts to select friends whom they share their drug experiences with, who use cocaine in what they say is a 'safe' way. And therefore we think that this selection becomes crystallized into the pattern of use itself and relates to variables such as 'route of administration' that Morningstar and Chitwood built into their index. I agree with you that our approach to definition is unorthodox. I would prefer to call it 'novel' rather than 'odd'. I feel our approach has a certain face validity: we are known and know ourselves by the friends we keep.

Edwards: I'd like to ask Marian Fischman whether, as a laboratory scientist, she finds the idea of what people are referring to as 'controlled use', a likely pattern of behaviour.

Fischman: Yes. A substantial number of volunteers who join my studies are people whom I would define as 'controlled users'—people who use cocaine occasionally, or regularly, but in relatively low doses—the weekend user, for example. Some of those people use cocaine in those patterns for years and don't get into trouble. This concept doesn't surprise me, having interviewed hundreds of people who are cocaine users.

Jones: My laboratory has had the same experience. Most laboratory studies of cocaine use in the USA are drawing from populations of similar 'controlled' cocaine users. Typically, our San Francisco group of research volunteers on average have been using cocaine for five years; smaller numbers have used it 15–20 years. The modal pattern is only 1–2 times per month; others use it once or twice a week. Some have histories of binges, varying in frequency over a 5–10 year period. But, in general, in our study and in most laboratory studies in the USA, prospective research subjects must convince the experimenters that they are controlled cocaine users. That means that none of us is studying out-of-control users in a controlled laboratory setting.

Benowitz: Do you have any sense of what proportion of the people who start to use cocaine become uncontrolled cocaine users? Is it a very small percentage, or is it the majority?

I would also like more information about the patterns of cocaine use of individuals: what percentage of cocaine users use weekly or every day? Of those who use it daily, do we know anything about their pattern of use within the day?

Jones: I don't know if anyone has precise numbers. In past years, when there was at any time an estimated 7-8 million cocaine users in the United States, they must have represented a constantly shifting group of users beginning and leaving. I believe some estimates are that as many as 50 million people have used cocaine on occasion. We are now given estimates of 336 000 who seem to be daily users (NIDA 1990). I would assume that that's the group where the compulsive users are, at least in the USA. I would not term people using cocaine once or twice weekly compulsive users.

Kleber: The numbers I draw from the NIDA Household Survey would be about 25 million who have ever used cocaine (rather than your figure of 50 million). Our estimate of current users (from NIDA data) is of approximately two million cocaine addicts, defined as those using cocaine at least 2-3 times per week. The large majority of those people would probably exhibit features covered under the DSM-III-R diagnosis of cocaine dependency where the drug use has become the crucial focus of their life and activities.

The important point here is that the data change over time. In the high school survey, for example, the number of people who enter the pool (that is, who have ever used cocaine) and go on to regular use has been changing over the last five or so years, and was substantially different in 1990 from 1985. Any number that one selects of how many enter the drug-use 'pipeline' and how many get 'into trouble' may vary with where we are in the epidemic.

Kaplan: The numbers in the San Francisco group (Murphy et al 1989) of course were small, initially—27 users. As I mentioned in the paper, those authors indicate four patterns of use. They also report the one case who continued from the initiation of cocaine use to heavy use—the typical heroin addict trajectory. Murphy et al considered this an exception rather than a pattern. But two of the four patterns include a 'heavy use' period; either it leads to abstinence, or (which is intriguing) it leads to a return to controlled use.

Edwards: Are you happy in applying statistical methods to data gathered through a 'snowballing' technique?

Kaplan: I am happy when I find numbers and people's descriptions—quantities and qualities—integrated in a coherent way. Of course, you are correct in emphasizing the play of chance in applying statistics to fieldwork studies. But there is much exciting work being done today by statisticians developing the new tools that will be effective in integrating fieldwork with mathematical modelling. The European Social Network Association has made this issue a research priority. The generalizability and representativeness of 'snowball' samples is of course the key problem. Now we are fortunate to have a new logic of inquiry that Karl van Meter (1990) has termed 'ascending' methodologies adapted for the study of small or local populations, in contrast to the more familiar logics adapted for general populations. Successive cross-classification of local samples provide confidence in the generalizability of local results. There are, obviously, problems in the calculation of general population estimates and the explanation of variance, but, as van Meter states, we seem to be at the threshold of some new breakthroughs that will reduce the play of chance in intensive studies such as Murphy et al (1989). With this as a methodological background, I have some confidence in quoting figures that seem to fit with other intensive studies.

Anthony: In our five-site Epidemiologic Catchment Area study in the USA in the early 1980s, we studied some 900–1000 subjects who reported using cocaine at least five times—obviously not applying as stringent an inclusion criterion as Dr Kaplan. Among these subjects, about 15% reported daily cocaine use lasting two weeks or more, so about 85% had used five times but had not gone on to daily use for a sustained period of at least two weeks.

We also asked what proportion of current cocaine users at the start of the survey were still using it one year later. There were about 20% still using. That is, first we asked: 'Have you used cocaine in the past year?' A year later, at follow-up, we asked these subjects if they had used cocaine during the two weeks just before the follow-up interview. Only about 20% said 'yes', but about 80% said 'no'. This implies a good degree of turnover in the active cocaine-using population within the general US population. If you went after the street-dwelling inhabitants in inner cities, I presume you would get larger values, but this is a different perspective on cocaine use.

Moore: You can get a sense of that by looking at how the proportions of chronic, intensive daily cocaine users (regular users) versus other users change over time. You can work out what fraction advance to chronic intensive use.

In our study of alcohol (Moore & Gerstein 1983), where we had good data on people's consumption patterns, both in the short run and over a long period, we found a wide and continuous distribution of drinking patterns, with most people drinking nothing or relatively little, and a few people drinking quite a lot.

The patterns of drinking—measured in terms of quantity consumed and activities paired with drinking—were not constant for individuals over time. Some people who were heavy drinkers became less heavy in their drinking over 10 years. Others who were light drinkers became moderate or heavy drinkers. So it did not seem that people were destined to be a particular type of drinker.

We also found that serious adverse consequences of drinking showed up in all parts of the distribution of consumption—though they were of different types and with lower probabilities at lower ends of consumption. (Some people who drank only occasionally were nonetheless victims of drunk driving, or arrested in drunken brawls. Only heavy drinkers died of cirrhosis.) Again, because there are so many people drinking at low levels, the infrequent drinkers were found to contribute a substantial amount to the overall alcohol problem. Thus one could conclude that for alcohol, at least, drug use is a highly variable phenomenon.

O'Brien: We are like the blind men who are examining an elephant; we are looking at very different ends of the same problem. Dr Kaplan at one end is using the 'snowball' procedure and is finding one group that may be very different from the people who answer an advertisement in a newspaper, such as Reese Jones or Marian Fischman employ to obtain volunteers for their studies. My end of the elephant seems quite different again. In Philadelphia the people who come to us, desperate for treatment, on average have been using cocaine for a relatively short time (three years or less). They usually cannot take cocaine on a daily basis, because when they start doing so they lose control, and so they tend to 'binge', taking progressively higher doses in a short period of time. On average they have used cocaine for 15–18 days out of the past 30 days. At the time of admission to treatment, they show a high frequency of psychiatric disorder.

There is an over-representation of African-Americans among our cocaine-dependent patients. We don't know whether differences among patients presenting with alcohol, opiate and cocaine dependence represent simply differences in drug availability, or whether there are biological differences that make some people tend to lose control of their cocaine use and get into psychiatric dysfunction and addictive patterns more readily. There are also differences in the way different groups administer cocaine. Most of our patients take it by smoking crack or by intravenous injection of cocaine hydrochloride. Few take it by the intranasal route and, if so, only at the beginning of their cocaine-using careers.

Negrete: However, an individual could be classified as one thing today and as something different some months or a few years later. Has any prospective study been made of this? Has anyone had the chance to follow a group over time? In Patricia Erickson's work (a cross-sectional, point-in-time study only) in Canada, it was found that 20% of a group of cocaine users could be defined as addicted (Erickson & Alexander 1989). I have been looking at the question of when cocaine users come for treatment myself. A self-selected group of volunteer subjects show a modal time of three years from the time they start to use cocaine, but some people are coming for treatment after 10, 12 or more years of use. Therefore I have to assume that somebody who has been more or less managing his habit for 8–10 years doesn't manage it any more. So what are we talking about? The percentage of users who turn into abusers, or uncontrolled users, is essentially a longitudinal development—something that changes over time.

Kalant: I am confused about the nature of the terminology, with terms such as 'controlled' and 'casual'. Are these meant to be descriptive of amounts and frequencies of cocaine use, or are they meant to describe cognitive mechanisms of voluntary intent with respect to when, where, under what circumstances and how much the user would use cocaine? It sounds to me like a mixture of different things—on the one hand a description of low amounts of use that have not yet given rise to any problem, or of a degree of deliberate voluntary control over use, and on the other hand a retrospective grouping of people who have already run into problems and who may have been (at an earlier stage) describable under one of the other terms. I would like someone to explain it in a way that says, under one system of nomenclature, what these things mean.

Kaplan: 'Controlled use' began as a user-defined category—the patient's own description. The categories of 'salience' and 'compulsive' were DSM-III-R categories (the diagnostic system recommended by the American Psychiatric Association that is heavily influenced by Professor Edwards' Drug Dependency Syndrome: see Kosten et al 1987). The clinically and socially relevant diagnosis and classification of patterns of drug use is an attempt to combine a lot of variables that are part of what these people self-report—that is, how much they are using cocaine, in what settings, intentions, and so on, combined with the descriptions that psychiatrists have obtained from clinical work. We are trying to put the patients' localized self-description together with the psychiatrists' 'universal' diagnostic system and make sense of it, using statistical methods and qualitative techniques.

Jones: I don't think there is yet a good answer to the key question of what is the natural history of patterns of human cocaine use, particularly the behaviours we term 'loss of control' or 'controlled'. Our measures of cocaine use are crude and are mostly based on self-reports with no independent validation. For example, the measure 'daily use' of cocaine in most survey data is about as fine a resolution as we have available. To know only that someone is a 'daily user' is not very helpful when considered from a pharmacological standpoint. There can certainly be 'controlled' daily use; for example, a typical pattern reported by some of our research volunteers is to come home from work, open up a beer, take a single snort or two of cocaine, then watch television for the evening and drink beer until onset of sleep. Such people never use cocaine during the working day, or ever use cocaine 'out of control'. That's one common type of 'daily use'. Is it controlled use? I suggest it is.

Another kind of daily use is often reported in survey data and seems inconsistent with my clinical experience. This is the cocaine user who says 'I have been using a gram or more of cocaine every day for months on end'. High dose cocaine use almost always seems to be cyclic. It comes and goes, for reasons not totally dependent on supply. Yet our best resolution of cocaine dosimetry that leads to public policy decisions is 'the daily dose'—not how much the dose is, or by what route, or if it's taken in or out of control, or all the other things that we want to know, and expect to know, if we are talking about tobacco or alcohol or any other psychoactive drug. As scientists we would be laughed at if we talked about another drug in the way we talk about cocaine dosimetry. Imagine if all tobacco smokers or all alcohol users, or all caffeine users, were lumped into a 'daily user' category without any attempt at a finer resolution and then we tried to understand the benefits or toxicity of those drugs.

Kleber: I both agree and disagree with you! In terms of what you see clinically, during the years that I have been running cocaine treatment clinics, it appeared to us that the 'daily user' was in less trouble than the binge user, at least in the pre-crack days. The daily user was often the one with the psychiatric problem (e.g. a bipolar, self-medicating to maintain the hypomanic phase), or someone self-medicating attention deficit disorder. As Chuck O'Brien said earlier, the person in trouble with cocaine is more likely to be a binge user, using cocaine 2–3 days a week, crashing, then staying clean for a couple of days, and then starting all over again. That is the quintessential cocaine addict. As far as I understand it, the NIDA definition of heavy cocaine abuser, or where the figure of two million addicts comes from, is some combination of a variety of things, including some individuals who meet DSM-III-R criteria and others defined as 'heavy' users who might not meet the dependence criteria. So it's a mishmash!

Des Jarlais: I think there is a strong argument for taking the pure ethnographic approach to the definitions of types of cocaine users. People using cocaine typically do it in a social setting; they depend on others in order to buy drugs, and they depend on others for social approval of their drug use. When the users themselves start making the distinctions between a casual user, a controlled user and an out-of-control user, they generally have a good basis for doing so.

Thus, if I am a controlled user, I have to know who is an out-of-control user, because that is somebody I don't want to give money to, to buy drugs for me, because the out-of-control user will probably use them himself and I shall never get the drugs or my money back. I also need to know who is a casual user, in terms of 'can I tell them that I use cocaine?'. Also, if someone is a casual user, that person is not likely to be a good source of drugs if I need to buy drugs, because casual users are unlikely to have good sources of supply. In fact, one definition that I have heard cocaine users use themselves is that a casual user is someone who has used cocaine but has never paid for it. Such users are not interested enough in cocaine to go out and buy it; but if someone offers it at a party, they will use it! Still, cocaine is not important enough to them to spend their own money on it.

Kalant: So the cocaine use is not initiated by them, and it depends on the circumstance—the presence of other people with the drug?

Des Jarlais: Yes, it's totally situational.

Kaplan: Like numerous other drug-regulated behaviours, such as needle-sharing. It is 'on the spot', situationally determined.

Des Jarlais: Although cocaine is not important enough to the casual users for them to go and spend a lot of money, if somebody offers it, they use it. They don't tend to suffer ill effects, nor do they get tremendously high on it; when you talk to them about it, they say 'I used it and it was OK'. So they noticed the pharmacological effect; it's not that the quality of drug was very poor, but it wasn't reinforcing enough for them to feel they must go out and buy it. Thus if we want to try to make distinctions among users and use patterns, there is an argument for using the distinctions that the people who invest a lot of time, effort and money in the drugs are using to differentiate among different types of users.

Edwards: A final comment, Dr Kaplan?

Kaplan: The 'snowball' method is like cocaine itself; it goes in and out of fashion. It is a reputable technique in the social sciences for locating rare and hidden populations that general surveys can't pick up. Our intention was exactly this: that by starting from the fieldwork of the ethnographer, we asked then how we could add some system to it in order to achieve the level of generalizability that could complement, and inform, the good work that the general population surveys are doing. We also wanted to develop a method that is, I would say, more policy-context sensitive than existing scientific methods. Policy makers need timely facts that represent the actual situation of drug use and are embedded in a framework of interpretation that can readily be implemented into political actions. The 'snowball' method provided such a possibility, producing not only some numbers, but qualitative descriptions of social worlds where cocaine was used. We are all good scientists, but as epidemiologists or in whatever functional role we are cast, there is a very practical need for information and for related policy statements that are reliable for 'all practical purposes'. Research using snowball methods is cheap, fast and throws a glimmer of light in a sea of darkness. And 'a sea of darkness' is what knowledge of cocaine was like in Europe, and it is still more or less that way; hardly anybody until very recently had ever seen a cocaine-using patient in a clinic outside a heroin treatment centre. Our research was an attempt to wade into the swamps—the streets of European cities—to discover the nature and extent of cocaine use in Europe.

References

Erickson PG, Alexander BK 1989 Cocaine and addictive liability. Social Pharmacol 3:249–270

Kosten TR, Rounsaville BJ, Babor TF, Spitzer RL, Williams JBW 1987 Substance use disorders in DSM III-R: the dependence syndrome across different psychoactive substances. Br J Psychiatry 151:834–843

Moore MH, Gerstein DR 1983 Alcohol and public policy: beyond the shadow of prohibition. National Academy of Sciences, Washington, DC

Morningstar PC, Chitwood DD 1984 Cocaine users view of themselves. Implicit behavior theory in context. Human Organization 43:307–318

Murphy SB, Reinarman C, Waldorf D 1989 An ll-year follow-up of a network of cocaine users. Br J Addict 84:427–436

NIDA 1990 National Household survey on drug abuse. (Reprinted in NIDA Notes, vol 6 no.1, winter 1990/91) US Department of Health and Human Services, Washington, DC

van Meter KM 1990 Sampling and cross-classification analysis in international social research. In: Øyen E (ed) Comparative methodology: theory and practice in international social research. Sage Publications, London, p 172–186

Molecular pharmacology of cocaine: a dopamine hypothesis and its implications

Michael J. Kuhar

Neuroscience Branch, Addiction Research Center, National Institute on Drug Abuse, P.O. Box 5180, Baltimore, MD 21224, USA

>*Abstract.* The reinforcing properties of cocaine have been related to cocaine binding at the dopamine transporter in mesolimbocortical neurons. The molecular properties of the transporter have been studied in a number of laboratories. While this 'dopamine hypothesis' is strongly supported in animal studies of drug self-administration, the extent of its involvement in human drug dependence has not been fully elucidated.
>
>*1992 Cocaine: scientific and social dimensions. Wiley, Chichester (Ciba Foundation Symposium 166) p 81–95*

Cocaine has been the subject of scientific investigation for more than 100 years. It continues to be an abused drug and recently there has been a serious worldwide epidemic of its use. The aim of this paper is to summarize findings on the molecular mechanisms of actions on cocaine that have been elucidated in the past several years. The implications of these findings will also be discussed.

The dopamine transporter: an apparent cocaine receptor

Beginning in 1980, various cocaine binding sites have been identified in the brain and other tissues of rodents and monkeys (Reith et al 1980, Kennedy & Hanbauer 1983, Schoemaker et al 1985, Calligaro & Eldefrawi 1987, Madras et al 1989). At least some of these binding sites appear to be re-uptake carriers or transporters for neurotransmitters. The function of these transporters is believed to be the inactivation of released neurotransmitter (Kuhar 1973). It is not surprising that cocaine binds to these transporters, because it had been known for many years that cocaine is a relatively potent inhibitor of neurotransmitter re-uptake; for example, it was shown by Harris & Baldessarini (1973) that cocaine inhibited ^{3}H-labelled dopamine uptake (Snyder & Coyle 1969, Horn 1990) into nigrostriatal tissues. While cocaine has many pharmacological effects, the effects that appear to be related to and predictive of its addictive properties are its reinforcing effects (Johanson & Fischman 1989). Further, while there are many

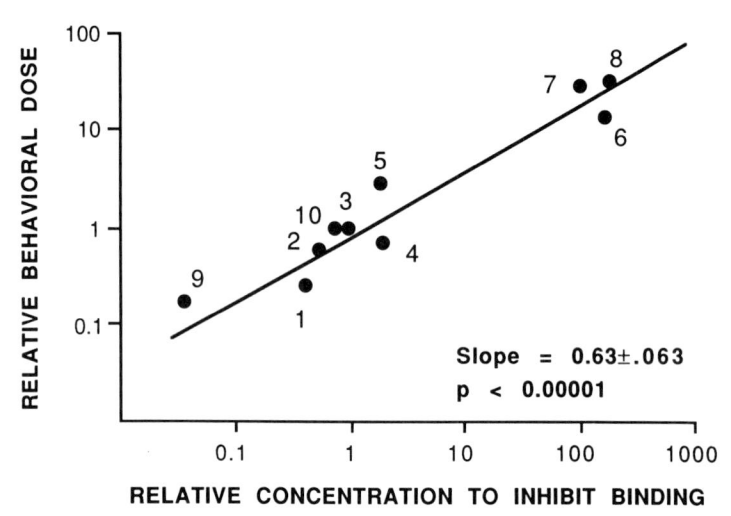

FIG. 1. Correlation between drug binding at the dopamine transporter and drug self-administration behaviour. The relative concentration of drug which inhibits binding (abscissa) reveals the relative affinity of various drugs (compared to cocaine) at the dopamine transporter. The relative behavioural dose is the dose (relative to cocaine) that causes drug self-administration behaviour. Cocaine has the value of one on both axes. Each point represents another drug; the positive correlation suggests a close relationship between drug binding to the dopamine transporter and the reinforcing properties of the drugs. (Modified from Ritz et al 1987.)

binding sites for cocaine, the only binding site that has been related to its reinforcing properties (Fig. 1) is the dopamine transporter (Ritz et al 1987, Bergman et al 1989). Thus, the dopamine transporter appears to be the 'receptor' site, or the initial site of action where the events resulting in the reinforcing effects of cocaine are initiated.

A large number of experimental results with animals from a variety of experimental disciplines are compatible with the notion that the dopamine transporter is a relevant cocaine receptor. For example, selective lesions of mesolimbic dopaminergic nerve terminals disrupt the self-administration of cocaine. Also, dopamine receptor blockers disrupt cocaine self-administration. These findings as well as many others have recently been summarized (Kuhar et al 1991).

Structure–activity studies

Because of its apparent role in cocaine addiction, many laboratories have investigated the properties of the dopamine transporter. Structure–activity relationships indicate very specific requirements for binding at the transporter and for initiating self-administration behaviour. First of all, the cocaine binding site at the dopamine transporter is stereospecific. Of the eight possible stereoisomers of cocaine, the naturally occurring (−) cocaine is clearly the most potent. The remaining isomers have potencies that are 1/60th to 1/600th of that of (−) cocaine (Carroll et al 1991).

The metabolites of cocaine have been known to be inactive for many years. Thus, ecgonine methyl ester and benzoyl ecgonine are inactive at the binding site (Ritz et al 1990). An interesting finding has been that removal of the ester linkage between the phenyl group and the tropane moiety results in compounds that are significantly more potent than cocaine; halogen substitution in the *para* position of the phenyl group results in further increases in potency (Reith et al 1986, Boja et al 1990).

The methyl group at the methoxy position can be substituted by much longer carbon chains without any significant loss of potency. Also, the nitrogen on the cocaine molecule can be moved to another position on the molecule without a great loss in potency (Ritz et al 1990, Carroll et al 1992).

Thus, binding at the dopamine transporter has very specific molecular requirements. In a sense, the binding site for cocaine is not optimally structured for cocaine, because removing the ester linkage between the phenyl ring and the tropane moiety results in compounds of higher affinity. Since some studies have shown that cocaine's inhibition of dopamine uptake is competitive (Krueger 1990), it is tempting to speculate that the phenyl ring on the cocaine molecule binds to a region similar to where the catechol ring of dopamine binds, and that the amino group of dopamine binds to a region similar to that where the nitrogen of the tropane moiety binds. Additional studies will be required to verify this notion.

These structure–activity studies provide some information on the pharmacophore (i.e. the binding site) for cocaine. But a more complete assessment of the cocaine binding site requires a better understanding of the dopamine transporter and its function. Thus, many laboratories have initiated molecular studies of the transporter.

Characterization of the transporter protein

By means of photoaffinity probes that are derivatives of GBR 12909 (a drug that binds to the dopamine transporter), the transporter has been shown to be a protein of an apparent molecular mass of 75 000–80 000 daltons (Da) (Grigoriadis et al 1989, Sallee et al 1989, Berger et al 1990). Also, the transporter appears to be a glycoprotein containing a carbohydrate moiety that is rich in sialic acid residues that are N-linked to the protein (Sallee et al 1989, Lew et al 1991a). Most recently, multiple dopamine transporter proteins have been identified, in that the molecular mass of the transporter from the nucleus accumbens of the rat forebrain appears to be slightly larger than that from the striatum (Fig. 2; Lew et al 1991b). While some laboratories have reported a

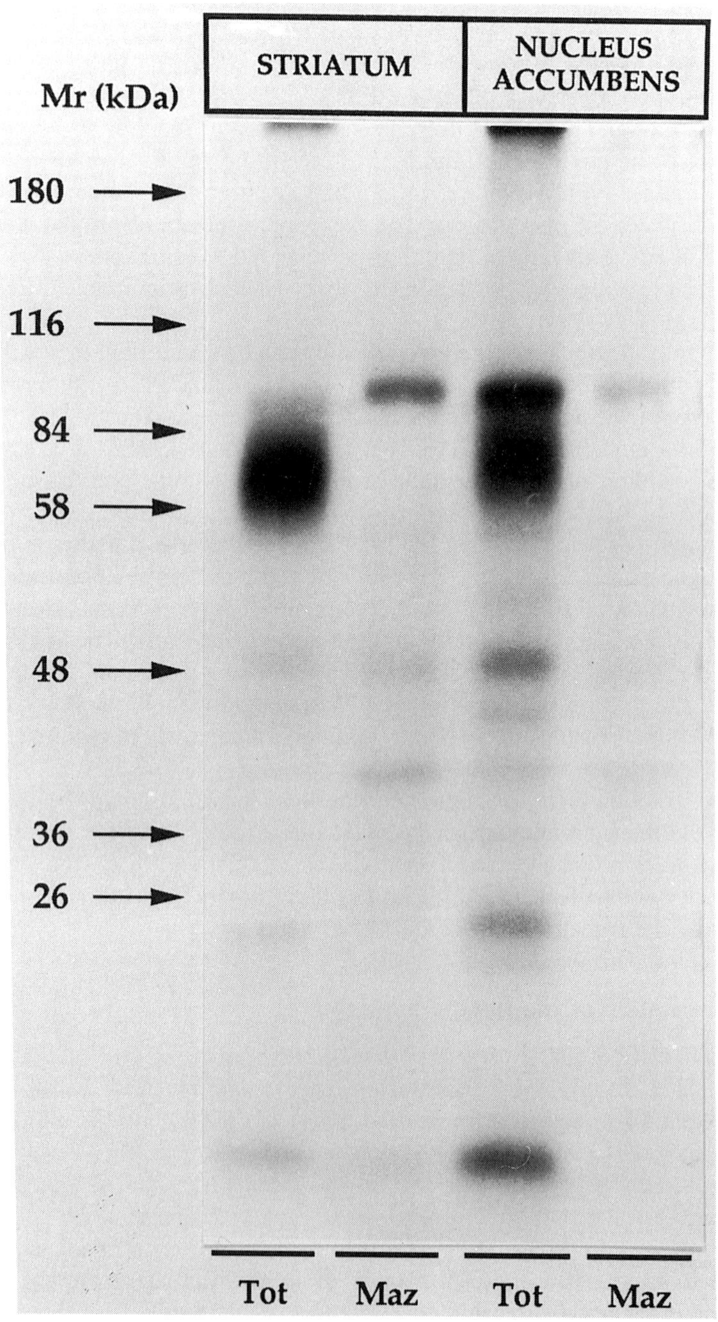
STRIATUM
NUCLEUS ACCUMBENS
Mr (kDa)
180
116
84
58
48
36
26
Tot
Maz
Tot
Maz

pharmacological difference between the transporter in the nucleus accumbens and that in the striatum, this has not been confirmed by others (Boja & Kuhar 1989). Thus, it is unclear whether or not this difference in apparent molecular mass has a functional significance. Also, it is unclear whether the apparent heterogeneity is due to different genes or whether it is due to differences in post-translational processing of the protein. Recent unpublished studies showing that deglycosylation reduces the differences in molecular mass suggest that at least part of the heterogeneity is due to differences in glycosylation.

Cloning of transporter proteins

While the gene for the dopamine transporter has not yet been cloned, transporters for other neurotransmitters have recently been cloned and work on the dopamine transporter is in progress. A cDNA (complementary DNA) for the GABA transporter (Guastella et al 1990) has been cloned; it suggests that the transporter is a protein of molecular mass of approximately 67 Da with 12 or 13 hydrophobic membrane-spanning regions. There are potential glycosylation sites as well as potential phosphorylation sites on the protein. Pacholczyk et al (1991) have recently cloned a cDNA for the noradrenaline (norepinephrine) transporter. The structure and properties of the predicted protein are similar to those described for the GABA transporter. Moreover, Pacholczyk et al (1991) have pointed out that there is significant homology between the human noradrenaline transporter and the human GABA transporter, where the overall identity of amino acids is 46%. Allowing for conservative amino acid substitutions, the similarity between these two transporters increases to 68%. These data indicate that the neurotransmitter transporters probably form a family of similar proteins. Thus, it is expected that the dopamine transporter will be a protein that has similar properties and is a member of this family. Because of the availability of cloning techniques that make it relatively easy to identify members of a family once similarities have been established, it seems likely that the dopamine transporter will be cloned in the near future.*
This should lead to a more thorough understanding of how the transporter

---

Note added since the symposium: The cloning and expression of a cDNA for a cocaine-sensitive dopamine transporter have been reported (Shimada et al 1991 Science [Wash DC] 254:576–578; Kilty et al 1991 Science [Wash DC] 254:578–579). Expression of this protein confers both dopamine uptake activity and cocaine analogue binding activity in cultured cells.

FIG. 2. (*opposite*) Evidence for multiple dopamine transporters: an autoradiograph of an SDS-PAGE gel on which proteins labelled with an iodinated irreversible probe (^{125}I-DEEP) for the dopamine transporter are identified. The broad bands of molecular mass about 75 kDa represent the dopamine transporter. The transporter from the rat nucleus accumbens has a slightly higher molecular mass than that from the striatum, suggesting a heterogeneity among dopamine transporter molecules. (See Lew et al 1991a,b for more details.)

functions and how cocaine affects it. The development of a direct, competitive or allosteric cocaine antagonist, if that is possible, may depend on having a complete picture of the transporter molecule.

Dopamine hypothesis and its implications

The dopamine hypothesis of the reinforcing properties of cocaine (for a recent review see Kuhar et al 1991) suggests that cocaine binds to the dopamine transporter of mesolimbocortical neurons, which results in the inhibition of dopamine re-uptake, the potentiation of dopaminergic transmission, and ultimately the behavioural phenomenon of reinforcement (Fig. 3). This model suggests potential medications for the treatment of cocaine abuse and dependence. For example, possibilities for substitution therapy would include using other uptake inhibitors, or direct dopamine receptor agonists. While substitution therapy with an uptake inhibitor like methylphenidate does not appear to be promising (Gawin et al 1985), other drugs or strategies might be useful.

Another possibility is the utilization of dopamine receptor blocking drugs as a potential treatment. I mentioned earlier that dopamine receptor blockers disrupt the self-administration of cocaine in experimental animals. However, the use of receptor blockers has not yielded promising results in human studies in all cases. Gawin et al (1989) showed that flupenthixol appears to cause a decrease in craving for cocaine and a large increase in the average time that patients were retained in treatment; however, the study was an 'open' trial and

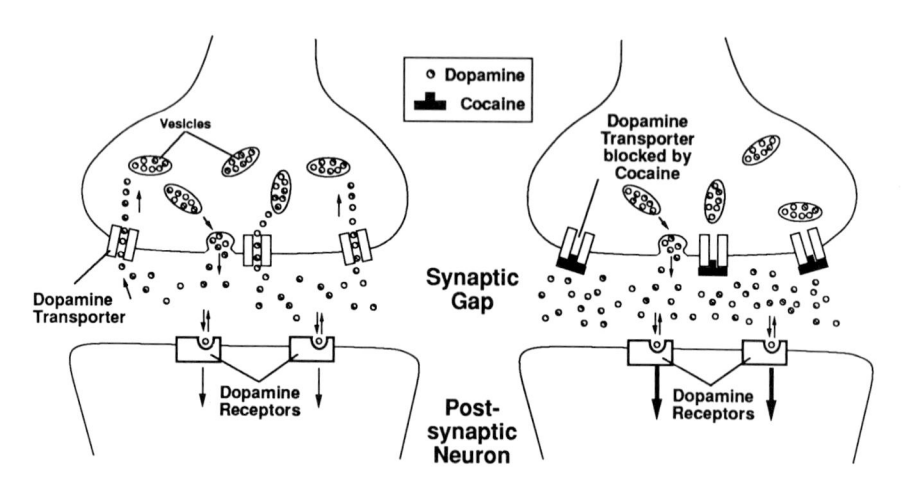

FIG. 3. The dopamine hypothesis of the reinforcing properties of cocaine. Cocaine binds to the dopamine transporter and blocks the re-uptake of dopamine in the mesolimbocortical pathway. This potentiates dopaminergic neurotransmission and, according to the hypothesis, initiates the sequence of events that ultimately cause the rewarding effects of the drug. (From Kuhar et al 1991.)

the authors noted the need for a double-blind follow-up study. While this study suggested the usefulness of dopamine receptor blockers, other studies did not find significant effects of these drugs. Gawin (1986) found that chlorpromazine and haloperidol (neuroleptic drugs which act by blocking dopamine receptors) did not block cocaine-induced euphoria and cocaine self-administration. Similarly, Sherer et al (1989) reported that haloperidol had no effect on cocaine-induced 'rush' (the rapid initial euphoria), but only a small effect on some subjective effects of the drug. Thus, these initial human studies suggest that blockade of the D_2 category of dopamine receptors does not affect the euphoric properties of cocaine. These results are in contrast to studies with amphetamines, where euphoria was apparently sensitive to the pretreatment of patients with dopamine receptor blockers (Gunne et al 1972). However, many subtypes of dopamine receptors (e.g. D_3-D_5) have recently been identified, and blockade of these additional subtypes has not been thoroughly studied in cocaine-abusing populations. Also, euphoria may not be the proper effect to study; the reinforcing effects of cocaine may be more relevant. Thus, a thorough evaluation of the dopamine hypothesis in humans has not been carried out, and the role of dopamine in mesolimbocortical neurons in human cocaine abuse remains to be elucidated.

Summary and conclusions

In the past several years, significant advances in our understanding of the molecular action of cocaine have been achieved. The dopamine transporter, rather than other binding sites for cocaine, has been identified as the potential initial site of action of the drug as regards its reinforcing properties. Detailed structure–activity studies have revealed the nature of the binding pharmacophore. Extensive studies of the transporter proteins, along with the cloning of the cDNA for the transporter (see footnote on p 85), will reveal much of the detail of cocaine's interaction with the dopamine transporter. These findings have implications for the development of medication for drug abusers. While the 'dopamine hypothesis' receives strong support from animal studies, the evidence produced thus far in human studies has not been especially supportive, and much remains to be done.

References

Berger P, Martenson R, Laing P, et al 1990 Photoaffinity labeling of the dopamine reuptake carrier protein using a novel high affinity ayidoderivative of GBR-12935. Soc Neurosci Abstr 16:13 (abstr 11.3)

Bergman J, Madras BK, Johnson SE, Spealman RD 1989 Effects of cocaine and related drugs in nonhuman primates. III. self-administration by squirrel monkeys. J Pharmacol Exp Ther 251:150–155

Boja JW, Kuhar MJ 1989 ^{3}H-Cocaine binding and inhibition of ^{3}H-dopamine uptake is similar in both rat striatum and nucleus accumbens. Eur J Pharmacol 173: 215–217

Boja JW, Carroll FI, Rahman MA, Philip A, Lewin AH, Kuhar MJ 1990 New, potent cocaine analogs: ligand binding and transport studies in rat striatum. Eur J Pharmacol 184:329–332

Calligaro DO, Eldefrawi ME 1987 Central and peripheral cocaine receptors. J Pharmacol Exp Ther 243:61–67

Carroll FI, Lewin AH, Abraham P, Parham K, Boja JW, Kuhar MJ 1991 Synthesis and ligand binding of cocaine isomers at the cocaine receptor. J Med Chem 34:883–886

Carroll FI, Lewin AH, Boja JW, Kuhar MJ 1992 Cocaine receptor: biochemical characterization and structure–activity relationships of cocaine analogs at the dopamine transporter. J Med Chem, in press

Gawin FH 1986 Neuroleptic reductions of cocaine-induced paranoia but not euphoria? Psychopharmacology 90:142–143

Gawin F, Riordan C, Kleber H 1985 Methylphenidate treatment of cocaine abusers without attention deficit disorder: a negative report. Am J Drug Alcohol Abuse 11:193–197

Gawin FH, Allen D, Humblestone B 1989 Outpatient treatment of 'crack' cocaine smoking with flupenthixol decanoate. A preliminary report. Arch Gen Psychiatry 46:322–325

Grigoriadis DE, Wilson AA, Lew R, Sharkey JS, Kuhar MJ 1989 Dopamine transport sites selectively labeled by a novel photoaffinity probe: ^{125}I-DEEP. J Neurosci 9:2664–2670

Guastella J, Nelson N, Nelson H et al 1990 Cloning and expression of a rat brain GABA transporter. Science (Wash DC) 249:1303–1306

Gunne LM, Anggard E, Jonsson LE 1972 Clinical trials with amphetamine-blocking drugs. Psychiatr Neurol Neurochir 75:225–226

Harris JE, Baldessarini RJ 1973 Uptake of [^{3}H]-catecholamines by homogenates of rat corpus striatum and cerebral cortex: effects of amphetamine analogues. Neuropharmacology 12:669–679

Horn AS 1990 Dopamine uptake: a review of progress in the last decade. Prog Neurobiol 34:387–400

Johanson C-E, Fischman MW 1989 The pharmacology of cocaine related to its abuse. Pharmacol Rev 41:3–52

Kennedy LT, Hanbauer I 1983 Sodium-sensitive cocaine binding to rat striatal membrane: possible relationship to dopamine uptake sites. J Neurochem 41:172–178

Kuhar MJ 1973 Neurotransmitter uptake: a tool in identifying neurotransmitter-specific pathways. Life Sci 13:1623–1634

Kuhar MJ, Ritz MC, Boja JW 1991 The dopamine hypothesis of the reinforcing properties of cocaine. Trends Neurosci 14:299–302

Krueger BK 1990 Kinetics and block of dopamine uptake in synaptosomes from rat caudate nucleus. J Neurochem 55:260–267

Lew R, Grigoriadis DE, Wilson A, Boja JW, Simantov R, Kuhar MJ 1991a Dopamine transporter: deglycosylation with exo- and endoglycosidases. Brain Res 539:239–246

Lew R, Vaughan R, Simantov R, Wilson A, Kuhar MJ 1991b Dopamine transporters in the nucleus accumbens and the striatum have different apparent molecular weights. Synapse 8:152–153

Madras BK, Fahey MA, Bergman J, Canfield DR, Spealman RD 1989 Effects of cocaine and related drugs in nonhuman primates. I. [^{3}H]Cocaine binding sites in caudate-putamen. J Pharmacol Exp Ther 251:131–141

Pacholczyk T, Blakely RD, Amara SG 1991 Expression cloning of a cocaine- and antidepressant-sensitive human noradrenaline transporter. Nature (Lond) 350:350–354

Reith MEA, Shershen H, Lajtha A 1980 Saturable [^{3}H]cocaine binding in central nervous system of mouse. Life Sci 27:1055–1062

Reith MEA, Meisler B, Shershen H, Lajtha A 1986 Structural requirements for cocaine congeners to interact with dopamine and serotonin uptake sites in mouse brain and to induce stereotyped behavior. Biochem Pharmacol 35:1123-1129
Ritz MC, Lamb RJ, Goldberg SR, Kuhar MJ 1987 Cocaine receptors on dopamine transporters are related to self-administration of cocaine. Science (Wash DC) 237:1219-1223
Ritz MC, Cone EJ, Kuhar MJ 1990 Cocaine inhibition of ligand binding at dopamine, norepinephrine and serotonin transporters: a structure–activity study. Life Sci 46:635-645
Sallee FR, Fogel EL, Schwartz E, Choi SM, Curran DP, Niznik HB 1989 Photoaffinity labeling of the mammalian dopamine transporters. FEBS (Fed Eur Biochem Soc) Lett 256:219-224
Schoemaker H, Pimoule C, Arbilla S, Scatton B, Javoy-Agid F, Langer SZ 1985 Sodium dependent [^{3}H]cocaine binding associated with dopamine uptake sites in the rat striatum and human putamen decrease after dopaminergic denervation and in Parkinson's disease. Naunyn-Schmiedebergs' Arch Pharmacol 329:227-235
Sherer MA, Kumor KM, Jaffe JH 1989 Effects of intravenous cocaine are partially attenuated by haloperidol. Psychiatry Res 27:117-125
Snyder SH, Coyle JT 1969 Regional differences in H^3-norepinephrine and H^3-dopamine uptake into rat brain homogenates. J Pharmacol Exp Ther 165:78-86

DISCUSSION

Balster: Our research relates very closely to what Mike Kuhar has described. We have been looking at the behavioural effects of various cocaine analogues and attempting to relate them to activities at the dopamine transporter (Balster et al 1992). We find that some of the phenyltropane analogues that he mentioned are extremely potent in inducing cocaine-like behavioural effects in rats. It now seems feasible to find analogues with up to 100-fold more potency than cocaine.

I am not quite as hopeful as Dr Kuhar that chemists won't learn to synthesize these analogues illicitly. We need to be aware that 'designer drugs' related to cocaine might become a public health issue.

Another potent analogue of cocaine is a metabolite called cocaethylene; it is the ethyl ester of cocaine that seems to be formed during the combined use of ethanol and cocaine (Hearn et al 1991). The molecule is probably *N*-demethylated and then, with the increased availability of an ethyl group from ethanol, forms the ethyl ester. We find cocaethylene to be only slightly less potent than cocaine (Woodward et al 1991); it therefore could very easily contribute to the pharmacological effects of cocaine used in combination with alcohol. This relates to what Dr Musto said earlier (p 11) about the medicated wine formulations of the turn of the century with low contents of cocaine which were in solutions containing about 15% absolute alcohol. Although the doses of cocaine in these products may have been small, there is a possibility that, in combination with the alcohol, cocaethylene may have been formed. This active metabolite may have contributed to the production of greater effects than would be predicted from the dose of cocaine alone.

Our work supports what Dr Kuhar says about a critical role for the dopamine transporter in the reinforcing and other behavioural effects of cocaine related to its use. Dopamine appears to play an essential role, but is it really the whole story? Cocaine has many other effects besides the inhibition of dopamine uptake. It will be interesting to see, in the future, whether the pharmacology of cocaine is isomorphic with that of more selective dopamine re-uptake blockers, of which several are available for study: drugs like GBR 12909, for example. Studies with these drugs will be a critical test of the hypothesis that this action at the dopamine transporter is a major part of cocaine's action.

Woolverton: We have done behavioural studies with GBR 12909 in rhesus monkeys. Monkeys readily self-administer this agent, and the discriminative stimulus effects are similar to those of cocaine. Although it is a highly potent dopamine re-uptake blocker, its potency in behavioural studies is relatively low. This is probably a pharmacokinetic issue, that GBR 12909 doesn't get into the brain very well. Nevertheless, behavioural data obtained with the compound support Dr Kuhar's statements.

Kalant: Given that cocaine also binds to sodium channels, at either their intracellular or their extracellular ends, how do you differentiate the binding sites that are related to the sodium channel and those sites that are dopamine transporter related? And what about other local anaesthetics that block sodium channels? Procaine, for example, I believe is to some extent self-administered by animal subjects?

Kuhar: Yes, some local anaesthetics, including procaine, are self-administered in monkeys, and they also block the dopamine transporter. In binding experiments, it is fairly easy to distinguish between the different cocaine binding sites; for example, by taking specific brain regions and using appropriate tissue incubation conditions, you can study binding at the dopamine transporter by comparison with other, different transporter sites. That isn't a problem.

Fibiger: I was very interested in the differences between the dopamine transporter in the nucleus accumbens and in the striatum. Could part of that difference be due to the fact that the nucleus accumbens contains a significant numbers of noradrenergic terminals, and that part of what you are measuring in the nucleus accumbens is the noradrenaline transporter on those terminals? Is it possible that you are not able to discriminate between dopamine and noradrenaline transporters on your gels?

Kuhar: I don't think so. The binding of ^{125}I-DEEP to that protein on the gel is not blocked by noradrenaline re-uptake inhibitors; it's blocked only by dopamine re-uptake inhibitors. So, from the pharmacological evidence, it appears to be a real dopamine transporter. Not only is the apparent molecular mass higher in the nucleus accumbens, it's also higher in the olfactory tubercle, which is part of the same mesolimbic pathway.

Negrete: You find a lack of correlation with changes in serotonin function.

Molecular biology of cocaine

Recently, however, I heard that serotonin *is* now considered to be a factor in cocaine's action. What is your view on this?

Kuhar: Cocaine does act at serotonin transporters, but the action there has been related not to the reinforcing properties of the drug, but to other effects. Some have related it to the seizure-producing effects of cocaine and its compounds. There is also older evidence that cocaine inhibition at serotonin transporters opposes the reinforcing properties of cocaine.

Woolverton: In fact, lesions of serotonergic systems in the brain, which deplete serotonin, can enhance the reinforcing effects of cocaine (Loh & Roberts 1990). This finding supports the idea that the serotonin-related component of cocaine's action may exert a negative influence on its self-administration.

Kleber: We know that cocaine affects the dopamine, serotonin and noradrenaline systems, and that drugs which affect only one of those systems are not nearly as reinforcing as cocaine. Thus pure dopamine agonists do not tend to be as reinforcing. So it is possible that even though serotonin itself, or noradrenaline, does not produce euphoria, there may be an interaction between these actions of cocaine and the dopaminergic effects, to achieve the great reinforcing actions of cocaine. This then may be another fruitful area for inquiry in relation to treatment, to do something that affects the serotonin or noradrenergic systems which may then affect the overall reinforcing effect.

Kuhar: When we first considered that interactions might be important we talked to several statisticians about our data. Analysis of the data suggested that there didn't appear to be any interaction. So far, there is no reason to believe that an interaction between different cocaine binding sites is important for reinforcement, but one can't completely rule it out.

Benowitz: Considering human intoxication with cocaine, where there is massive systemic release of catecholamines and hypertension, is there some direct catecholamine-releasing effect of cocaine that occurs as a consequence of blocking of the dopamine transporter, or by some other mechanism? Does systemic and peripheral blockade of noradrenaline uptake add to the systemic toxicity of cocaine?

Kuhar: I think there must be a systemic blockade of noradrenaline uptake which probably has a lot to do with the cardiovascular effects. Is cocaine a catecholamine releaser? Some evidence has been published suggesting that it is, but the current view of others is that cocaine is nowhere near as effective as amphetamine as a releaser. Amphetamine is an uptake blocker and a releaser, whereas cocaine is an uptake blocker but not a releaser, or at least not a very good releaser.

Benowitz: So what is the explanation for the sometimes massively elevated systemic catecholamine concentrations seen in intoxicated cocaine users? Is that all via blocking of dopamine re-uptake?

Kuhar: No. It could be due to inhibition of the inactivation of noradrenaline from sympathetic nerve terminals, at least in part. I don't know if that could account for the entire effect.

Benowitz: You can give people other catecholamine uptake blockers and you don't see tremendously elevated systemic catecholamine levels, so it seems there must be some release mechanism as well.

Kuhar: It's possible that cocaine is more of a releaser at sympathetic nerve terminals for noradrenaline than at central synapses for dopamine. But I don't know of any study where this is compared.

Fibiger: It is worth remembering that anatomically, dopaminergic perikarya are innervated both by serotonergic and by cholinergic neurons, and therefore it's quite conceivable that cocaine's ultimate actions will be influenced by both serotonergic and cholinergic tone in the brain. Such interactions could easily occur, despite the fact that cocaine probably doesn't affect cholinergic systems directly.

Balster: Most of the attention in studies of the neural and behavioural basis of cocaine abuse have focused on postsynaptic changes that might account for some of the psychiatric sequelae, or various other phenomena such as tolerance and dependence. With your knowledge of transporters in general, Dr Kuhar, how amenable do you think these molecules are to up- and down-regulation and other changes that would occur as a consequence of repeated cocaine abuse—changes that could account for the behavioural and neuropsychiatric sequelae?

Kuhar: The classical neurotransmitter receptor will up- and down-regulate (i.e. increase and decrease in number), depending on whether agonists or antagonists are present chronically. Experiments with the dopamine transporter and chronic cocaine administration have been disappointing, in the sense that the transporter does not appear to up- and down-regulate. One study (Wiener et al 1989) says that the monoamine oxidase (MAO) inhibitor, deprenyl, up-regulates the dopamine transporter after chronic administration. But up- and down-regulation of the transporter are not easy to demonstrate. What is impressive is the up-regulation and down-regulation of postsynaptic dopamine receptors after you block the transporter. Giving cocaine chronically has a powerful effect on the neuronal circuitry, because it does affect the dopamine receptors; they change markedly.

Kleber: Didn't Dr Nora Volkow find that on positron emission tomography (PET) scanning, changes in dopamine receptors persisted for 3–6 months?

O'Brien: No; her study showed that in the first week after cessation of cocaine, the uptake of N-methyl spiperone by dopamine receptors is suppressed, but one is not sure what that means. Then at one month and at three months, the uptake appeared normal (Volkow et al 1990).

Woolverton: We have also found down-regulation of CNS dopamine receptors and the dopamine transporter in rats (Kleven et al 1990) and monkeys (Farfel et al 1990), primarily of D_1 dopamine receptors, two weeks after the last injection of cocaine.

Fibiger: Even though chronic treatment with cocaine may not directly affect the dopamine transporter, it's also now evident from microdialysis studies in rats that chronically administered cocaine enhances the ability of subsequent injections of cocaine to increase extracellular concentrations of dopamine. So, while data from the binding studies may not reflect it, in the living brain long-term cocaine administration clearly has lasting effects on some dopaminergic systems.

Edwards: Let me put a broader question. We come from different disciplines, but will probably all stand in awe of the elegance of Dr Kuhar's work. The question I want to put at this point is not to be interpreted as destructive. I should like to know why the US government funds these basic researchers. I know why they fund epidemiologists, because policy makers need these data. They fund treatment research because everyone wants ill people to be made better. Are they funding this basic work because the researchers have persuaded the funding agencies that its elegance and its beauty is like music, and American society should have beautiful scientific music, or is it because of a belief in the near or distant practical utility of what is being discovered?

Kleber: I will give you two answers to that. One relates to John Enders, who learned to grow virus in monkey tissue, and from that came the polio vaccine. If you don't fund Enders, you don't get Salk, Sabin and all of this. So, by investing in the basic science, somewhere down the line you achieve some applied results. The other example, that keeps us all hoping, is the development of methadone maintenance for the treatment of heroin dependence. Here you have a pharmacological treatment which, combined with appropriate counselling and so on, can ameliorate (not cure) the psychosocial pathology that goes along with the condition of opiate addiction. These two examples keep me telling the US government that we must continue funding people to do not just Dr Kuhar's type of work, but also Dr Anthony's epidemiological work. We clearly need both.

Jaffe: I agree with Dr Kleber. There is also the need to feel that we have left no stone unturned, even if we have few expectations initially of what we shall find under the stone.

Perhaps something *will* turn up. There is inevitably a political aspect: the policy makers want to be seen as supportive of basic research. A Sabin vaccine or a penicillin could come up even when it is unexpected. If you had sufficient resources and were never called on to make exceedingly difficult choices, you could fund things that seem very far afield. In the US we have been blessed with the kind of support that allows drug abuse research to go in a wide variety of directions, including into areas that are very basic but do not seem likely to contribute to the social solution in the near term. The basic work being done now on cocaine may not yield any practical applications until this epidemic has run its course. But there will, no doubt, be other drug problems, and something coming from the present work may well prove useful then.

Jones: I personally think we should support Dr Kuhar and others doing similar elegant science that may some day help us understand how the brain works.

But methadone substitution for other opiates may not be the best example of something with which to justify the value of basic research. It did not come out of basic science research. Methadone maintenance was the idea of a clinician who probably had the wrong model in mind, but it turned out to be useful. Nevertheless, methadone was an opiate analgesic drug that was taken off the shelf, because its pharmacokinetics offered a useful profile, not because it was any less addicting than heroin.

Jaffe: But how did such drugs get *on* the shelf in the first place? The researchers were working on the wrong model; they were trying to solve the problem of heroin addiction by finding a non-addictive analgesic. It is clear now that such an analgesic couldn't have an impact on the people who were currently manufacturing and distributing heroin. It was the wrong model, but the search for a non-addictive analgesic turned up a wide variety of interesting pharmacological agents, including naloxone and naltrexone, and pointed clearly to the existence of distinct receptors. It was the development of naloxone that made possible the discovery of the opiate receptors. The decision to fund basic research 20 years ago, when I was formulating policy under Richard Nixon, although it couldn't have a major impact on the heroin epidemic of that time, resulted in the tools being available for others to discover opiate receptors, and the endogenous opiate ligands—major developments in neuroscience.

Jones: I agree, but so far the problem is that understanding the opiate receptor, although elegant science, has not done very much for the problems of opiate addicts!

Jaffe: I didn't intend to imply that the discovery of the opiate receptor has done anything for the opiate addiction problem thus far, but recent work suggesting that naltrexone may be useful in alcoholism indicates that it may be many years before we accurately gauge the value of investments in basic research.

References

Balster RL, Carroll FI, Graham JH et al 1992 Potent substituted-3β-phenyltropane analogs of cocaine have cocaine-like discriminative stimulus effects. Drug Alcohol Depend, in press

Farfel GM, Kleven MS, Perry BD, Woolverton WL, Seiden LS 1990 Effects of repeated cocaine injections on D1 and D2 binding sites and dopamine reuptake sites in rhesus monkey caudate. Soc Neurosci Abstr 16:13

Hearn WL, Flynn DD, Hime GW et al 1991 Cocaethylene: a unique cocaine metabolite displays high affinity for the dopamine transporter. J Neurochem 56:698–701

Kleven MS, Perry BD, Woolverton WL, Seiden LS 1990 Effects of repeated injections of cocaine on D1 and D2 dopamine receptors in rat brain. Brain Res 532:265–270

Loh EA, Roberts DCS 1990 Break points on a progressive ratio schedule reinforced by intravenous cocaine increase following depletion of forebrain serotonin. Psychopharmacology 101:262–266

Volkow ND, Fowler JS, Wolf AP et al 1990 Effects of chronic cocaine abuse on postsynaptic dopamine receptors. Am J Psychiatry 147:719–724

Wiener HL, Hashim A, Lajtha A, Sershen H 1989 Chronic L-deprenyl-induced up-regulation of the dopamine uptake carrier. Eur J Pharmacol 163:191–194

Woodward JJ, Mansbach RS, Carroll FI, Balster RL 1991 Cocaethylene inhibits dopamine uptake and produces cocaine-like actions in drug discrimination studies. Eur J Pharmacol 197:235–236

The neurobiology of cocaine-induced reinforcement

H. C. Fibiger*, A. G. Phillips** and E. E. Brown*

*Division of Neurological Sciences, Department of Psychiatry and **Department of Psychology, University of British Columbia, Vancouver, BC, Canada, V6T 1Z3

Abstract. Cocaine has potent pharmacological actions on a number of monoaminergic systems in the brain, including those that use noradrenaline, dopamine and serotonin as neurotransmitters. There is growing evidence that cocaine's effects on dopaminergic neurons, particularly those that make up the mesolimbic system, are closely associated with its rewarding properties. For example, low doses of dopamine receptor antagonists reliably influence cocaine self-administration, whereas noradrenaline and serotonin receptor antagonists are without consistent effects. Similarly, selective lesions of dopaminergic terminals in the nucleus accumbens, a major target of the mesolimbic dopamine projection, disrupt cocaine self-administration in a manner that is consistent with loss of cocaine-induced reward. The introduction of *in vivo* brain microdialysis as a tool with which to investigate the neurochemical correlates of motivated behaviour has provided new opportunities for investigating the role of dopamine in the nucleus accumbens in the acquisition and maintenance of cocaine self-administration. Although the body of literature that has been generated by this approach appears to contain some important inconsistencies, these probably reflect the use of inappropriate microdialysis conditions by some investigators. A critical review of the literature suggests that microdialysis results are generally consistent with a role for mesolimbic dopamine in cocaine-induced reward, although it does not seem to be the case that animals will work to maintain consistent increases in extracellular concentrations of dopamine in the nucleus accumbens in all experimental conditions. Elucidation of the complete neural circuitry of cocaine-induced reward remains an important priority for future research.

1992 Cocaine: scientific and social dimensions. Wiley, Chichester (Ciba Foundation Symposium 166) p 96–124

The intravenous self-administration procedure developed by Weeks (1962) has been used widely to study the rewarding properties of a variety of psychoactive drugs. When used in combination with brain lesions or pharmacological probes, this approach has generated considerable knowledge about the neuroanatomical and neurochemical substrates that mediate cocaine's ability to function as a positive reinforcer. One strategy that has been employed widely to identify the neurochemical mechanisms by which cocaine may produce its rewarding effects is to examine the effect of selective neurotransmitter receptor antagonists on responding for intravenous cocaine. This approach has generated widespread consensus that dopaminergic, but not noradrenergic, mechanisms mediate the ability of cocaine to sustain high rates of bar-pressing for intravenous infusions. For example, many investigators have demonstrated that low doses of a variety of dopamine receptor antagonists, including pimozide, haloperidol, sulpiride, α-flupenthixol, chlorpromazine and SCH 23390 increase the rate of responding for intravenous cocaine (De Wit & Wise 1977, Ettenberg et al 1982, Roberts & Vickers 1984, Koob et al 1987). One interpretation of these results is that low doses of dopamine receptor antagonists produce a partial receptor blockade so that higher doses of cocaine are required to maintain the preferred level of occupancy of postsynaptic receptors by dopamine. In contrast, neither α-adrenergic nor β-adrenergic receptor antagonists have been demonstrated to alter cocaine self-administration (Wilson & Schuster 1974, De Wit & Wise 1977, Woolverton 1987).

There are other interpretations for the robust ability of low doses of neuroleptics to increase rates of responding for intravenous cocaine. One that has been favoured by some investigators is that dopamine receptor antagonists may enhance cocaine self-administration by antagonizing the rate-reducing effects of this drug on operant responding without changing its rewarding effects. According to this interpretation, the reason that low doses of neuroleptics increase the rate of responding for cocaine is that this psychomotor stimulant produces competing responses in the animal that are incompatible with higher rates of self-administration. Neuroleptics selectively block these competing responses and thereby enable the animal to work for cocaine at higher rates of responding. There is considerable evidence for this interpretation and in a recent comprehensive review Johanson & Fischman (1989) favoured the view that dopamine receptor antagonists 'exert their effect by antagonizing effects of cocaine unrelated to its reinforcement.' However, more recent data continue to argue for a reward-related interpretation of the effects of neuroleptics on intravenous cocaine self-administration. For example, Roberts et al (1989) used a progressive ratio schedule of reinforcement to study the effects of the neuroleptic drug haloperidol on intravenous cocaine self-administration in rats. In this procedure, the first operant response each day produced a drug infusion, after which the requirements of the schedule increased with each subsequent reinforcement until the operant behaviour extinguished. It was found that a relatively low dose of haloperidol (0.05 mg/kg), which had previously been shown to produce an increase in responding for cocaine on a continuous reinforcement (CRF) schedule (Roberts & Vickers 1984), substantially reduced the final ratio completed; that is to say, haloperidol significantly decreased the breaking point (defined as the final schedule of reinforcement that was completed) maintained by intravenous cocaine (Fig. 1). These findings are not easily accommodated by simple rate-reduction antagonism hypotheses but are

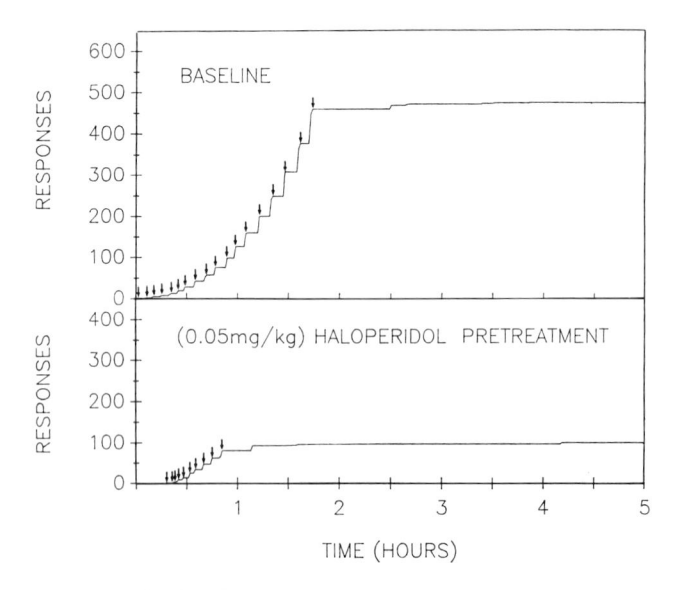

FIG. 1. Event record of a five-hour cocaine self-administration session for a rat responding under a progressive ratio schedule of reinforcement. The effect of haloperidol pretreatment (0.05 mg/kg, 60 min prior to the session) on responding is shown in the bottom portion of the figure. *Vertical increments* represent level responses. *Arrows* indicate the time of the cocaine injections. (From Roberts 1991, with permission.)

quite consistent with formulations suggesting that neuroleptics block or attenuate the rewarding effects of cocaine. In summary, it would seem prudent not to adopt an 'either/or' position with respect to the mechanisms by which dopamine receptor antagonists influence the self-administration of cocaine. There is evidence to indicate that dopamine receptor antagonists can, depending on the experimental conditions, influence the rate of cocaine self-administration by blocking its rewarding effects, by blocking its rate-reducing effects, or by some combination of these. Additional research is required to determine the precise circumstances under which either mechanism predominates.

Lesion studies have been particularly useful in identifying the anatomical and chemical substrates of cocaine-induced reward. In the first of such studies, we trained rats to self-administer cocaine intravenously (Roberts et al 1977). After stable rates of responding had been obtained, the animals received bilateral 6-hydroxydopamine (6-OHDA) lesions of the nucleus accumbens, which produced large and selective decreases in the concentration of dopamine within this forebrain nucleus. In animals with extensive reductions in dopamine in the nucleus accumbens there was a substantial decrease in the rate of lever pressing for intravenous cocaine. Similar lesions of the major ascending noradrenergic projections to the telencephalon were without effect. In a similar study, Lyness et al (1979) found that 6-OHDA lesions of the nucleus accumbens also greatly reduced rates of responding for intravenous injections of d-amphetamine.

Subsequently, we analysed the pattern of cocaine self-administration after 6-OHDA lesions of the nucleus accumbens (Roberts et al 1980). On the first day that cocaine was made available after the 6-OHDA lesions, some animals responded rapidly during the early part of the three-hour session. The rate of responding then decreased gradually within the first session until there was little or no responding by the end of the three hours. Similar patterns were obtained on the following days; however, the number of responses in the first part of the session was reduced and responding ceased earlier in the session. The high rate of responding for intravenous cocaine early in the first post-lesion session indicated that the subsequent reduction in cocaine self-administration was not due to lesion-induced performance deficits. Perhaps more importantly, the pattern of cocaine self-administration after the 6-OHDA lesions resembled an extinction effect, characterized by high rates of responding when the reinforcer is first removed, followed by a gradual attenuation in the rate of responding as the animals learn that the operant response no longer results in the delivery of a reward. These findings argue strongly that extensive lesions of the dopaminergic innervation of the nucleus accumbens produced by 6-OHDA result in an attenuation or blockade of the rewarding effects of intravenous cocaine.

Using a more sophisticated behavioural paradigm, Dworkin & Smith (1988) have provided further evidence that 6-OHDA lesions of the nucleus accumbens specifically decrease the rewarding effects of intravenous cocaine. They trained rats to respond for cocaine, food and water on a concurrent chained fixed-ratio schedule of reinforcement. After acquisition, 6-OHDA lesions of the nucleus accumbens did not alter responding for food or water, but flattened the dose–effect curve for cocaine self-administration. These results were interpreted to indicate that the lesions specifically attenuated the rewarding effects of cocaine. Koob and co-workers (1987) have used a progressive ratio procedure to examine the effects of 6-OHDA lesions of the nucleus accumbens on cocaine self-administration. They found that such lesions significantly decreased the highest ratio for which rats would respond to obtain cocaine. The anatomical specificity of this effect was demonstrated by the failure of similar lesions of the dorsal striatum to influence responding.

In interpreting these results it is important to emphasize that changes in the breaking point are not necessarily accompanied by alterations in the rate of responding for a drug on simple schedules of reinforcement. Thus, while we failed to note changes in the rate of responding for apomorphine after 6-OHDA lesions of the nucleus accumbens (Roberts et al 1977), in a subsequent study Roberts et al (1989) found that these same lesions produced substantial increases in the breaking point maintained by intravenous apomorphine. The data obtained using the progressive ratio schedule are what might be expected if such lesions resulted in denervation-induced supersensitivity of postsynaptic dopamine receptors. The latter findings serve to emphasize that significant motivational influences on drug intake may be missed if the rate of drug self-administration is used as the only dependent variable.

Although these lesion studies are highly consistent with the hypothesis that dopaminergic mechanisms in the nucleus accumbens mediate at least some of the rewarding properties of intravenous cocaine, other observations indicate that this is only part of the story. For example, Roberts & Koob (1982) found that while 6-OHDA lesions of the ventral tegmental area (VTA), the origin of the meso-accumbens dopamine projection, produced substantial decreases in the rate of lever pressing for intravenous cocaine, the correlation between dopamine depletion in the nucleus accumbens and the degree of change in cocaine intake was not significant. Indeed, several rats that had substantial depletions in accumbens dopamine showed near normal rates of responding for cocaine. The authors speculated that dopaminergic projections from the VTA to other structures, or a combination of structures, may mediate the rewarding properties of intravenous cocaine. In this regard, it is interesting that Goeders & Smith (1983) find that rats self-administer cocaine directly into the medial prefrontal cortex, but not into either the nucleus accumbens or VTA. In an attempt to examine the extent to which the rewarding properties of systemically administered cocaine are mediated by dopaminergic terminals in the medial prefrontal cortex, we investigated the effects of 6-OHDA lesions in this structure on the rate and pattern of intravenous cocaine self-administration (Martin-Iverson et al 1986). Despite producing substantial depletions of dopamine in the medial prefrontal cortex, the 6-OHDA lesions did not affect either the rate or pattern of intravenous cocaine self-administration. These data indicate that although rats may respond for infusions of cocaine directly into the medial prefrontal cortex, dopamine terminals in this structure do not appear to contribute significantly to the rewarding action of intravenously administered cocaine. Leccese and Lyness (1987) have confirmed this in rats self-administering d-amphetamine. Specifically, they found that 6-OHDA lesions of the medial prefrontal cortex failed to alter either the acquisition or maintenance of intravenous self-administration of d-amphetamine. However, bearing in mind the limitations associated with simple rate measures of cocaine self-administration (see above), it would be worthwhile to reinvestigate the role of the medial prefrontal cortex using other approaches such as the progressive ratio procedure.

The advent of *in vivo* microdialysis has dramatically increased current understanding of the neurochemical actions of cocaine. However, the microdialysis technique is not without limitations, one being that it does not directly measure neurotransmitter release. Rather, microdialysis samples from the brain's interstitial space, and the neurotransmitters present in the interstitial fluid do not necessarily reflect synaptic release. For example, a portion of the dopamine present in dialysate shortly after the implantation of a dialysis probe is due to tissue damage, and is not under classical neuronal control (Westerink

& De Vries 1988, Santiago & Westerink 1990). This confounding factor clearly limits the value of experiments conducted shortly after the implantation of the probe. An additional shortcoming of many dialysis studies is that they are conducted in anaesthetized rats. Anaesthesia can profoundly alter brain chemistry (Bertorelli et al 1990, Osborne et al 1990, Damsma & Fibiger 1991), and it is not surprising, therefore, that data obtained by *in vivo* microdialysis are affected by anaesthesia (Stahle et al 1990, Opacka-Juffry et al 1991). Despite these potential methodological problems, microdialysis has proven to be invaluable in the study of the neurochemistry of cocaine, particularly as it relates to the rewarding properties of this psychomotor stimulant.

The ability of cocaine to increase interstitial concentrations of dopamine in the rat striatum has been well documented (Church et al 1987, Di Chiara & Imperato 1988, Hurd & Ungerstedt 1989). Moreover, a linear relationship between extracellular cocaine and dopamine concentrations in the rat striatum has been demonstrated after peripheral administration of the drug (Hurd et al 1988, Nicolaysen et al 1988). These studies suggest that the short-lived behavioural and neurochemical effects of cocaine are a direct function of the rapid pharmacokinetics of this drug.

As shown in Fig. 2, the local application of cocaine through the dialysis probe into the striatum can also produce dose-dependent increases in interstitial dopamine (Hurd & Ungerstedt 1989, Nomikos et al 1990). Nomikos et al (1990)

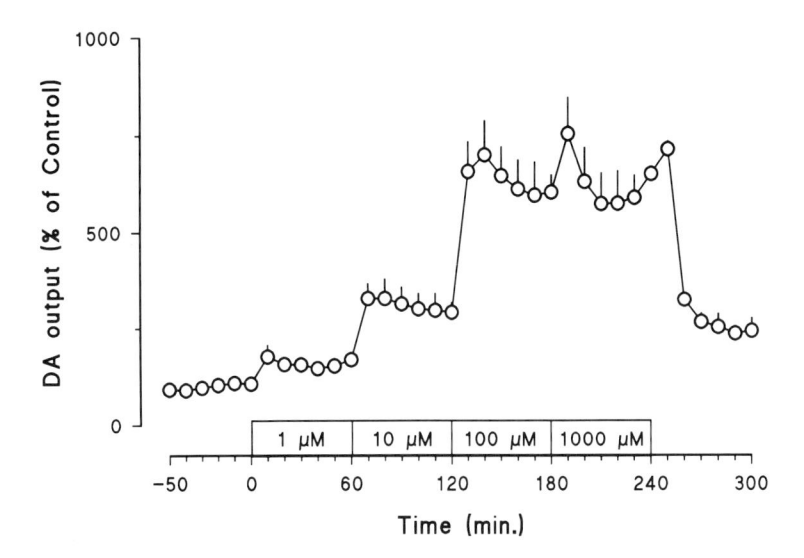

FIG. 2. Effect of local application of 1, 10, 100 and 1000 μM cocaine on extracellular striatal dopamine concentrations. Values represent the group mean $(n=4) \pm $ SEM. Percentage values of dialysate concentrations are based on an average of six samples before the initiation of cocaine application. (Adapted from Nomikos et al 1990.)

further characterized this cocaine-induced increase by demonstrating that it is almost totally action potential dependent, indicating that cocaine affects dopamine *in vivo* by inhibiting uptake, not by inducing amphetamine-like release. In addition to its action at dopaminergic terminals, cocaine increases extracellular dopamine in the VTA (Bradberry & Roth 1989). This finding may account for the ability of cocaine to decrease the firing of VTA dopaminergic neurons (Einhorn et al 1988, Lacey et al 1990), as an increase in dopamine in the VTA would result in greater activation of somatodendritic autoreceptors.

Given the importance of the nucleus accumbens in the reinforcing properties of cocaine, its actions within this limbic structure have been the focus of much research (Di Chiara & Imperato 1988, Bradberry & Roth 1989, Moghaddam & Bunney 1989, Pettit & Justice 1989, Brown et al 1991). Di Chiara and Imperato (1988) have suggested that drugs of abuse, including cocaine, preferentially increase extracellular concentrations of dopamine in the mesolimbic system. This study did not, however, examine the effect of cocaine on dopamine in the medial prefrontal cortex, an area that has also been implicated in the rewarding properties of cocaine (Goeders & Smith 1983). In this regard, Moghaddam and Bunney (1989) found that a moderate dose of cocaine (1 mg/kg, i.v.) produced a selective increase in interstitial dopamine concentrations in the nucleus accumbens, while no change in dopamine in the medial prefrontal cortex was observed. Larger doses of cocaine (2 mg/kg, i.v.) did increase interstitial dopamine in the medial prefrontal cortex, but to a lesser degree than the increase observed in the nucleus accumbens. Interestingly, these authors reported that *d*-amphetamine (1 mg/kg, i.v.) produced similar increases in the nucleus accumbens and the medial prefrontal cortex. These microdialysis data provide indirect support for the self-administration results of Martin-Iverson et al (1986) which indicated that 6-OHDA lesions of the medial prefrontal cortex did not alter the intravenous self-administration of cocaine. There is evidence that behaviourally equivalent doses of amphetamine and cocaine produce comparable increases in extracellular dopamine in the medial prefrontal cortex (Maisonneuve et al 1990). This study illustrates that large doses of cocaine can increase dopamine concentrations in the medial prefrontal cortex, but does not indicate how these doses would affect dopamine in the nucleus accumbens. It should be noted that both of the aforementioned studies were conducted in acutely implanted preparations, in which the dopamine collected in the dialysate reflects both neuronal activity and neuronal damage. Given this shortcoming, a study conducted using a dialysis preparation with tetrodotoxin (TTX)-sensitive and Ca^{2+}-dependent dialysate dopamine, examining the effects of various doses of cocaine in both of these areas, would be of great value.

Chronic administration of cocaine produces behavioural sensitization to the locomotor stimulant effects of this drug (see Post & Contel 1983 for review). Recent dialysis studies have shown that this sensitization is accompanied by an enhanced increase in interstitial dopamine concentrations produced by cocaine

(Akimoto et al 1989, Kalivas & Duffy 1990, Pettit et al 1990). Pettit et al (1990) found that the increase in extracellular dopamine is accompanied by an increase in the concentration of extracellular cocaine, suggesting that pharmacokinetic changes play an important factor in the enhanced effects of cocaine. However, they also note that the increase in extracellular cocaine cannot fully account for the enhanced dopaminergic response. From these findings it appears that the neurochemical changes associated with cocaine sensitization are both metabolic and neuronal.

The sensitization studies discussed above examined the effect of a cocaine challenge on interstitial dopamine concentrations in animals that had previously received repeated injections of cocaine. An additional aspect of cocaine sensitization involves the classical conditioning of cocaine's unconditioned neurochemical effects with specific environmental stimuli (Tatum & Seevers 1929, Barr et al 1983, Stewart et al 1984). Stewart et al (1984) have proposed that the conditioned stimuli associated with stimulants such as cocaine produce neural states that resemble those produced by the drugs themselves. Given the importance of dopaminergic transmission in the nucleus accumbens in the unconditioned effects of cocaine, *in vivo* microdialysis experiments have recently been conducted in this laboratory to assess the ability of environmental stimuli specifically paired with cocaine to affect interstitial concentrations of dopamine in this nucleus. Although the acute administration of cocaine (10 mg/kg, i.p.) produced a dramatic increase in dopamine in the nucleus accumbens, exposure of the conditioned rats to the environment in which they had previously received cocaine did not produce an increase in dopamine that was significantly different from the pseudoconditioned controls (Fig. 3). The absence of a conditioned neurochemical event is contrasted by the significant increase in locomotion in rats that received cocaine under the same schedule of conditioning (Fig. 4). These data do not support the hypothesis that conditioned stimuli associated with cocaine arouse similar neural states as the drug itself. However, it should be remembered that absence of evidence cannot be equated with evidence of absence, and it is possible that microdialysis is not sufficiently sensitive to detect the neurochemical changes associated with environmentally specific cocaine-conditioning. This limitation aside, these data are in agreement with a previous neurochemical study of cocaine that failed to find a difference in tissue dopamine turnover between conditioned and pseudoconditioned subjects upon presentation of the conditioned environment (Barr et al 1983). Moreover, several investigators have reported that while dopamine receptor antagonists block both the acute unconditioned behavioural effects of cocaine and the development of environment-specific conditioning, they do not attenuate the conditioned locomotor effects of cocaine and other psychomotor stimulants (Beninger & Hanh 1983, Beninger & Hertz 1986, Weiss et al 1989). Taken together, these data suggest that although the development of cocaine-induced environment-specific conditioning is dopamine

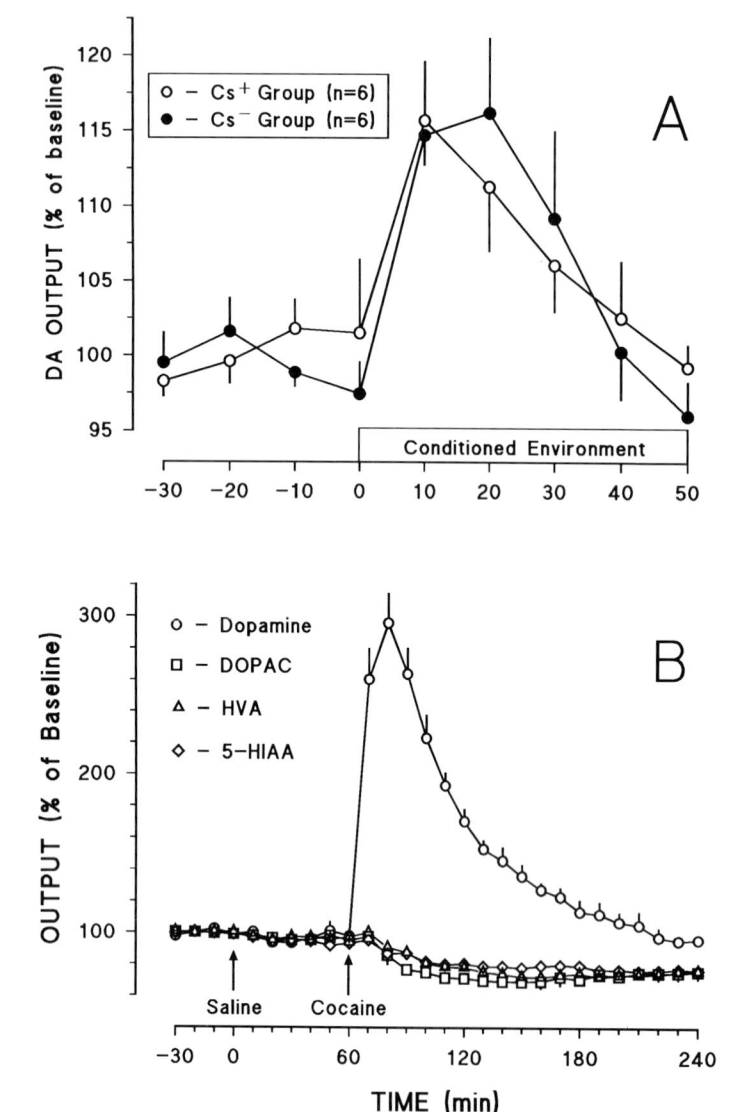

FIG. 3. A. Interstitial concentrations of dopamine in the nucleus accumbens as measured by *in vivo* brain microdialysis, before and during exposure to an environment paired with cocaine (Cs$^+$ group, $n=6$) or saline (Cs$^-$ group, $n=6$). Values represent group means ± SEM. Testing was conducted 48 h after the last conditioning session. During the training portion of the experiment, conditioned subjects (Cs$^+$ group) received cocaine (10 mg/kg, i.p.) immediately before being placed into the distinct environment for 30 min; 4.5 h after the cocaine injection, subjects were injected with saline and returned to their home cages. This procedure was repeated for 10 days. Pseudoconditioned subjects (Cs$^-$ group) were treated in a similar manner; however, they received saline before being

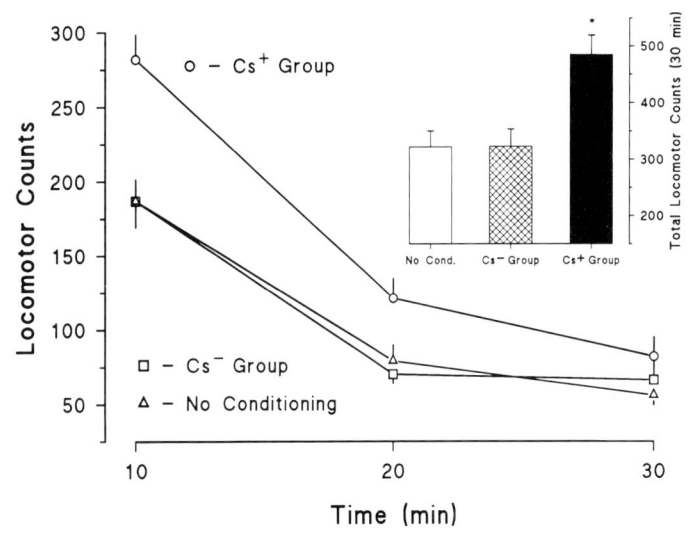

FIG. 4. Locomotor activity counts of conditioned (Cs$^+$ group, $n = 10$), pseudoconditioned (Cs$^-$ group, $n = 10$) and control (No Conditioning, $n = 10$) rats. Values represent groups means ± SEM. Testing was conducted 48 h after the last conditioning sessions. *Inset*: Total activity counts for the conditioned, pseudoconditioned and control subjects over the 30 min test session. During the training portion of the experiment, conditioned subjects received cocaine (10 mg/kg, i.p.) immediately before being placed into the locomotor apparatus for 30 min. Four hours after being removed from the locomotor apparatus these rats were injected with saline and returned to their home cages. This procedure was repeated for 10 days. Pseudoconditioned subjects were treated in a similar manner except that they received saline before being placed in the locomotor box and cocaine before being returned to their home cage. Control subjects received the same manipulations, except they received only saline injections throughout the training period.

dependent, the neurochemical events associated with the expression of the conditioned response are not.

Given the extensive use of the self-administration paradigm to assess the rewarding properties of cocaine, an examination of interstitial dopamine levels during the self-administration of cocaine is of obvious interest. Hurd et al (1989) reported that cocaine self-administration produces an increase in extracellular dopamine in rats that were naive to the paradigm; however, rats that had self-administered for nine to ten days before the dialysis experiment exhibited no increase in dopamine during the self-administration session, even though they responded for large amounts of cocaine. These surprising results are in direct

---

placed in the distinct environment and cocaine before being returned to their home cages. B. The effect of the acute administration of saline (1 ml/kg) and cocaine (10 mg/kg, i.p.) on microdialysis output of dopamine in the nucleus accumbens ($n = 4$). Values represent the group mean ($n = 4$) ± SEM. Percentage values of dialysate concentrations were based on an average of three samples before the injection of saline.

opposition to two studies by Pettit and Justice (1989, 1991) in which animals that had previous experience of self-administering cocaine exhibited robust increases in interstitial dopamine during self-administration. Moreover, the aforementioned sensitization studies provide evidence for an increased response to cocaine following previous exposure. One possible explanation for this discrepancy is that Hurd et al (1989) sampled from the posterior accumbens while Pettit and Justice (1989, 1991) implanted their probes within the anterior accumbens. However, it seems more likely that differences in the dialysis procedure account for these conflicting results. When implanted acutely, the type of probe (CMA/10) used by Hurd et al (1989) results in dialysate dopamine reported to be only 45% TTX-sensitive (Santiago & Westerink 1990), suggesting that neuronal damage accounts for a large portion of the recovered dopamine. As the type of probe used by Pettit and Justice has a smaller diameter than the CMA/10 it might produce less tissue damage and provide a dopamine signal that is more physiological in origin. In their initial study, Pettit and Justice (1989) presented data which suggest that animals titrate, or adjust, their responding to maintain a specific elevated level of dopamine within the nucleus accumbens. Although individual rats appeared to maintain different dopamine concentrations, the level that each animal maintained appeared to be stable.

A subsequent study examined the effect of dose manipulation on self-administration behaviour and interstitial dopamine concentrations in the nucleus accumbens (Pettit & Justice 1991). As the dose of cocaine was increased, the

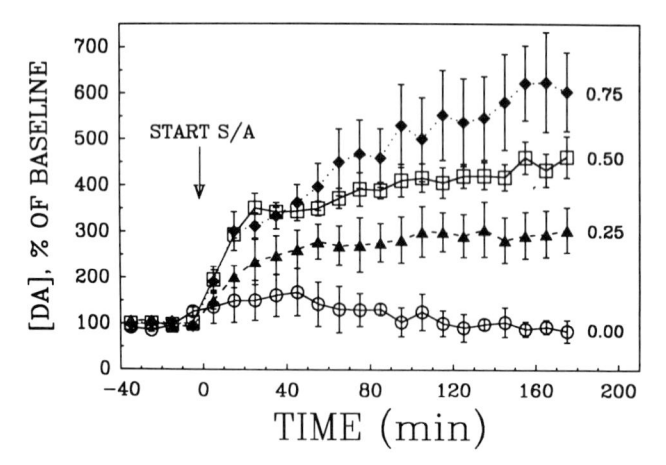

FIG. 5. The extracellular concentrations of dopamine in the nucleus accumbens during the self-administration of 0.25, 0.50 and 0.75 mg/infusion doses of cocaine ($n=6$). The dopamine concentration in the nucleus accumbens was increased and maintained at higher levels as the dose of cocaine was increased in the self-administration paradigm. Open circles represent the dopamine concentrations that were observed during extinction conditions in a subset of animals ($n=3$). The arrow depicts the beginning of the self-administration (S/A) period. Vertical bars represent the SEM. (From Pettit & Justice 1991, with permission.)

rate of responding for the drug decreased; however, the decrease in responding did not fully compensate for the increase in dose. That is, as the dose of cocaine was increased the total amount of cocaine consumed increased. As a result, the interstitial concentrations of dopamine in the nucleus accumbens were maintained at higher levels during the administration of the higher doses of cocaine (Fig. 5). This finding suggests that animals do not titrate the amount of cocaine they self-administer to maintain a specific elevated level of dopamine in the nucleus accumbens. Moreover, it argues against a simple relationship between extracellular dopamine concentrations in the nucleus accumbens and reward. Although the reasons for this disparity are unclear, an additional factor that may influence the self-administration of cocaine relates to its ability to affect serotonin (Richelson & Pfenning 1984, Ritz et al 1987). Selective lesions of serotonergic neurons in the medial forebrain bundle or in the amygdala increase the breaking point for cocaine on a progressive ratio schedule (Loh & Roberts 1990), suggesting that depletions of forebrain serotonin increase the incentive value of cocaine. Furthermore, the administration of fluoxetine, a specific serotonin re-uptake inhibitor, decreased the breaking points reached in rats on a progressive ratio schedule for intravenous cocaine. The actions of cocaine on serotonin may, therefore, influence the self-administration of this compound. At present, there are no published reports using microdialysis to assess potential actions of cocaine on serotonin. Clearly, microdialysis studies of transmitters other than dopamine will be important for a more comprehensive understanding of the *in vivo* actions of cocaine. An additional factor that should be recognized is that the doses of cocaine used by Pettit and Justice (1991) are on the descending portion of the dose–response curve, where non-reward-related aspects of cocaine become evident (Woods et al 1987, Johanson & Fischman 1989). It may be overambitious to attempt to correlate neurochemistry with behaviour (the rate of responding in this case), when the factors influencing the behaviour are poorly understood. Given that the rate of responding for intravenous infusions is a product of both the reward- and non-reward-related actions of cocaine over the range of doses examined by Pettit and Justice (1991), the neurochemical results may simply reflect this complex interaction.

Concluding remarks

The evidence reviewed here indicates that there are dopaminergic components in the neural circuitries that mediate the motoric and hedonic properties of cocaine. While the nucleus accumbens appears to play an important role in mediating its reinforcing effects, there are data which indicate that animals do not work for cocaine to produce fixed increases in extracellular dopamine concentrations in this structure and that dopaminergic mechanisms in other brain regions may also be involved. An important task for future research will be to identify the complete neural circuitry of cocaine-induced reward. Efforts in this direction have already been initiated by Koob and co-workers, who have examined the role of the efferent projections of the accumbens to the ventral pallidum in cocaine self-administration (Hubner & Koob 1990). Because this projection is in part GABAergic, microdialysis studies of the ventral pallidum during cocaine self-administration would be of considerable interest. Finally, there is recent evidence that cocaine can activate the expression of the protooncogene c-*fos* in subpopulations of neurons in certain brain regions (Young et al 1991). *Fos* immunocytochemical detection, used in combination either with retrograde tracing techniques (Robertson et al 1990) or with *in situ* hybridization, holds very considerable promise for unravelling the detailed biochemical neuroanatomy of cocaine's actions in the central nervous system.

Acknowledgements

Work conducted in the authors' laboratories was supported by the Medical Research Council of Canada (PG-23). The excellent secretarial assistance of Sandra Sturgeon is gratefully acknowledged.

References

Akimoto K, Hamamura T, Otsuki S 1989 Subchronic cocaine treatment enhances cocaine-induced dopamine efflux, studied by in vivo intracerebral dialysis. Brain Res 490:339–344

Barr GA, Sharpless NS, Cooper S, Schiff SR, Paredes W, Bridger WG 1983 Classical conditioning, decay and extinction of cocaine-induced hyperactivity and stereotypy. Life Sci 33:1341–1351

Beninger RJ, Hanh BL 1983 Pimozide blocks establishment but not expression of amphetamine-produced environment-specific conditioning. Science (Wash DC) 220:1304–1306

Beninger RJ, Hertz RS 1986 Pimozide blocks establishment but not expression of cocaine-produced environment-specific conditioning. Life Sci 38:1425–1431

Bertorelli R, Hallström A, Hurd YL, Carlsson A, Consolo S, Ungerstedt U 1990 Anaesthesia effects on in vivo acetylcholine transmission, comparisons of radioenzymatic and HPLC assays. Eur J Pharmacol 175:79–83

Bradberry CW, Roth RH 1989 Cocaine increases extracellular dopamine in rat nucleus accumbens and ventral tegmental area as shown by in vivo microdialysis. Neurosci Lett 103:97–102

Brown EE, Finlay JM, Wong JTF, Damsma G, Fibiger HC 1991 Behavioral and neurochemical interactions between cocaine and buprenorphine: implications for the pharmacotherapy of cocaine abuse. J Pharmacol Exp Ther 256:119–126

Church WH, Justice JB, Byrd LD 1987 Extracellular dopamine in rat striatum following uptake inhibition by cocaine, nomifensine, and benztropine. Eur J Pharmacol 139:345–348

Damsma G, Fibiger HC 1991 The effects of anaesthesia and hypothermia on interstitial concentrations of acetylcholine and choline in rat striatum. Life Sci 48:2469–2474

De Wit H, Wise RA 1977 Blockade of cocaine reinforcement in rats with the dopamine receptor blocker pimozide but not with the noradrenergic blockers phentolamine or phenoxybenzamine. Can J Psychol 32:195–203

Di Chiara G, Imperato A 1988 Drugs abused by humans preferentially increase synaptic dopamine concentrations in the mesolimbic system of freely moving rats. Proc Natl Acad Sci USA 85:5274–5278

Dworkin SI, Smith JE 1988 Neurobehavioral pharmacology of cocaine. In: Clouet D, Asghar K, Brown R (eds) Mechanisms of cocaine abuse and toxicity. (National Institute on Drug Abuse Research Monograph 88) US Government Printing Office, Washington, DC

Einhorn LC, Johansen PA, White FJ 1988 Electrophysiological effects of cocaine in the mesoaccumbens dopamine system: studies in the ventral tegmental area. J Neurosci 8:100–112

Ettenberg A, Pettit HO, Bloom FE, Koob GF 1982 Heroin and cocaine intravenous self-administration in rats: mediation by separate neural systems. Psychopharmacology 78:204–209

Goeders NE, Smith JE 1983 Cortical dopaminergic involvement in cocaine reinforcement. Science (Wash DC) 21:773–775

Hubner CB, Koob GF 1990 The ventral pallidum plays a role in mediating cocaine and heroin self-administration in the rat. Brain Res 508:20–29

Hurd YL, Ungerstedt U 1989 Cocaine: an in vivo microdialysis evaluation of its acute action on dopaminergic transmission in rat striatum. Synapse 3:48–54

Hurd YL, Kehr J, Ungerstedt U 1988 In vivo microdialysis as a technique to monitor drug transport: correlation of extracellular cocaine levels and dopamine overflow in the rat brain. J Neurochem 51:1314–1316

Hurd YL, Weiss F, Koob GF, And N-E, Ungerstedt U 1979 Cocaine reinforcement and extracellular dopamine overflow in rat nucleus accumbens: an *in vivo* microdialysis study. Brain Res 498:199–203

Johanson C-E, Fischman MW 1989 The pharmacology of cocaine related to its abuse. Pharmacol Rev 41:3–52

Kalivas PW, Duffy P 1990 The effects of acute and daily cocaine treatment on extracellular dopamine in the nucleus accumbens. Synapse 5:48–58

Koob GF, Le HT, Creese I 1987 D-1 receptor antagonist SCH 23390 increases cocaine self-administration in the rat. Neurosci Lett 78:315–321

Lacey MG, Mercuri NB, North RA 1990 Actions of cocaine on rat dopaminergic neurones *in vitro*. Br J Pharmacol 99:731–735

Leccese AP, Lyness WH 1987 Lesions of dopamine neurons in the medial prefrontal cortex: effects on self-administration of amphetamine and dopamine synthesis in the brain of the rat. Neuropharmacology 26:1303–1308

Loh EH, Roberts DCS 1990 Break-points on a progressive ratio schedule reinforced by intravenous cocaine increase following depletion of forebrain serotonin. Psychopharmacology 101:262–266

Lyness WH, Friedle NM, Moore KE 1979 Destruction of dopaminergic nerve terminals in nucleus accumbens: effects of d-amphetamine self-administration. Pharmacol Biochem Behav 11:553–556

Maisonneuve IM, Keller RW, Glick SD 1990 Similar effects of D-amphetamine and cocaine on extracellular dopamine levels in medial prefrontal cortex of rats. Brain Res 535:221–226

Martin-Iverson MT, Szostak C, Fibiger HC 1986 6-Hydroxydopamine lesions of the medial prefrontal cortex fail to influence intravenous self-administration of cocaine. Psychopharmacology 88:310–314

Moghaddam B, Bunney BS 1989 Differential effect of cocaine on extracellular dopamine levels in rat prefrontal cortex and nucleus accumbens: comparison to amphetamine. Synapse 4:156–161

Nicolaysen LC, Pan H-T, Justice JB Jr 1988 Extracellular cocaine and dopamine concentrations are linearly related in rat striatum. Brain Res 456:317–323

Nomikos GG, Damsma G, Wenkstern D, Fibiger HC 1990 In vivo characterization of locally applied dopamine uptake inhibitors by striatal microdialysis. Synapse 6:106–112

Opacka-Juffry J, Ahier RG, Cremer JE 1991 Nomifensine-induced increase in extracellular striatal dopamine is enhanced by isoflurane anaesthesia. Synapse 7:169–171

Osborne PG, O'Connor WT, Drew KL, Ungerstedt U 1990 An in vivo microdialysis characterization of extracellular dopamine and GABA in dorsolateral striatum of awake freely moving and halothane anaesthetised rats. J Neurosci Meth 34:99–105

Pettit HO, Justice JB Jr 1989 Dopamine in the nucleus accumbens during cocaine self-administration as studied by in vivo microdialysis. Pharmacol Biochem Behav 34:899–904

Pettit HO, Justice JB Jr 1991 Effect of dose on cocaine self-administration behavior and dopamine levels in the nucleus accumbens. Brain Res 539:94–102

Pettit HO, Pan H-T, Parsons LH, Justice JB Jr 1990 Extracellular concentrations of cocaine and dopamine are enhanced during chronic cocaine administration. J Neurochem 55:798–804

Post RM, Contel NR 1983 Human and animal studies of cocaine: implications for development of behavioral pathology. In: Creese I (ed) Stimulants: neurochemical, behavioral and clinical perspective. Raven Press, New York, p 163–203

Richelson E, Pfenning M 1984 Blockade by antidepressants and related compounds of biogenic amine uptake into rat brain synaptosomes: most antidepressants selectively block norepinephrine uptake. Eur J Pharmacol 104:277–286

Ritz MC, Lamb RJ, Goldberg SR, Kuhar MJ 1987 Cocaine receptors on dopamine transporters are related to self-administration of cocaine. Science (Wash DC) 237:1219–1223

Roberts DCS 1991 Neural substrates mediating cocaine reinforcement. In: Lakoski JM, Galloway MP, White FJ (eds) Cocaine: pharmacology, physiology and clinical strategies. CRC Press, Boca Raton, FL

Roberts DCS, Koob GF 1982 Disruption of cocaine self-administration following 6-hydroxydopamine lesions of the ventral tegmental area in rats. Pharmacol Biochem Behav 17:902–904

Roberts DCS, Vickers G 1984 Atypical neuroleptics increase self-administration of cocaine: an evaluation of a behavioral screen for antipsychotic activity. Psychopharmacology 81:135–139

Roberts DCS, Corcoran ME, Fibiger HC 1977 On the role of ascending catecholaminergic systems in intravenous self-administration of cocaine. Pharmacol Biochem Behav 6:615–620

Roberts DCS, Koob GF, Klonoff P, Fibiger HC 1980 Extinction and recovery of cocaine self-administration following 6-hydroxydopamine lesions of the nucleus accumbens. Pharmacol Biochem Behav 12:781–787

Roberts DCS, Loh EA, Vickers G 1989 Self-administration of cocaine on a progressive ratio schedule in rats: dose-response relationship and effect of haloperidol pretreatment. Psychopharmacology 97:535–538

Robertson GS, Vincent SR, Fibiger HC 1990 Striatonigral projection neurons contain D_1 dopamine receptor-activated c-*fos*. Brain Res 523:288–290

Santiago M, Westerink BHC 1990 Characterization of the in vivo release of dopamine as recorded by different types of intracerebral microdialysis probes. Naunyn-Schmiedeberg's Arch Pharmacol 342:407–414

Stahle L, Collin A-K, Ungerstedt U 1990 Effects of halothane anaesthesia on extracellular levels of dopamine, dihydroxyphenylacetic acid, homovanillic acid and 5-hydroxyindolacetic acid in rat striatum: a microdialysis study. Naunyn-Schmiedeberg's Arch Pharmacol 342:136–140

Stewart J, de Wit H, Eikelboom R 1984 Role of unconditioned and conditioned drug effects in the self-administration of opiates and stimulants. Psychol Rev 91:251–268

Tatum AL, Seevers MH 1929 Experimental cocaine addiction. J Pharmacol Exp Ther 36:401–410

Weeks JR 1962 Experimental morphine addiction: method for automatic intravenous injections in unrestrained rats. Science (Wash DC) 138:143–144

Weiss SRB, Post RM, Pert A, Woodward R, Murman D 1989 Context-dependent cocaine sensitization: differential effect of haloperidol on development versus expression. Pharmacol Biochem Behav 34:655–661

Westerink BHC, De Vries JB 1988 Characterization of in vivo dopamine release as determined by brain microdialysis after acute and subchronic implantation: methodological aspects. J Neurochem 51:683–687

Wilson MC, Schuster CR 1974 Aminergic influences on intravenous cocaine self-administration by rhesus monkeys. Pharmacol Biochem Behav 2:563–571

Woolverton WL 1987 Evaluation of the role of norepinephrine in the reinforcing effects of psychomotor stimulants in rhesus monkeys. Pharmacol Biochem Behav 26:835–839

Woods JH, Winger GD, France CP 1987 Reinforcing and discriminative stimulus effects of cocaine: analysis of pharmacological mechanisms. In: Fisher S, Raskin A, Uhlenhuth EH (eds) Cocaine: clinical and biobehavioral aspects. Oxford University Press, New York, p 21–65

Young ST, Porrino LJ, Iadarola MJ 1991 Cocaine induces striatal c-fos immunoreactive proteins via dopaminergic D_1 receptors. Proc Natl Acad Sci USA 88:1291–1295

DISCUSSION

O'Brien: Dr Fibiger, can you reconcile your data with the microdialysis data published by Kalivas & Duffy (1990)? They showed sensitization (progressive increases in dopamine in the region of the nucleus accumbens in rats) with repeated intraperitoneal injections of the same dose of cocaine. After 5–7 days of giving cocaine injections, they injected saline. After saline, they found an increase in dopamine in the same brain area—not as high as after cocaine injections, but still an apparent conditioned effect. This would tend to support the hypothesis. Although there were no behavioural data, there was an apparent biochemical conditioning effect.

Fibiger: Our results would not agree with that. I don't believe, though, that Kalivas' group has studied conditioning *per se*. Most of his work, including that recently published by Kalivas & Duffy (1990), has been on sensitization. I am not aware of any study where he specifically looked at conditioned effects of cocaine. We certainly don't see any such effect.

I should add that our data are consistent with Dr Rick Beninger's work. He has demonstrated that it's quite easy to block the unconditioned locomotor stimulant effects of cocaine with a neuroleptic such as pimozide, but that cocaine-induced conditioned locomotion is much more resistant to attenuation by dopamine receptor antagonists (Beninger & Herz 1986). This result agrees with our data which suggest that the conditioned locomotor effects are not dopaminergically mediated.

Balster: Are you using results from Dr Justice's lab. to argue against the dopamine hypothesis for cocaine's actions? It is true that Pettit & Justice (1991) have reported levels of extracellular dopamine that are different at different cocaine doses, reflecting poor titration (i.e. subjects do not adjust their self-administration of different doses of cocaine to produce constant levels of dopaminergic activation). We know from experiments with other drugs that 'dosage titration' doesn't work very well; for example, with alcohol and drinking, if you increase the concentration of alcohol in the beverage, higher doses of alcohol are typically consumed. Thus, it is likely in Justice's experiments that higher self-administered doses of cocaine, leading to higher brain concentrations of cocaine and correspondingly higher levels of dopaminergic activation, simply reflect this difficulty of dosage titration, not an indictment of the dopamine hypothesis. The aspect of their evidence that supports the dopamine hypothesis is the remarkable stability of dopamine levels in the synapse within sessions, showing that the animals carefully regulated the intra-injection interval to produce a constant level of dopamine over one or two hours.

Fibiger: I don't view Justice's data as being substantially inconsistent with the dopamine hypothesis. However, his results are not compatible with the notion that animals will invariably work to increase extracellular dopamine concentrations in the brain by exactly $X\%$, across a variety of conditions. Clearly, it is not going to be as simple as that.

Kleber: Do your data support the view (which I raised earlier with Mike Kuhar) that all three neurotransmitter systems (noradrenergic, serotonergic and dopaminergic) are involved in the action of cocaine, and that this may be more fruitful for the search for pharmacological treatment for cocaine abuse than to search simply for drugs that interfere with dopamine?

Fibiger: Dr Roberts found that lesions of serotonergic neurons do change the breakpoint of cocaine self-administration (Loh & Roberts 1990). This suggests that neurotransmitter systems other than dopamine are also involved. We can only speculate about exactly how this occurs. It may be due to direct effects of the drug on serotonergic neurons. Alternatively, as I mentioned earlier, dopaminergic neurons are innervated by serotonergic neurons, and if you remove that innervation, the normal regulation of the dopaminergic neurons may be altered. I agree, therefore, that other transmitter systems will be involved in regulating the rate and pattern of cocaine consumption. From what I know about the brain, it would be foolish to think that it would be any other way.

Kleber: Do your findings refute the hypothesis of Drs Dackis and Gold (1985) that dopamine depletion is the basis for the craving after the cessation of cocaine use?

Fibiger: Our data don't really address that hypothesis in a direct manner. Nevertheless, to the extent that conditioned stimuli produce cocaine craving, it is worth noting that there was no difference in extracellular dopamine

Neurobiology of cocaine-induced reinforcement 113

concentrations between the cocaine conditioned and pseudoconditioned groups. This is not consistent with a form of the dopamine depletion hypothesis.

Negrete: This was extracellular dopamine, but the proponents of the dopamine depletion theory were not suggesting that; they hypothesized that presynaptic, intracellular dopamine was depleted.

Fibiger: That is so, but the only way presynaptic, intracellular dopamine can be translated into function is by the amount released extracellularly.

Woolverton: But Justice's group didn't see any dips in extracellular dopamine concentration in the animals that were self-administering cocaine; they continued to take cocaine without any such falls in dopamine concentration in the accumbens.

Fibiger: Yes. But the problem there may be the time resolution of microdialysis. We are forced to look at five-minute samples, and there could be fluctuations within that period.

Woolverton: It seems likely that you would have seen one fall, even on a random basis, with so many samples, if it had occurred.

Fibiger: Perhaps. As I said, I don't think our data speak clearly to the dopamine depletion hypothesis. I also know that Dr Justice has data which do to some extent support the dopamine depletion hypothesis (Parsons et al 1991). However, those data clearly indicate that the situation is much more complicated than the simple form of the hypothesis would suggest.

Kleber: Dr Bozarth and Dr Wise (1981) have shown connections between the ventral tegmental area (VTA) and the nucleus accumbens. Does the point that lesions in the VTA don't have the same effect as those placed in the nucleus accumbens mean that these connections are *not* a critical element in the reinforcing process? If the VTA is not involved, do you have alternative explanations of why buprenorphine may be effective in treating cocaine addicts? Could the VTA and its connections to the nucleus accumbens be another fruitful area for research into possible therapeutic intervention?

Fibiger: The input to the dopaminergic neurons in the ventral tegmental area may be very important. Some work is addressing this question, but for the most part it is purely anatomical. There is less biochemical neuroanatomy being done, and this is needed to determine not only the sources of the inputs, but the neurotransmitters contained in each of these inputs.

Kalant: I wonder if one can really reject the possibility that the different dopamine levels that you are finding with different cocaine dosages represent an effect, rather than a causal mechanism, of cocaine self-administration. The fact that the animals maintain self-administration at different dosages of cocaine, presumably producing different cocaine concentrations at its site of action, but resulting in different sustained levels of dopamine, would surely argue for the dopamine level being a consequence of, rather than a mechanism for maintaining, cocaine self-administration. I am wondering whether this doesn't fit better with, say, the finding that rats would self-administer cocaine into the medial prefrontal cortex and *not* into the nucleus accumbens, but would self-administer amphetamine into the accumbens and not into the medial prefrontal cortex (Goeders & Smith 1983). With the self-administration of alcohol, which is presumably also tapping into a reinforcement system, there was very little effect of dopaminergic blockers on consumption, and yet a very significant reduction by opiate blockers (Linseman 1989, 1990).

Fibiger: To my knowledge, intracerebral studies with cocaine microinjections into the prefrontal cortex by Goeders & Smith (1983) have not been replicated by other workers. The fact is that if the dopaminergic innervation of the frontal cortex is destroyed by 6-hydroxydopamine lesions, intravenous cocaine self-administration is not affected (Martin-Iverson et al 1986). So, if Goeders & Smith are right, the intracerebral injections of cocaine must reinforce behaviour in some way that is different from systemically administered cocaine.

With regard to the first part of your comment, rats do to a large extent 'titrate' the amount of cocaine that they self-administer. That is, the total consumption of cocaine per unit time does not vary that much. The animals compensate for higher doses per injection by decreasing the rate of lever pressing. However, in terms of extracellular concentrations of dopamine in the nucleus accumbens, it is evident that animals do not compensate completely for the effects of higher doses (Parson et al 1991).

Kalant: Wouldn't that also tend to dissociate the dopamine level from the reinforcement obtained with cocaine?

Fibiger: To me, it says that the relationship is not going to be very simple, but I don't think it eliminates the hypothesis that dopamine is importantly involved in the reinforcing effects of cocaine.

Kalant: But it at least requires an important modifier.

Fibiger: I agree. There was discussion earlier about postsynaptic mechanisms, and already in microdialysis studies we can often demonstrate clear dissociations between behaviour and dopamine chemistry. For example, if you inject a stimulant drug and record locomotor activity and stereotypy early in the post-injection period, as well as measure dopamine release, then typically you obtain a nice correlation between the increase in dopamine release and the increase in behaviour. That relationship often starts to fall apart after 30 or 60 minutes. The dopamine levels stay high and the behavioural output may gradually fall. This suggests to me that there are rapid compensatory mechanisms, perhaps postsynaptic, that come into play that influence the behavioural output so that it decreases, even in the presence of the maintained high dopamine concentrations. That is, compensatory postsynaptic mechanisms must be engaged fairly quickly, which cause the earlier strong relationship between extracellular dopamine concentrations and behaviour to disintegrate after a short period of time.

Kuhar: On this issue of whether more than dopamine is involved in reinforcement, we are in a way talking about two different things. When I said earlier that we have no evidence for the involvement of other neurotransmitter systems, I was talking about the initial site of action of cocaine. But the final behaviour depends on a chain of neurons, and therefore several other neurons are involved in the action of cocaine. I was referring only to the initial site of action where cocaine first binds to set everything else off. After that first binding, many other events occur, but, so far as I know, it is only the dopamine transporter site that has been correlated with reinforcement.

Fibiger: I agree.

Balster: A useful concept might be that dopamine is necessary but perhaps not sufficient as an explanation for cocaine's effects.

Negrete: On the question of the neuroleptic haloperidol reducing the self-administering of cocaine, are you quite satisfied that it is not an effect on the motor system of the animal, that will not permit the rat to press the bar lever?

Fibiger: Yes, we are quite sure about that, because, at low doses, neuroleptics *increase* cocaine self-administration. This would be very difficult to explain on the basis of motoric incapacity produced by low doses of haloperidol. On the other hand, at high enough doses of haloperidol, animals won't respond at all for cocaine, and this may indeed be due to a neuroleptic-induced motor deficit.

Negrete: According to Woods et al (1987), increasing doses of haloperidol proportionately reduced self-administration, so there remains a doubt there.

A clinical question: why do we not find a similar effect in patients, in whom we cannot control their cocaine-taking behaviour by giving them haloperidol?

Fibiger: That's a complicated question. In the clinical context, however, it may be important that you are generally dealing with very experienced cocaine users. What I have shown is that the behaviourally conditioned effects of cocaine are not dopaminergically mediated. Perhaps, if one examined the effects of haloperidol on a drug (cocaine)-naive individual's initial response to his first injection of the stimulant, one might see a strong attenuation of the rewarding effects. However, in an experienced cocaine user, it may be quite different.

Woolverton: It is possible that conditioned effects play an important role for the more experienced user and that these are not easily modified by haloperidol.

Balster: The poor results with haloperidol described by Dr Negrete may be important as we begin to think about the use of dopamine blockers, or antipsychotic drugs in general, as possible treatments for cocaine abuse. One of the findings from animal research is that antipsychotics such as haloperidol actually increase the rates of cocaine self-administration, for reasons that Dr Fibiger has explained. But in many situations these increases are hard to explain simply on the basis of a reduced potency of cocaine. There is reason to suspect, from animal experiments, that haloperidol and other antipsychotic drugs might increase the *efficacy* of cocaine as a reinforcer. It is important to remember that cocaine is also a haloperidol antagonist, so cocaine could be expected to reverse the dysphoric or other aversive effects of antipsychotic drugs; therefore, patients treated for cocaine abuse with an unpleasant antipsychotic medication might turn to cocaine as a treatment for their treatment!

Kleber: It is difficult to persuade a non-psychotic person to take haloperidol, or other antipsychotics; cocaine reverses that dysphoria.

I would like to bring in here the question of the effects of the cocaine levels obtained in the blood in humans with different routes of administration. Relating these levels to what we see clinically, the intranasal user is taking cocaine every 30 minutes; the crack smoker or intravenous injector is taking it every 15 minutes or so. However, judging from the plasma levels (see Fischman 1988), although the smoker is taking more cocaine at 15 minutes, he still has at that time as much cocaine in his blood as the individual who has been snorting it (intranasal route) and has reached a peak. It is as if the brain is compensating for the decrease in blood level. So one should really be looking for changes in dopamine levels, rather than simply enough dopamine.

Fischman: Although we measure and present data on venous levels of cocaine, the absolute amount of cocaine in the blood, or even in the brain, is not the relevant value. It is the rate of change of cocaine level on the ascending limb of the cocaine curve that probably determines response to drug (see Fig. 1). And when we talk about rates of change, it is clearly not venous levels that are important, but brain levels. We assume that venous levels can give us an inexact profile of brain levels, and take venous blood samples because they are the least invasive measure we can make which is also relevant.

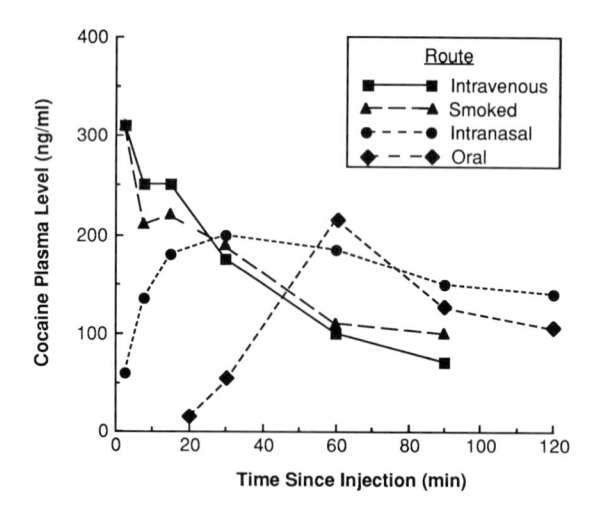

FIG. 1 (*Fischman*). Plasma levels of cocaine after administration via the intravenous, smoked, intranasal and oral routes. (Figure redrawn from Fischman 1988 and reproduced by permission of Physicians Postgraduate Press, Inc from *The Journal of Clinical Psychiatry*, 1988, volume 49 [no.2, supplement], p 7–10. ©1988 Physicians Postgraduate Press.)

Kleber: Therefore, one of the problems that Mike Kuhar and Chris Fibiger are having is that they are measuring absolute levels of dopamine, and perhaps that's not the critical issue; what is important may be the relative rates of change in these levels.

Kuhar: The rate of change in the quantity of neurotransmitter could be important; for example, you could be having a rapid desensitization of dopamine receptors. Many different things are almost certainly going on.

Kleber: That might explain some of the inability to explain experimentally what we know clinically happens all the time, namely the continued use of cocaine even when blood levels are high, and why the dopamine theory isn't adequate, because we are not looking at the rate of changes of dopamine in the brain. We are measuring absolute levels of dopamine.

Fibiger: Unfortunately, the temporal resolution of microdialysis isn't good enough to answer that question. If and when *in vivo* voltammetry becomes a more proven procedure, its better temporal resolution will enable us to ask those questions directly.

Jaffe: The curves of plasma cocaine levels represent venous levels; they don't represent arterial cocaine levels very well. And they don't really reflect brain levels of cocaine, because brain levels, after an intravenous dose, can be as much as seven times higher than venous levels. We shall not discover the importance of rate of change until somebody looks at the rate of change of cocaine levels in the brain.

Fischman: My subjects aren't very enthusiastic about volunteering for that!

Jaffe: On the subject of haloperidol, we persuaded some cocaine users to participate in an experiment (Sherer et al 1989) in which they were pretreated with haloperidol (about 0.1 mg/kg; the dose was 8 mg, injected intramuscularly). They were then challenged with cocaine (i.v. injection, 20–30 min later). We saw none of the hypothesized increases in efficacy; the changes in subjective effects were in the direction of an attenuation of the euphoria-inducing effects— the 'high'. We concluded that we had not waited long enough before injecting the cocaine. Here again, the issue is: how quickly does haloperidol get into the brain? We had probably not reached equilibrium. Our subjects did not report dysphoria in the first hour or two after the intramuscular haloperidol, so there was no dysphoria to attenuate. We did not see any attenuation of the phenomenon of 'rush' (i.e. the first, often intensely pleasurable sensation that subjects refer to as 'rush' was as intense and as long whether the subjects were pretreated with placebo or haloperidol), which we did observe with another pharmacological intervention—pretreatment with the calcium channel blocker, nifedipine (Muntaner et al 1991). This suggests that the intravenous bolus of cocaine produces a very rapid rise in brain cocaine levels which may be sufficient to overcome the effects of brain levels of haloperidol that you are likely to achieve with chronic (intramuscular) administration. Given that people take cocaine by routes that produce sharp increases in brain levels (intravenous injection, or smoked), it's likely that at most feasible levels of any blocker there will be a transient override of the blockade. And even though the duration of any reinforcing effects so produced is short, it may be sufficient to sustain self-administration. Even when people are taking modest levels of naltrexone (an opioid antagonist) chronically, if you give a big enough dose of an opioid such as morphine, there may be a transient effect; they can detect the opiate effect. This may be sufficient to produce a reinforcing effect.

Negrete: But 8 mg of haloperidol injected intramuscularly is a sizeable clinical dose; it should be enough to cause noticeable sedation.

Jaffe: In fact, the subjects weren't even sure that they had received haloperidol; nor were we. (That part of the study was double-blind: neither the observers nor the subjects were aware of what pretreatment had been given at the time the cocaine injection was given.) There were slight changes; they looked a little calmer (there's a certain anxiety about the cocaine injection procedure at the time of the experiment). We did see an unusual percentage of subjects developing extrapyramidal effects (e.g. involuntary twisting of neck muscles); these generally appeared after about 22 hours. Does this suggest that this is when the peak brain levels of haloperidol occur, or does it mean that that's when you get a decline in haloperidol level, after a peak? I have been told by a colleague that PET (positron emission tomography) scanning of volunteer subjects after they had received haloperidol indicates that the peak levels in brain may occur at 8–10 hours or later; the peak is certainly not at the 20–30 minutes which we used as the pretreatment time, which does coincide with the peak plasma levels of haloperidol. So, to conclude, there was some attenuation of the effects of cocaine, but it was not dramatic and there was no attenuation of the 'rush'.

Fibiger: There are animal data that may be relevant to your study. Another procedure commonly used to look at the rewarding effects of cocaine is the 'place preference' procedure, in which animals have been shown to prefer to spend time in an environment previously associated with injections of the drug. It has been shown that haloperidol does not block the ability of systemically administered cocaine to produce place preference in rats, at doses of haloperidol that block the locomotor stimulatory effects of cocaine. These results suggest that there is more to cocaine than dopamine, and this may be consistent with the clinical observations; perhaps place preference is tapping into some sort of a 'rush' phenomenon, as opposed to other aspects of cocaine's reinforcing effects.

Kuhar: We have thought a lot about Jerry Jaffe's experiment. The point is that the dopamine hypothesis comes from animal data, where one measures reinforcement. How that is related to rush and euphoria in humans, we don't know. Some people say that they are not closely related, so maybe rush and euphoria are not the right things to measure. Maybe we should be looking specifically at reinforcement in humans.

Another point is that haloperidol blocks D_2 dopamine receptors. But there are many kinds of dopamine receptors; maybe, in humans, it will be a different dopamine receptor that we have to block to block the effects of cocaine. Perhaps we haven't blocked the right dopamine receptor, or combination of receptors, to disrupt cocaine's effects.

Kaplan: I would have expected that the finding by Goeders and Smith of cortical involvement in cocaine reinforcement would have everybody in the animal area rushing to look at cortex, particularly because of its place in human behaviour. Shouldn't you be starting to look at cortex rather than the mid-brain for new experiments? Or at least to try to replicate the work of Goeders and Smith (1983)?

Fibiger: In my laboratory, we went to the cortex of the rat and came up with nothing (Martin-Iverson et al 1986).

Des Jarlais: All this discussion of neurochemistry makes me increasingly pessimistic about the possibility of developing a substitution type of treatment for cocaine dependence. The neurochemistry of the opiates is complicated enough, but we have there a relatively easy replacement of long-acting methadone for short-acting heroin. In trying to develop some form of substitution that will deal not only with dopamine but with several other neurotransmitter systems, combined with the fact that cocaine is a re-uptake blocker, rather than simply acting on a receptor, we seem unlikely to find anything as straightforward as methadone for treating cocaine dependence.

Negrete: On the question of routes of administration, in relation to patterns of use, and the particular question of smoking coca paste, which I discussed earlier, the major difference in the use of concentrated cocaine preparations in South and North America is that the preferred pattern in South America is smoking; there is almost no snorting (inhalation). Since peak blood concentrations, and the rapid change in brain levels, are the factors most responsible for the user's behaviour, this particular pattern of use is the characteristic of cocainism in South America. The number of people involved is large. In 1989, 5.3% of males between 12 and 50 years of age in Lima reported having smoked coca paste. These are people who are exposing themselves to the experience of *immediate* and strong reinforcement. Their behaviour is likely to be more affected than that of the majority of cocaine users in North America, who prefer to absorb the drug through the nasal mucosa.

Strang: Something I don't understand is whether one regards smoking (whether of crack or of *pasta*) as injecting cocaine without the needle and syringe. The implication has been that many of the behaviour patterns are associated with the rapid onset of the drug effect, and that the patterns of behaviour aren't the same with different speeds of onset. I can understand how a different route gives a different delivery system, so you can have a different rush, a different speed of onset; but I can't see how a different delivery system gives a different decay, or a different elimination of the drug. Once it's there, whatever the route by which it reaches the brain, and once you have reached peak level, surely you then see the same elimination of the drug, irrespective of the original route of administration?

Kleber: You have two ways of metabolizing cocaine, by enzymes in the liver and by certain enzymes in the blood. The route of administration may affect the relative amount of metabolism by these two methods.

Jaffe: You have to consider the two directions—going into the brain and coming out. If you use a route that gets a bolus of cocaine into the brain (e.g. the intravenous route), within a minute or so it's almost all coming out, with nothing continuing to come in. Whereas with, say, a large oral dose of cocaine, some is going into the brain and the level continues to increase as more drug is absorbed into the bloodstream. Some cocaine is also coming out; but more is still going in, so at some point there may be a relatively steady level which is then followed by a slow decrease. So the route could well determine the rate at which brain cocaine levels fall.

Strang: I can understand how 'snorting' would be different from injecting, but I was thinking about injecting cocaine versus free-basing or crack-smoking, where you have the same effect of an almost instantaneous entry of cocaine into the blood and brain.

Jaffe: There is a difference, in that with smoking you by-pass the right side of the heart.

Negrete: Yes. It takes double the time for intravenously injected cocaine to reach the brain; it is eight seconds from the lung, and 16 seconds when it is injected in the arm.

Jaffe: The net effect of the intravenous route compared to inhalation is more dilution of a given dose.

Jones: Smoking cocaine is *not* equivalent to taking an intravenous dose; smoking is a far more efficient way of getting a drug into the brain. By smoking a smaller delivered dose (smaller in the sense of the amount that gets into the body) the dose going into lung, with its tremendous surface area, is almost instantly absorbed; it then goes into left heart, and thence directly to brain. The same amount of cocaine if injected into an arm vein has to follow a far more circuitous route before arriving at the brain sites of action. It isn't that the metabolism of smoked cocaine is so different, but probably what is more important is that when it is smoked there is less time and opportunity for distribution into other tissues before the cocaine reaches the brain. An experienced cocaine smoker can take in a relatively small amount of cocaine (as compared to an equipotent intravenous dose) and deliver it in a more concentrated bolus to brain. After the first pass, the brain cocaine levels probably fall more rapidly after smoking than after intravenous injection. What may be important to maximize the desired mood change is a sudden rise in brain level, and there's no way of mimicking that smoking route, short of a carotid artery injection or direct brain injection!

Neurobiology of cocaine-induced reinforcement

Strang: Yet the opposite argument is made for heroin, that using heroin by smoking is a less efficient delivery system, and you need a larger dose to get the same hit.

Jones: A larger dose in the pipe is needed, but much is pyrolized and otherwise lost before it gets to the lungs, so a smaller dose is delivered. Many ex-cocaine smokers tell me that the reason people stop smoking cocaine is that it's a terrible waste; you use up a lot of cocaine.

Jaffe: One should not confuse the issue of the efficiency of cocaine use (effects/dollars spent) with how much drug is needed to produce a given biological effect. Coca free base can be got into vapour form without too much destruction. Whereas with the kind of heroin that is ordinarily injected, if you try to heat it, you destroy a lot of it in the process of getting it vaporized so that it can enter the lung and brain.

So there are two ways in which we need to conceptualize efficiency. How much vaporized cocaine must be put into the body (the lung) to get a given peak brain level? And how much cocaine must be put in the apparatus to get a given amount into the lung? That has to do with the efficiency with which you arrange the apparatus, and the form of drug. You can smoke cocaine hydrochloride; you don't have to make free base. But in doing so you destroy a tremendous amount of the cocaine hydrochloride in the process of getting a little bit of active cocaine into the lung.

O'Brien: There is a merchandizing advantage of crack. As Dr Jaffe points out, the vapour point of alkaloid cocaine is only about 100 °C, whereas cocaine HCl is vaporized at 200 °C, so you pyrolize a lot of it when you heat it. In contrast, it is easy to vaporize free base (alkaloidal cocaine). The sellers of the free base (crack) sell very small quantities which give a quick and brief 'high'. In Philadelphia and other East Coast cities, crack can be sold for $5 a chip; in some cases they sell it for $2 or $3, on 'sale'. Thus a lot of young users can begin with only a small amount of money. But the 'high' lasts only a brief period, even though it gets to the brain very efficiently.

Kalant: There is a common misconception in relation to the difference between the speeds of attainment of peak concentration after inhalation and after intravenous injection. Lung-to-brain circulation times, and arm-to-brain circulation times, are based not on measurement of the actual amount getting there, but on the shortest time for the first amount of indicator to be detectable. That doesn't tell you anything about the build-up of concentration. If you use a drug marker, you give enough to ensure that there is as rapid as possible an absorption, and all that you are concerned with is when the first bit gets to the brain. The actual *amount* from an inhaled dose will be diluted and spread through a considerably larger volume of blood, because the circulation time through the apical capillaries of the lung will be different from that through the hilar capillaries. And you will probably get a less effective bolus by inhalation than by intravenous injection of an actual bolus of a defined volume. There has been some mythology about the relative effectiveness of a build-up of brain levels of drug by the two routes.

Fischman: We have collected behavioural data from both cocaine smokers and intravenous users of cocaine which might provide information about choice of the route of administration. A subgroup of my cocaine-using research subjects have had experience with both the smoked and intravenous routes of administration. Most of these people tell us that their preferred route of administration is intravenous. My assumption is that they prefer the intravenous route because it is the least expensive way to get the most cocaine to their brains quickly. In other words, it is an efficient way to get the maximal cocaine effect. In the laboratory, as I shall describe in my paper (p 165), I give these subjects repeated opportunities to choose between intravenous injections of cocaine or puffs of cocaine from a pipe, with the venous levels obtained via the two doses controlled for. We find that these subjects generally choose to smoke cocaine under these conditions—many, when the choice is between 25 mg smoked cocaine and 32 mg intravenous cocaine; virtually all when the choice is between 50 mg smoked cocaine and 32 mg intravenous cocaine.

All subjects have an intravenous catheter in place during the session, so they are not avoiding the needle 'stick'. We assume it has to do with the rapidity with which the initial amounts of cocaine reach the brain.

Jaffe: Actually, we have seen a similar thing with tobacco smoking. Although needles have been around for 100 years, and you can get nicotine in pure form rather easily, most people prefer to smoke it in the form of tobacco! Even if you manipulate the dose of nicotine to mimic what cigarette smokers seem to get from smoking, with i.v. nicotine (or even with, I think, larger doses of i.v. nicotine), subjects report that satisfaction is greater with inhaled nicotine. It's an exact parallel in many respects.

Jones: Harold Kalant is probably right about what's going on in terms of the cocaine distribution, but what we see is similar to what Marian Fischman described. With the smoked route, if one considers the dose actually absorbed, about half of the amount of cocaine taken by smoking produces about twice the effects, at least as measured by heart rate and pupil diameter change. That is, 20 mg of cocaine absorbed (absorption as measured by benzoylecgonine levels in plasma) produces the effect of 40 mg of cocaine injected intravenously over one minute. So whether it's a matter of the rate of change of cocaine level in brain, or something else, the subjects both behaviourally and in terms of physiological response get more kick from less drug actually entering the body. I think the same could be said for nicotine in a similar situation where smoking and intravenous administration are compared.

Benowitz: We have studied the influence of the rate of dosing on the effects of infusions of nicotine in people. Three mg of nicotine given intravenously over 10 minutes does not produce the same intensity of subjective effects as does 1 mg nicotine absorbed via cigarette smoke over the same period of time.

When one smokes or inhales a drug, a relatively small dose of the drug is delivered into the lungs quickly. The pulmonary circulation is such that blood sweeps through the lungs in a second or two. A drug gets from the lung into the brain within about 10 seconds (Benowitz 1990). The other thing about smoking is that one can obtain small doses from each inhalation and then titrate to a cumulative dose to achieve the desired subjective effects. Thus, the total dose needed to achieve a particular effect may be substantially less if one smokes and titrates the dose, than if the drug is taken intravenously.

Edwards: To round off at this point, I would like to ask Dave Musto to tell us something about the history of 'faith in science'. When did people dealing with addictions first believe that science, rather than morality or the law, could help solve these problems?

Musto: A faith in science characterized the early stages of morphine's, heroin's and cocaine's popularity. The drugs' commercial production as well as isolation was the result of scientific advance and, when people first started using them, their value and even their safety dominated popular opinion. As problems arose, the answer was thought also to lie in further scientific research. The hope was to preserve the undoubted value of the drugs while providing an effective treatment for the occasional personal catastrophe. In the first decade or two of this century, immunology seemed to hold the solution to addiction, or so a number of scientific studies suggested.

Then, at least in the United States, a great change in attitude occurred after World War I. The question of drug use passed beyond moderation to intolerance. No drug use was acceptable. The answer to the drug problem was no longer in some complex medical treatment, in a new round of scientific research, but in abstention. The use of drugs for non-medical purposes became immoral, not just unwise or even possibly rewarding. Research faded, faith in medical treatment was given up. Maintenance, once tolerated, became unacceptable except in clear cases of terminal illness or iatrogenic addiction. Of course, one must grant that the medical treatments—based on erroneous notions of physiology and biochemistry—were, in fact, worthless, but there was little effort to discover better ones.

So I agree with you: faith in science and faith in law enforcement are each deep convictions that endure for long periods and are not easy companions. That is why I am worried about the future of research in the United States, because the hope that science will discover the answer to drug addiction, so prominent in the 1970s, is fading as we turn more and more to the criminal justice system. Anger at drugs and the drug user is insistent and demanding, and views research and treatment as slow and uncertain.

References

Beninger RJ, Herz RS 1986 Pimozide blocks establishment but not expression of cocaine-produced environment-specific conditioning. Life Sci 38:1425–1431

Benowitz NL 1990 Clinical pharmacology of inhaled drugs of abuse: implications in understanding nicotine dependence. In: Chiang CN, Hawks RL (eds) Research findings on smoking of abused substances. (National Institute on Drug Abuse Research Monograph 99) US Government Printing Office, Washington, DC, p 12–29

Bozarth MA, Wise RA 1981 Heroin reward is dependent on a dopaminergic substrate. Life Sci 29:1881–1886

Dackis CA, Gold MS 1985 New concepts in cocaine addiction: the dopamine depletion hypothesis. Neurosci Biobehav Rev 9:469–477

Fischman MW 1988 Behavioral pharmacology of cocaine. J Clin Psychiatry 49(2) (suppl): 7–10

Goeders NE, Smith JE 1983 Cortical dopaminergic involvement in cocaine reinforcement. Science (Wash DC) 221:773–775

Kalivas PW, Duffy P 1990 The effects of acute and daily cocaine treatment on extracellular dopamine in the nucleus accumbens. Synapse 5:48–58

Linseman MA 1989 Central versus peripheral mediation of opioid effects on alcohol consumption in free-feeding rats. Pharmacol Biochem Behav 33:407–413

Linseman MA 1990 Effects of dopaminergic agents on alcohol consumption by rats in a limited access paradigm. Psychopharmacology 100:195–200

Loh EA, Roberts DCS 1990 Break-points on a progressive ratio schedule reinforced by intravenous cocaine increase following depletion of forebrain serotonin. Psychopharmacology 101:262–266

Martin-Iverson MT, Szostak C, Fibiger HC 1986 6-Hydroxydopamine lesions of the medial prefrontal cortex fail to influence intravenous self-administration of cocaine. Psychopharmacology 88:310–314

Muntaner C, Kumor K, Nagoshi C, Jaffe JH 1991 Effects of nifedipine pretreatment on subjective and cardiovascular responses to cocaine. Psychopharmacology 105:37–41

Parsons LH, Smith AD, Justice JB 1991 Basal extracellular dopamine is decreased in the rat nucleus accumbens during abstinence from chronic cocaine. Synapse 9:60–65

Pettit HO, Justice JO Jr 1991 Effect of dose on cocaine self-administration behavior and dopamine levels in the nucleus accumbens. Brain Res 539:94–102

Sherer MA, Kumor KM, Jaffe JH 1989 Effects of intravenous cocaine are partially attenuated by haloperidol. Psychiatry Res 27:117–125

Woods JH, Winger GD, France CP 1987 Reinforcing and discriminative stimulus effects of cocaine: analysis of pharmacological mechanisms. In: Fisher S, Raskin A, Uhlenhuth EH (eds) Cocaine, clinical and behavioral aspects. Oxford University Press, New York, p 21–65

How toxic is cocaine?

Neal L. Benowitz

Division of Clinical Pharmacology and Experimental Therapeutics, San Francisco General Hospital Medical Center, and the Departments of Medicine and Psychiatry, University of California, San Francisco, CA 94110, USA

Abstract. The toxicities of cocaine are far-ranging. They include sudden death, acute medical and psychiatric illness, infectious complications, reproductive disturbances, trauma, criminal activities and societal disruption, including child neglect and abuse and lost job productivity. This chapter focuses on the medical complications. Medical complications in general reflect the intense sympathomimetic activities of cocaine ('sympathetic neural storm'). Psychiatric complications include acute anxiety or panic and paranoid psychosis. Cardiovascular complications include arrhythmias and sudden death, acute myocardial infarction, myocarditis, dissecting aneurysm and bowel infarction. Neurological complications include seizure, intracerebral haemorrhage and brain injury due to hyperthermia and/or seizures, and headache. The incidence of medical complications has been estimated using two databases collected prospectively in the United States. In 1989 and 1990 cocaine ranked first in total encounters, major medical complications and drug-related deaths. An attempt was made to assess the intrinsic toxicity of cocaine by computing the incidence of adverse health outcomes per population of drug abusers. Rates of emergency department visits and deaths were 15.1 and 0.5 respectively, per 1000 persons using drugs in the past year. The magnitude of the cocaine problem, while considerable, is relatively small compared with that of cigarette smoking or alcohol abuse.

1992 Cocaine: scientific and social dimensions. Wiley, Chichester (Ciba Foundation Symposium 166) p 125–148

Cocaine has been used medicinally as a local anaesthetic and abused as a central nervous system stimulant for many years. As late as the 1970s, cocaine was not considered to be a highly dangerous drug or even a drug with a great propensity to cause physical dependence. For example, in 1973 the Council on Drug Abuse opined 'The morbidity associated with cocaine use does not appear to be great and there are virtually no confirmed deaths from cocaine overdose' (Strategy Council on Drug Abuse 1973). Since 1980, however, there has been a steady rise (now at a plateau in the USA) in cocaine-related deaths and other medical complications, as well as other health and welfare problems including trauma (such as motor vehicle accidents and homicide), child neglect and abuse, loss of job productivity, and criminal activity. This review will focus primarily on medical complications of cocaine abuse. I shall briefly review the clinical pharmacology of cocaine, discuss the mechanisms and nature of medical complications of cocaine, and then compare the incidence of cocaine-related medical toxicity with that of other drugs of abuse.

Clinical pharmacology of cocaine

To understand mechanisms of toxicity, we need to understand the human pharmacology of cocaine as it is usually abused. As of 1989, in the USA cocaine was most commonly smoked, less commonly taken by injection, and less often abused by sniffing (National Institute on Drug Abuse 1990). Cocaine can be obtained as the crystalline salt—cocaine hydrochloride—or as cocaine base. Cocaine base, usually in pellet or chunk (crack) form, is preferred for smoking because it is more volatile and vaporizes at a lower temperature than does cocaine hydrochloride. Smoking or intravenous injection of cocaine results in rapid delivery of the drug into the systemic blood circulation which, in turn, results in rapid delivery to the brain. Cocaine concentrations in venous blood peak sooner after smoking or i.v. cocaine than after administration by other routes (Jones 1990) (Fig. 1). Peak arterial concentrations of cocaine are several times higher than are maximal venous concentrations after smoking or i.v. dosing. After sniffing or oral ingestion, the absorption of cocaine is prolonged over 30–60 minutes and the effects are less intense than those observed after smoking or intravenous injection. Although cocaine is not generally abused by the oral route, oral absorption is a significant route of dosing as a cause of toxicity. Cocaine is

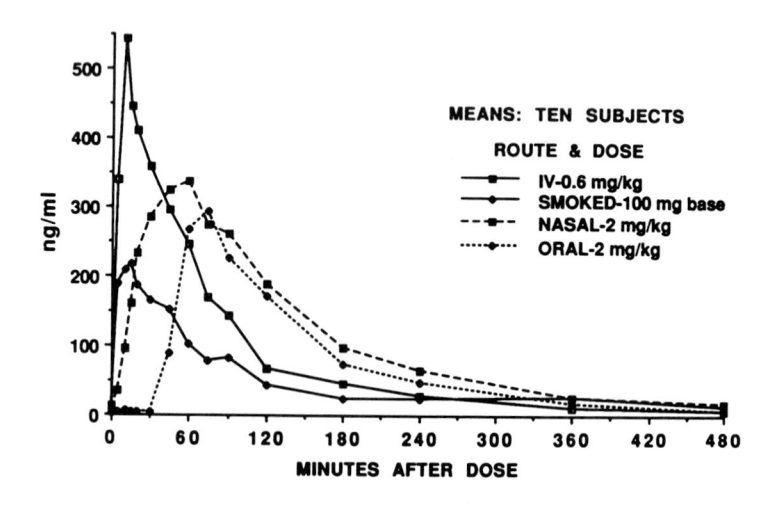

FIG. 1. Plasma levels of cocaine after dosing by different routes. (From Jones 1990, with permission.)

well absorbed orally. Its bioavailability is 30–40%, the remainder being eliminated by first-pass metabolism. Significant poisoning from oral cocaine has been observed after the rupture of cocaine-filled condoms or plastic bags, which are sometimes swallowed by smugglers or street dealers trying to avoid police detection (Fishbain & Wetli 1981), or in children who have swallowed cocaine in mother's milk, or cocaine that was applied to the face as a local anaesthetic after facial trauma.

Cocaine is extensively and rapidly hydrolysed by esterases in the blood, liver and other organs. The major metabolites are ecgonine methyl ester, benzoylecgonine and ecgonine (Fig. 2). These metabolites are relatively inactive compared with cocaine. Hepatic metabolism to norcocaine, which is pharmacologically active, accounts for only a small fraction (2–6%) of total elimination. Persons with deficient plasma cholinesterase activity might be expected to metabolize cocaine more slowly and, thus, may be at a higher risk for adverse effects. Renal excretion of cocaine is only a minor path of elimination, accounting for 5–10% of the dose, depending on urine pH. Cocaine is a weak base and higher concentrations are found in acid than in alkaline urine.

After intravenous injection, cocaine has a plasma half-life averaging 60 minutes. The transient nature of the effects of cocaine reported by users is due primarily to redistribution of the drug out of the brain and into other tissues. Systemic effects and plasma levels may be sustained for longer periods because of continued absorption after oral administration. After nasal dosing, cocaine levels may remain high for several hours, as a result of local vasoconstriction

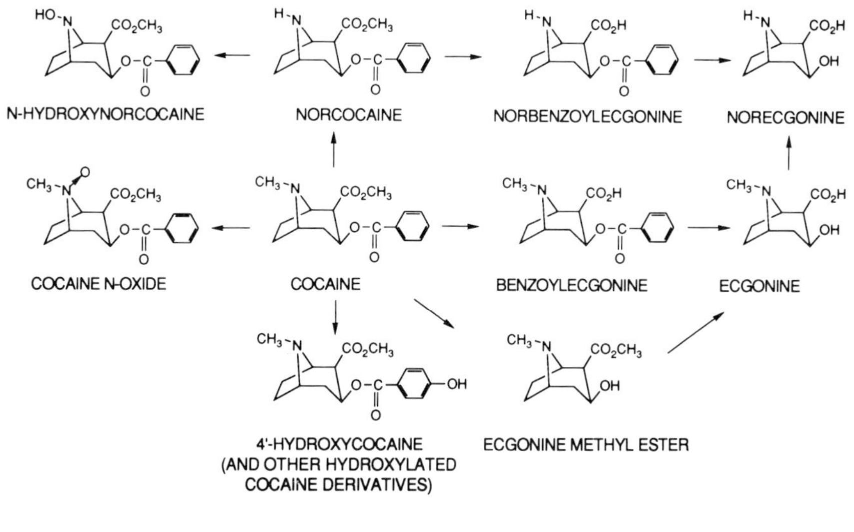

FIG. 2. Chemical structures of cocaine and major metabolites.

and resultant delayed absorption. Benzoylecgonine, the major metabolite of cocaine, has a half-life of about seven hours; ecgonine methyl ester has a half-life of about four hours.

Heating of cocaine, as occurs in smoking, results in the generation of cocaine-related breakdown products, primarily anhydroecgonine methyl ester (also called methylecgonidine). Anhydroecgonine methyl ester can be found in substantial concentrations in the urine of cocaine smokers but not after injection or sniffing of cocaine (Jacob et al 1990). The pharmacological contribution of anhydroecgonine methyl ester to cocaine's effects or toxicity is as yet unknown.

The primary effects of cocaine in people are euphoria and central nervous system (CNS) stimulation, as well as activation of the peripheral sympathetic nervous system, with tachycardia and blood pressure elevation. Cocaine is a potent local anaesthetic and vasoconstrictor, which results in the characteristic numbing of the nose in cocaine sniffers, and the pale and bloodless mucosa that is desirable for nose and throat surgery.

Tolerance develops quickly and completely to the euphoric and other subjective effects of cocaine (Foltin & Fischman 1991). Tolerance develops only incompletely to the cardiovascular effects of cocaine (Ambre et al 1988). Thus, a situation may evolve in which cocaine is repeatedly used to seek the cocaine 'high', with the consequence being progressive cardiovascular toxicity.

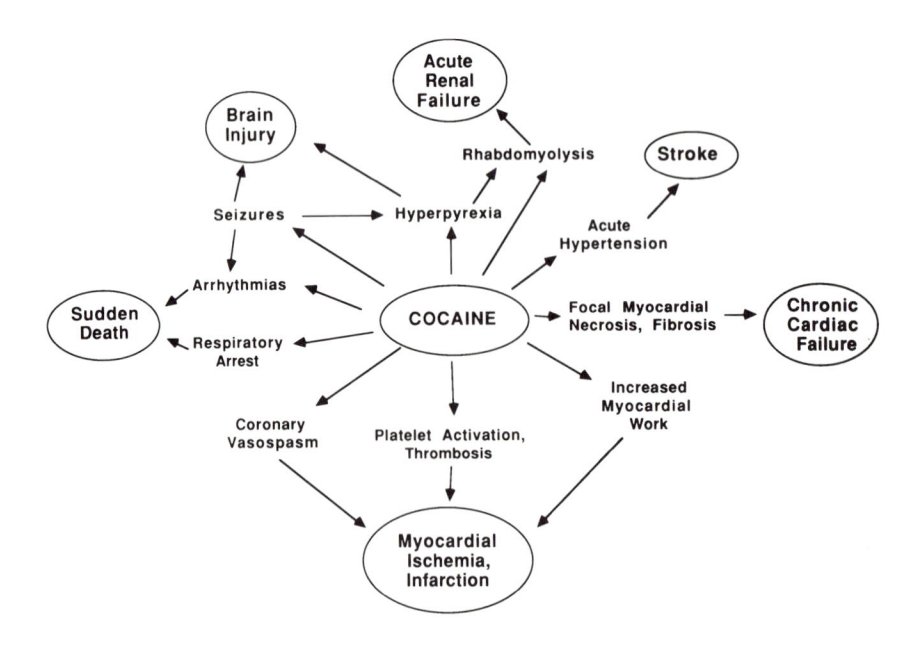

FIG. 3 Pathophysiology of medical complications of cocaine abuse (except for reproductive complications).

Mechanisms of cocaine toxicity

The manifestations of cocaine toxicity can be best appreciated if the mechanisms of action are understood. These include: (1) blockade of the neuronal re-uptake of catecholamines; (2) CNS stimulation with release of dopamine and systemic activation of the sympathetic nervous system; (3) release and/or blockade of uptake of serotonin; and (4) a local anaesthetic effect, due to blockade of fast sodium channels. The latter effect may result in neural and myocardial depression after large overdoses of cocaine. A scheme depicting the pathogenesis of many of the medical complications of cocaine intoxication is presented in Fig. 3.

Manifestations of cocaine toxicity

Cocaine intoxication and an overview of the medical complications

The following is an illustrative case. A 24-year-old man was found on a street kerb with a plastic bag in his mouth. He had swallowed cocaine that had been contained in that bag to avoid apprehension by the police. He was confused, frightened and hypervigilant. Blood pressure was 210/138 mm Hg, heart rate, 120; the pupils were widely dilated. An hour later he developed generalized convulsions, hypotension and hyperthermia (temperature 40.5 °C). He survived but was left with permanent brain injury, manifested by severe deficits in attention, memory and motor control.

Most of the manifestations of cocaine intoxication can be explained by excessive central and sympathetic neural stimulation. Autonomic and neuromuscular effects include tachycardia, hypertension, hyperthermia, mydriasis, seizures, respiratory arrest and cardiovascular collapse. Central nervous system stimulation results in behavioural and psychiatric abnormalities such as hyperactivity, irritability, insomnia, mood lability, agitation, psychosis (often paranoid), delirium, stupor and coma. Other psychiatric disturbances include acute anxiety, panic attacks or agitated delirium. Cocaine is a common cause for visits to emergency departments in US hospitals, especially in inner cities. Two surveys of patient complaints and symptoms in emergency departments found that chest pain, anxiety and altered mental status were particularly common (Table 1) (Brody et al 1990, Derlet & Albertson 1989).

Because cocaine has a relatively short half-life, acute intoxication usually resolves within six hours. Chronic intoxication may present as paranoid schizophrenia and may last for many days. After the cessation of chronic use, cocaine abusers may suffer fatigue, hypersomnia, hyperphagia, and depression lasting for days to weeks (Gawin & Kleber 1986).

A number of medical complications that may be life-threatening have been reported with cocaine intoxication (Table 2) (Mueller et al 1990). Many of these

TABLE 1 Cocaine-related emergency visits in the USA: results of two surveys

Atlanta survey[a] (n = 233) Complaints/symptoms		Sacramento survey[b] (n = 137) Complaints/symptoms	
Chest pain	39%[c]	Altered mental status	29%
Anxiety	22%	Chest pain	15%
Short of breath	22%	Syncope	14%
Palpitations	21%	Suicide	9%
Dizziness	13%	Palpitations	9%
Headache	12%	Seizures	9%
Psychosis	9%		
Confusion	9%		

[a]Brody et al 1990.
[b]Derlet & Albertson 1989.
[c]Percentage of total number of cocaine-related visits. In the Atlanta series, the total exceeds 100% because multiple complaints of patients are counted separately. In the Sacramento series, the total is less than 100% because the less common complaints are not listed.

involve excessive sympathetic neural stimulation. They include severe hypertension that may be complicated by stroke or dissecting aneurysm, cardiac arrhythmias that may include ventricular fibrillation, and sudden death. In addition, the vasoconstriction may lead to ischaemia of the heart, kidney and gastrointestinal tract. Other common major complications involve the central nervous system. The most important ones are headache that may be due to hypertension or to a migraine-like mechanism, seizures and stroke. Three types of toxicity have been of considerable interest, are illustrative of general mechanisms of cocaine toxicity, and will be discussed in more detail: cocaine-related deaths, cardiovascular disease, and reproductive disturbances.

Cocaine-related deaths

Most deaths directly due to the pharmacological effects of cocaine are sudden and occur within a few hours of cocaine intoxication. Death is believed to result most commonly from cardiac arrhythmias due to massive catecholamine release, with or without acute myocardial ischaemia. At autopsy, a number of sudden death cases after cocaine abuse have had evidence of significant coronary artery disease, supporting the idea that many deaths occur secondary to acute cardiac ischaemia (Mittleman & Wetli 1987). Cocaine concentrations in blood at autopsy are on average lower in people with coexisting coronary artery disease who died from cocaine intoxication than those without heart disease, which is consistent with the existence of a susceptible population. Many cocaine victims are seen to convulse prior to death. Convulsions *per se* can cause catecholamine release

TABLE 2   Medical complications of cocaine intoxication and abuse

Cardiovascular	Respiratory
Hypertension	Pneumomediastinum
Intracranial haemorrhage	Pneumothorax
Aortic dissection/rupture	Pulmonary oedema
Arrhythmias	Respiratory arrest
Sinus tachycardia	
Supraventricular tachycardia	*Metabolic and other*
Ventricular tachyarrhythmias	
Organ ischaemia	Hyperthermia
Myocardial ischaemia and infarction	Rhabdomyolysis (muscle breakdown)
Renal infarction	
Intestinal infarction	*Reproductive*
Limb ischaemia	
Myocarditis	Obstetric
Shock	Spontaneous abortion
Sudden death	Placental abruption
	Placenta praevia
Central nervous system	Premature rupture of the membranes
	Fetal
Headache	Intrauterine growth retardation
Seizures	Congenital malformations
Transient focal neurological deficits	Neonatal
Stroke	'Crack baby syndrome'
Subarachnoid haemorrhage	Cerebral infarction
Intracranial haemorrhage	Delayed neurobehavioural
Cerebral infarction	development
Embolic (endocarditis)	
Toxic encephalopathy/coma	*Infectious*[a]
Neurological complications	
	Acquired immune deficiency syndrome (AIDS)
	Infectious endocarditis
	Hepatitis B
	Wound botulism
	Tetanus

[a]Transmitted by contaminated needles or syringes.

and can produce life-threatening arrhythmias. Respiratory arrest may occur with very high levels of cocaine, presumably as a result of direct central nervous system depression. Finally, in some cases of sudden death there is intracerebral haemorrhage or a ruptured aorta—well-known complications of cocaine-induced hypertension.

A review of US medical examiners' (coroners') cases where cocaine was found in the deceased person suggests that more cocaine-related deaths may be due to trauma than to intoxication *per se* (Tardiff et al 1989). A series of 935 such cases from New York City in 1986 showed the top causes of death to be homicide

(37.5%), acute narcotism (combination of cocaine and heroin, 12.0%), other natural causes (11.1%) and suicide (6.6%). Direct cocaine intoxication, including cocaine overdose, occlusive coronary artery disease, cerebral haemorrhage and ruptured aorta, accounted for 11.6% of the deaths.

Of particular interest in helping us to understand the toxicology of cocaine are deaths due to 'excited delirium', reported initially in Dade County, Florida (Wetli & Fishbain 1985), but subsequently in other parts of the United States as well. Seven cases were described in which intense paranoia was followed by bizarre and violent behaviour, accompanied by hyperthermia. These people died suddenly, often while in police custody. Blood levels of cocaine were lower than those measured in cases of typical cocaine intoxication. Other cases of death due to hyperthermia from cocaine intoxication have been reported, raising the speculation that cocaine may produce a variant of the neuroleptic malignant syndrome (Kosten & Kleber 1988). Neuroleptic malignant syndrome is a potentially life-threatening complication of antipsychotic drug therapy, characterized by hyperthermia, autonomic instability and muscular rigidity.

Cardiovascular complications of cocaine abuse

Myocardial infarction due to cocaine has become commonplace in major urban medical centres in the USA (Isner & Chokshi 1991). Mechanisms of cocaine-induced myocardial infarction are believed to include one or more of (1) increased myocardial work with demand for oxygen and other nutrients that exceeds the supply; (2) coronary vasospasm; and (3) thrombosis. The blood pressure- and heart rate-elevating effects of cocaine markedly increase myocardial oxygen consumption, and, in people with underlying coronary heart disease who cannot adequately increase their coronary blood flow, promote angina or myocardial infarction. Coronary vasoconstriction has been documented in volunteer research patients receiving low doses of cocaine (Lange et al 1989). Coronary vasospasm has been observed in patients with cocaine-induced myocardial infarction (Zimmerman et al 1987). Cocaine enhances platelet aggregation *in vitro*, and many patients with cocaine-induced myocardial infarction have evidence of coronary thrombosis on angiography (Patel et al 1988, Togna et al 1985). It is noteworthy that myocardial infarction may develop from hours to days after the time of the last dose of cocaine, probably reflecting the variable time course of development of thrombosis, possibly at the site of the vasospasm. A study of ambulatory electrocardiographic monitoring of regular cocaine users undergoing detoxification showed persistent evidence of ST segment elevation, presumably reflecting coronary spasm, during the first weeks of withdrawal (Nademanee et al 1989). Chronic cocaine treatment of dogs results in enhanced coronary artery constrictor responses to endogenous vasoactive substances (Jones & Tackett 1990). The mechanisms for persistent or recurring coronary spasm after chronic cocaine intake are unknown.

Ischaemic complications may affect organs other than the heart as well. Renal and intestinal infarction have been described and may be life-threatening. Ischaemic limbs have occurred after the accidental intra-arterial injection of cocaine, resulting in a cool, pale and painful limb.

As already discussed, arrhythmias are common during cocaine intoxication and may be a consequence of sympathetic neural stimulation, myocardial ischaemia, or myocarditis. Sympathetic stimulation as the cause of arrhythmias is to be expected in the early phase of intoxication, when there is clinical evidence of other pharmacological actions of cocaine. Myocardial ischaemia and myocarditis tend to be manifest later in the course of intoxication, when cocaine has already been eliminated from the body.

The most common arrhythmia during cocaine intoxication is sinus tachycardia. Other arrhythmias that have been reported in cocaine users include atrial tachycardia and fibrillation, accelerated idioventricular rhythm, and ventricular tachycardia. Of note is that the electrocardiogram during cocaine intoxication occasionally shows wide complex tachycardia, which may represent sinus tachycardia with impaired cardiac conduction due to the local anaesthetic effects of cocaine (Kabas et al 1990). Ventricular fibrillation due to intense sympathetic stimulation is presumed to be the cause of many of the sudden deaths in cocaine users, although asystole, presumably related to its local anaesthetic actions, has also been observed.

Reproductive disturbances and neonatal effects

Surveys of pregnant women in inner city areas of the United States report rates of maternal cocaine use as high as 30%, although the usual figure is 10–20% (Zuckerman et al 1989). Maternal cocaine use can affect reproduction by adversely affecting the pregnancy, may directly injure the developing fetus, and/or may produce behavioural and developmental abnormalities in the neonate. Indirect toxicities of cocaine, which cannot be discussed further in this paper but which may present severe adverse health consequences for children, include child neglect and abuse, loss of family structure, as well as an increased risk of AIDS (acquired immune deficiency syndrome) and other congenitally acquired, sexually transmitted diseases. In addition, there are the economic burdens of prolonged hospitalization of newborns and of foster care.

Cocaine-associated obstetrical complications include an increased incidence of spontaneous abortion, abruption of the placenta, placenta praevia, and premature rupture of the membranes (Chasnoff et al 1989a,b). These complications, as well as fetal toxicities such as intrauterine growth retardation, are believed to result from the sympathomimetic effects of cocaine. Cocaine produces maternal and fetal hypertension and constricts uterine blood vessels, reducing uterine blood flow and presumably resulting in fetal ischaemia and hypoxia (Fig. 4). This pathophysiology has been supported by research in the

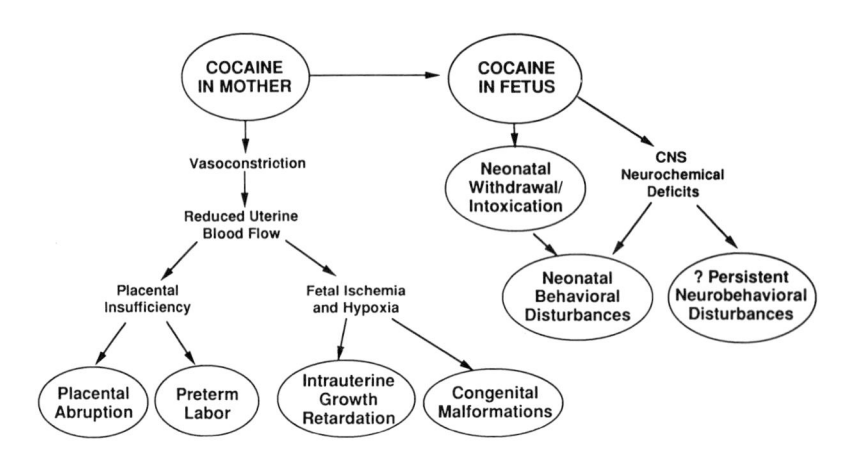

FIG. 4. Pathophysiology of reproductive disturbances due to cocaine abuse.

pregnant sheep, where intravenous cocaine given to the mother reduced uterine blood flow and fetal arterial oxygen tension (Woods et al 1987). In contrast, injection of cocaine directly into the fetus, while increasing fetal blood pressure and heart rate, did not result in changes in fetal oxygenation. These findings support the idea that maternal utero-placental circulatory disturbances are responsible for fetal hypoxaemia. Likewise, placental ischaemia is likely to be the cause of abruption of the placenta.

Congenital malformations, including those of the genitourinary tract and neural defects, have been reported in small surveys to be more frequent in babies of cocaine-using mothers than expected in babies of normal pregnancies (Chasnoff et al 1988), and have been demonstrated in mice (Finnell et al 1990). The mechanism of congenital malformation is unclear but could also be related to vascular insufficiency during critical stages of fetal development (Van Allen 1981).

Infants born to cocaine-abusing mothers may exhibit neurobehavioural abnormalities including abnormal sleep–wake cycles, tremulousness, poor feeding, hypotonia or hypertonia, and hyperreflexia (Oro & Dixon 1987). This syndrome in varying degrees may last for as long as eight to ten weeks. Of note, EEGs taken in neonates during the first week of life show a high percentage of abnormality (Doberczak et al 1988). Cocaine may be detected in the blood and urine of newborns of cocaine-using mothers. However, the rate and patterns of cocaine elimination from the human neonate have not yet been determined. The neonatal cocaine ('crack baby') syndrome could be a manifestation of cocaine intoxication and/or cocaine withdrawal. Cerebral infarction, possibly related to excessive vasoconstriction, has also been reported to occur with greater than expected frequency in babies of cocaine-abusing mothers.

Infants of such cocaine-abusing mothers may display irritability, agitation and delayed development (Oro & Dixon 1987). There is concern about delayed development and persistent neurobehavioural deficiencies. Such abnormalities could represent a toxic effect of cocaine *per se*, or result from a deficient home environment. Animal studies have shown that cocaine exposure *in vitro* retards neural development in the brain and may result in persistent neurochemical and behavioural deficits (Church & Overbeck 1990, Dow-Edwards et al 1990).

It should be recognized in any discussion of reproductive abnormalities related to cocaine abuse that there are many potential confounding factors to conclusions about causality. Confounding may arise from higher rates of cigarette smoking, alcohol and other drug abuse, poor prenatal health care, malnutrition, etc., all of which are associated with cocaine abuse and have also been associated with reproductive disturbances.

How toxic is cocaine?

Substance abuse is widely acknowledged to be a major health and social problem, and cocaine abuse is considered to be an important contributor to the substance abuse problem. This paper has focused so far on medical complications of cocaine abuse. An attempt will now be made to quantify the risks of such toxicity in cocaine users, in comparison to other drugs. It should be noted that because of the nature of the databases, other medical toxic effects of cocaine abuse, such as reproductive disturbances, neonatal complications, infectious complications and trauma, and non-medical 'toxicity' and societal costs, such as criminal activities, child neglect or lost job productivity, are not included in the relative risk estimations. Thus, any conclusions as to 'How toxic is cocaine?' will underestimate the full magnitude of the problem and cost to society.

In addition, the toxicity of cocaine appears to have changed over time. Medical complications were reported infrequently in the 1970s when cocaine use was mostly by sniffing among middle-class young people in the United States. Subsequently, cocaine use, presumably in higher doses, via intravenous injection or smoking, among people of lower socioeconomic class, many of whom are polydrug abusers, has become more toxic. Thus, my comments on the toxicity of cocaine address the toxicity of current use patterns in the United States and cannot necessarily be interpreted as describing the intrinsic toxicity of the drug.

The incidence of medical complications of cocaine use was evaluated using two databases collected prospectively in the United States. The Drug Abuse Warning Network (DAWN) collects reports from emergency departments in hospitals and medical examiners' offices throughout the United States on drug-related encounters and deaths, respectively (National Institute on Drug Abuse 1990). In 1989, 153 650 drug abuse episodes were reported from 770 hospitals in 21 cities, and 7162 drug abuse deaths were recorded in 87 medical examiners' offices in 27 areas in the USA. Limitations of the DAWN data include the

TABLE 3 Most frequent drugs in emergency department visits and medical examiner cases in the USA (1989 Dawn Report)

Drug	Most frequently mentioned drugs — No. of mentions	% total episodes	Medical Examiner data — No. of drug-related deaths	% total
Cocaine	61 665	40.1	3618[a]	50.5
Alcohol in combination	46 735	30.4	2778	38.8
Heroin/morphine	20 566	13.4	2743[b]	38.3
Codeine	—	—	840	11.7
Marijuana/hashish	9867	6.4	—	—
Acetaminophen	6456	4.2	—	—
Aspirin	5048	3.3	—	—
PCP/PCP combination	4899	3.2	—	—
Diazepam	4874	3.2	—	—

[a] In cocaine-related deaths—multiple drugs involved in 74% of cases.
[b] Includes opiates not specified as to type.

possibilities that emergency department staff miss drug-related episodes, that only occurrences that result in emergency department visits are identified, and that reports of drug use are based on self-report, often without toxicological confirmation. Several emergency department visits by the same person are also counted as separate occurrences. Data from medical examiners' offices may be judged to be drug related on the basis of either positive toxicology or circumstantial evidence. Also, as multiple drug use is very common, particularly in cocaine abusers, it cannot always be established which drug is the specific cause of death.

Relevant findings of the 1989 DAWN Report are summarized in Table 3. Cocaine ranked first in both total drug abuse episodes (61 665, 40.1%) and in drug-related deaths (3618, 50.5%). Alcohol in combination with other drugs (30.4% of encounters, 38.8% of deaths) and heroin/morphine (13.4%, 38.3%) were the next most highly ranked in these categories. Of note, 74% of cocaine deaths involved the co-ingestion of other drugs, primarily alcohol, opioids or cannabinoids (Fig. 5). Thus, toxicological investigations must consider the toxicity of cocaine combined with other drugs of abuse, particularly alcohol and heroin.

A second source of information that was reviewed was the 1990 Annual Report of the American Association of Poison Centers (AAPC) (Litovitz et al 1991). The AAPC surveyed 72 Poison Centers covering an area corresponding to 76.8% of the US population. In 1990, 1 713 462 human exposure cases were analysed. The limitations of this database are that only spontaneous calls from affected individuals or health care personnel to Poison Centers are available for analysis.

How toxic is cocaine?

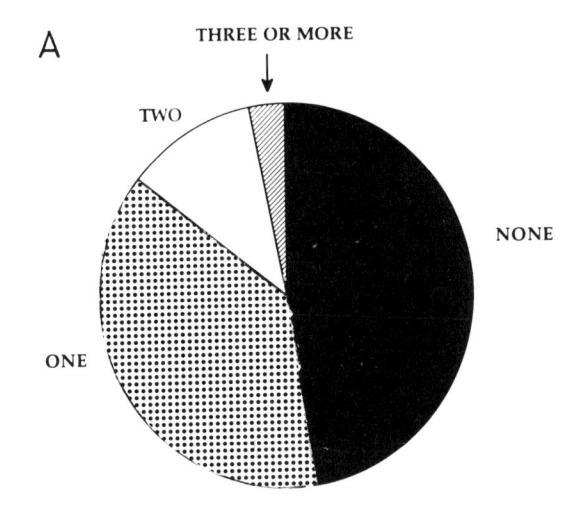

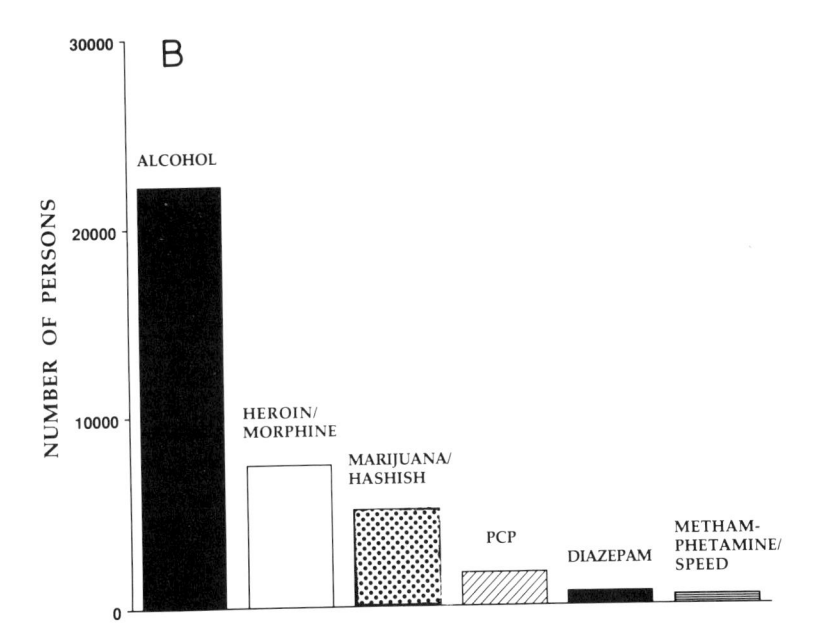

FIG. 5. Pie chart (A) shows proportions of cocaine episodes involving other drugs. Bar graph (B) shows the numbers of cocaine episodes in which other drugs were concomitantly abused. PCP, phencyclidine. Based on 1989 DAWN report (National Institute on Drug Abuse 1990).

TABLE 4 American Poison Center consultations and outcomes involving drugs of abuse (1990 AAPC Annual Report)

Drug	Total no. of exposures	Treated in health care facility	Outcome Moderate[a]	Major[a]	Death[a]	(Death rate per 1000 exposures)
Cocaine	2431	2261	319	82	32	(13.2)
Heroin	527	486	107	36	9	(17.0)
Amphetamines	4340	2840	337	46	6	(1.4)
Phencyclidine	267	242	54	13	2	(7.5)
Marijuana	716	503	51	8	1	(1.4)
LSD	1025	828	138	9	0	(0)

[a]Moderate outcome: symptoms that are pronounced, prolonged and/or systemic, usually requiring treatment.
Major outcome: symptoms that are life-threatening or resulted in residual disability or disfigurement.
Death as a result of the exposure or a direct complication of the exposure.
LSD, lysergic acid diethylamide.

How toxic is cocaine?

TABLE 5 Prevalence of drug use in USA according to NIDA National Household Surveys (1988 and 1990) on drug abuse

Cocaine	Year	Use in past year (%) Male	Female	Total	Use in past year (1000s of population)[a] Male	Female	Total	Mean
Cocaine	1990	4.3	2.0	3.1	4130	2117	6247	7227
	1988	5.6	2.8	4.1	5276	2932	8208	
PCP	1990	0.2	0.1	0.2	155	152	307	342
	1988	0.3	0.1	0.2	257	120	377	
Hallucinogens (PCP, LSD, etc)	1990	1.7	0.6	1.1	1591	676	2266	2676
	1988	2.4	0.8	1.6	2238	847	3085	
Marijuana	1990	12.1	8.4	10.2	11 656	8798	20 454	20 776
	1988	13.4	8.1	10.6	12 724	8375	21 099	
Cigarettes	1990	35.3	29.0	32.0	34 056	30 416	64 472	66 151
	1988	38.2	30.5	34.2	36 276	31 555	67 831	

[a]Estimate considering the total noninstitutionalized civilian population of the United States. PCP, phencyclidine. LSD, lysergic acid diethylamide.

Thus, the true incidence of drug abuse cases is greater than that reported in the AAPC survey. Cocaine-related medical problems that can be handled by health care personnel without Poison Center consultation also will not be recorded. As with the DAWN database, drug use is primarily by self-report, without toxicological confirmation in most cases. Because Poison Control Centers tend to be consulted on the management of more severe intoxications, the fraction of cases with serious complications is likely to be higher in the AAPC survey than in the DAWN data.

Data from the 1990 AAPC Annual Report are shown in Table 4. Among substances of abuse, cocaine was implicated in more major medical complications and deaths than any other. Case fatality rates (that is, deaths per 1000 exposures) were highest for heroin (17.0) and cocaine (13.2); both rates were considerably higher than those for any other drugs surveyed. Both the DAWN and the AAPC databases indicate that cocaine is a major cause of mortality and morbidity among drug abusers in the United States.

To assess the incidence of adverse health effects per population of drug users, the 1989 DAWN database was compared with data from the 1988 and 1990 NIDA National Household Surveys on Drug Abuse (National Institute on Drug Abuse 1989, 1991). These were surveys of 8814 (1988) and 9259 (1990) households in the United States in 1988 and 1990, respectively. The data were derived from direct interviews in the home as well as self-administered questionnaires. Household members aged 12 and older were included. Households were selected using a random sampling procedure controlled for

TABLE 6 Rates of emergency department mentions and medical examiner cases in 1989 per 1000 persons using drugs in the past year in the USA

Drug	ED mentions (per 1000 users)[a]	Medical examiner cases (per 1000 users)[b]
Cocaine	15.1	0.50
Phencyclidine	23.7	0.62
Marijuana	1.0	0.01
Cigarettes	—	(6.3)[c]

[a]Based on DAWN weighted emergency department (ED) estimates and NIDA household use survey data, as described in the text.
[b]Based on an unknown fraction of the US population, hence values underestimate true rate.
[c]Based on 420 000 deaths among the entire United States population.

the race-ethnicity and age of household members, and samples were obtained from various parts of the same areas. The estimates of drug abuse are probably underestimates because certain high-use populations, such as people in jails and the homeless, as well as people in military installations, college dormitories and hotels, are excluded.

Results from the 1988 and 1990 surveys for selected drugs of abuse are shown in Table 5. Among illicit drugs, the rate of cocaine use within the past year was second only to that of marijuana. An average of 3.1% (6.2 million) and 10.2% (20.5 million) of the US population used cocaine and marijuana, respectively, during 1990.

The population rates of emergency department visits were estimated from the 1989 DAWN weighted emergency department estimates (weighted to estimate the number of emergency department visits in the entire coterminous USA—i.e. excluding Alaska and Hawaii) and the household use survey data (Table 6). It is estimated that 15.1 of every 1000 people who used cocaine in 1989 were seen in an emergency room for a drug-related problem. The rate is even higher for phencyclidine (23.7), but much lower for marijuana/hashish (1.0). No weighted national data for medical examiner cases are available, but an idea of the relative death rates for different illicit drugs can be obtained using the DAWN medical examiner and the household use survey data. Cocaine and phencyclidine use were associated with comparable rates of death, which were 50 times or more greater than that associated with marijuana use.

Of considerable interest, however, is the contrast between cocaine and cigarette smoking. Taking the household data for cigarette use and the current US estimate of 420 000 tobacco-related deaths per year, the yearly death rate for tobacco (6.3 per 1000 smokers) is tenfold higher than that for cocaine or phencyclidine. Even considering that the medical examiner data underestimate total mortality and that many of the health and societal costs of cocaine are not included in the population rate estimates, cigarette smoking is still likely to be considerably more toxic per individual 'user'. Of course, smoking-related deaths occur after many years of cigarette smoking, whereas cocaine deaths are usually related to acute intoxication and affect a younger age group.

Conclusions

Cocaine abusers pay a considerable price for their habit. Cocaine abuse is associated with sudden death and a number of life-threatening complications involving many organ systems. Cocaine abuse is also associated with significant reproductive disturbances, psychiatric problems and other adverse effects on health. Currently in the USA, cocaine abuse is associated with more emergency department visits and more deaths than is any other illicit drug of abuse. The rates of emergency department visits and of death associated with cocaine use (excluding AIDS and trauma) are substantial and far exceed those of the most commonly abused illicit drug, marijuana. However, it is sobering to view cocaine abuse in the context of the abuse of licit drugs. Both the total number of deaths and the rate of deaths are far greater for cigarette smoking than for cocaine.

Acknowledgements

Research supported in part by grants DA01696 and DA02829 from the National Institute on Drug Abuse. The author thanks Ms Kaye Welch for preparation of the manuscript.

References

Ambre JJ, Belknap SM, Nelson J, Ruo TI, Shin S, Atkinson AA Jr 1988 Acute tolerance to cocaine in humans. Clin Pharmacol Ther 44:1–8

Brody SL, Slovis CM, Wrenn KD 1990 Cocaine-related medical problems: consecutive series of 233 patients. Am J Med 88:325–331

Chasnoff IJ, Chisum GM, Kaplan WE 1988 Maternal cocaine use and genitourinary tract malformations. Teratology 37:201–204

Chasnoff IJ, Griffith DR, MacGregor S, Dirkes K, Burns KA 1989a Temporal patterns of cocaine use in pregnancy. JAMA (J Am Med Assoc) 261:1741–1744

Chasnoff IJ, Lewis DE, Griffith DR, Willey S 1989b Cocaine and pregnancy: clinical and toxicological implications for the neonate. Clin Chem 35:1276–1278

Church MW, Overbeck GW 1990 Prenatal cocaine exposure in the Long-Evans rat. II. Dose-dependent effects on offspring behavior. Neurotoxicol Teratol 12:335–343

Derlet RW, Albertson TE 1989 Emergency department presentation of cocaine intoxication. Ann Emerg Med 18:182–186

Doberczak TM, Shanzer S, Senie RT, Kandall SR 1988 Neonatal neurologic and electroencephalographic effects of intrauterine cocaine exposure. J Pediatr 133:354–358

Dow-Edwards DL, Freed LA, Fico TA 1990 Structural and functional effects of prenatal cocaine exposure in adult rat brain. Dev Brain Res 57:263–268

Finnell RH, Toloyan S, Van Waes M, Kalivas PW 1990 Preliminary evidence for a cocaine-induced embryopathy in mice. Toxicol Appl Pharmacol 103:228–237

Fishbain DA, Wetli CV 1981 Cocaine intoxication, delirium, and death in a body packer. Ann Emerg Med 10:531–532

Foltin RW, Fischman MW 1991 Smoked and intravenous cocaine in humans: acute tolerance, cardiovascular and subjective effects. J Pharmacol Exp Ther 257:247-261

Gawin FH, Kleber HD 1986 Abstinence symptomatology and psychiatric diagnosis in cocaine abusers. Arch Gen Psychiatry 43:107-113

Isner JM, Chokshi SK 1991 Cardiac complications of cocaine abuse. Annu Rev Med 42:133-138

Jacob P III, Jones RT, Benowitz NL, Shulgin AT, Lewis ER, Elias-Baker BA 1990 Cocaine smokers excrete a pyrolysis product, anhydroecgonine methyl ester (methylecgonidine). J Toxicol Clin Toxicol 28:121-125

Jones LF, Tackett RL 1990 Chronic cocaine treatment enhances the responsiveness of the left anterior descending coronary artery and the femoral artery to vasoactive substances. J Pharmacol Exp Ther 255:1366-1370

Jones RT 1990 The pharmacology of cocaine smoking in humans. In: Chiang CN, Hawks RL (eds) Research findings on smoking of abused substances. (National Institute on Drug Abuse Research Monograph 99) US Government Printing Office, Washington, DC, p 30-41

Kabas JS, Blanchard SM, Matsuyama Y et al 1990 Cocaine-mediated impairment of cardiac conduction in the dog: a potential mechanism for sudden death after cocaine. J Pharmacol Exp Ther 252:185-191

Kosten TR, Kleber HD 1988 Rapid death during cocaine abuse: a variant of the neuroleptic malignant syndrome? Am J Drug Alcohol Abuse 14:335-346

Lange RA, Cigarroa RG, Yancy CW Jr et al 1989 Cocaine-induced coronary-artery vasoconstriction. N Engl J Med 321:1557-1562

Litovitz TL, Bailey KM, Schmitz BF, Holm KC, Klein-Schwartz W 1991 1990 Annual Report of the American Association of Poison Control Centers National Data Collection System. Am J Emerg Med 9:461-509

Mittleman RE, Wetli CV 1987 Cocaine and sudden 'natural' death. J Forensic Sci 32:11-19

Mueller PD, Benowitz NL, Olson KR 1990 Cocaine. Emerg Med Clin North Am 8:481-493

Nademanee K, Gorelick DA, Josephson MA et al 1989 Myocardial ischemia during cocaine withdrawal. Ann Intern Med 111:876-880

National Institute on Drug Abuse 1989 National Household Survey on Drug Abuse: 1988 Population Estimates. DHHS Publication No. (ADM) 891636. Alcohol, Drug Abuse, and Mental Health Administration, Washington, DC

National Institute on Drug Abuse 1990 Statistical Series. Annual Data 1989: Data from the Drug Abuse Warning Network Series 1, No. 9. DHHS Publication No. (ADM) 901717. Alcohol, Drug Abuse, and Mental Health Administration, Washington, DC

National Institute on Drug Abuse 1991 National Household Survey on Drug Abuse: 1990 Population Estimates. DHHS Publication No. (ADM) 911732. Alcohol, Drug Abuse, and Mental Health Administration, Washington, DC

Oro S, Dixon SD 1987 Perinatal cocaine and methamphetamine exposure. Maternal and neonatal correlates. J Pediatr 111:571-578

Patel R, Haider B, Ahmed S, Regan TJ 1988 Cocaine-related myocardial infarction: high prevalence of occlusive coronary thrombi without significant obstructive atherosclerosis. Circulation 78:1739 (abstr)

Strategy Council on Drug Abuse 1973 Federal strategy for drug abuse and drug traffic prevention. US Government Printing Office, Washington, DC

Tardiff K, Gross E, Wu J, Stajic M, Millman R 1989 Analysis of cocaine-positive fatalities. J Forensic Sci 34:53-63

Togna G, Tempesta E, Togna AR, Dolci N, Cebo B, Caprino L 1985 Platelet responsiveness and biosynthesis of thromboxane and prostacyclin in response to in vitro cocaine treatment. Haemostasis 15:100–107
Van Allen MI 1981 Fetal vascular disruptions: mechanisms and some resulting birth defects. Pediatr Ann 10:31–50
Wetli CV, Fishbain DA 1985 Cocaine-induced psychosis and sudden death in recreational cocaine users. J Forensic Sci 30:873–880
Woods JR Jr, Plessinger MA, Clark KE 1987 Effect of cocaine on uterine blood flow and fetal oxygenation. JAMA (J Am Med Assoc) 257:957–961
Zimmerman FH, Gustafson GM, Kemp HG 1987 Recurrent myocardial infarction associated with cocaine abuse in a young man with normal coronary arteries: evidence for coronary artery spasm culminating in thrombosis. J Am Coll Cardiol 9:964–968
Zuckerman B, Frank DA, Hingson R et al 1989 Effects of maternal marijuana and cocaine use on fetal growth. N Engl J Med 320:762–768

DISCUSSION

Negrete: Dr Benowitz, I am interested in the question of cardiac lesions, which we originally assumed were of two kinds, either ischaemic lesions (temporary or otherwise) or conduction lesions—the slowing down of interventricular conduction and other kinds of arrhythmia. But last year there was a convincing pathological report on 'cocaine' myocarditis—straightforward myocarditis (Maillet et al 1991). Is there such a thing? Also, clinicians have sometimes used propranolol for the accelerated pulse and borderline hypertension that some of our cocaine patients present. I assume that this is no longer recommended?

Benowitz: There is good evidence for myocarditis developing during intoxication with cocaine (Peng et al 1989, Karch & Billingham 1988). Conditions associated with very high circulating levels of catecholamines (the prototypic human condition is a pheochromocytoma, a tumour that secretes catecholamines) produce myocarditis with areas of focal necrosis, as well as contraction band necrosis. This is very much the picture seen in sudden deaths associated with cocaine. It is also seen with electrocution, and has been reported in people dying in aeroplane crashes. This type of myocardial injury may be a common response to massive catecholamine release. In addition to acute myocarditis, there are also a few instances of chronic cocaine abusers who have developed chronic myocardial scarring. The result may be a chronic dilated cardiomyopathy with congestive heart failure (Wiener et al 1986, Hogya & Wolfson 1990).

The reason for concern about propranolol is related to the high circulating concentrations of adrenaline (epinephrine) in cocaine-intoxicated people. If one gives propranolol in the presence of adrenaline, β-mediated vasodilatation is blocked, leaving unopposed α-adrenergic vasoconstriction. The result is aggravation of hypertension. There have been cases where cocaine-intoxicated patients have been given propranolol, which slowed the heart rate, but worsened the hypertension (Ramoska & Sacchetti 1985), which can lead to stroke and other complications. Thus if one needs to use β-blockers to treat cocaine-induced tachycardia or other arrhythmias, one should use a $β_1$-specific blocker such as metoprolol that works on the heart but not on the blood vessels.

Edwards: How confident are you of a unicausal explanation of cocaine toxicity in these probably often rather deprived, multi-problem young mothers, and how far is there evidence for a parallel toxicity in animal experiments?

Benowitz: In humans it's not possible to draw conclusions about unicausality, because most cocaine abusers also abuse alcohol or tobacco, or have poor prenatal care or are malnourished, or have some combination of these factors. It is felt however that some of the suspected cocaine-related toxicities—for example, the sorts of congenital malformations, or the clinical features of the 'crack baby' syndrome—have characteristics that are somewhat different from those that result from the effects of alcohol or tobacco.

In animal studies, fetal injury—brain abnormalities, congenital abnormalities— can be induced in rodents, by feeding cocaine to the pregnant rat or mouse (Dow-Edwards et al 1990, Finnell et al 1990). Some of the aspects of the pathophysiology, such as changes in uterine blood flow and fetal ischaemia, have been well documented in experimental animals (Woods et al 1987). The relative contribution of cocaine compared to that of other drugs in producing a particular fetal or neonatal toxicity is however hard to sort out.

Almond: Your comparison of cocaine use with cigarette smoking might seem to the casual listener to cancel out many of the points you made about its adverse consequences. I think it is therefore worth emphasizing the point you made briefly in your paper: that the cocaine-related incidents are affecting very young people, 20-year-olds and teenagers. The measure of comparison that is used with AIDS is 'lost years of expected life'. If you used that measure, you perhaps wouldn't get quite such a contrast between cigarette smoking and cocaine.

Benowitz: That is a very good point.

Maynard: If one is trying to measure the cost of cocaine use, whether you take the life-years approach, or the loss of GNP (gross national product), I think both measures have government health warnings associated with them! If you take the lost life years, it's clear that tobacco and alcohol, *even when* young people dying from drugs are taken into account, are much more efficient ways of killing people and removing life years. But even when you do these life-years calculations, or look at the GNP lost from premature death, you have to ask: 'so what?' It is an interesting but useless statistic, because the policy-maker wants to know the answer to a different question—not what the loss is, but what investments in which areas will reduce the loss. Should money be invested in health promotion, or in law enforcement activities? If you begin to look at costs in this way, you have to take great care.

Jaffe: What we are considering here primarily, and what was covered in Neal Benowitz's talk, is 'medical' toxicity. But with all the psychoactive drugs one has to deal with another form of toxicity that may not show up in emergency rooms or the coroner's office. I can conceive of a drug whose effects might be such that *other* people show up in the emergency room and in the coroner's office, not the people who use the drugs!

Cocaine is one of those drugs. It induces a kind of irritability and aggression and paranoia. I am not sure that this is a major issue, but conceptually we have to look at the behavioural consequences of drug use when trying to assess how society ought to respond to the drug. Marijuana has low toxicity, in terms of its biological activity on most organ systems, but in some of the ways it affects people's relationships and behaviour, it has a different and less predictable range of toxicities. For cocaine we must consider the wider range of issues as well as the more medical aspects.

Kalant: The DAWN (Drug Abuse Warning Network) data, and any emergency department data, always reflect not only the actual toxicity of the drug, but the degree of concern or alarm of the person who has used it. Twenty or so years ago there was a much higher percentage of cannabis cases than now, because people were experiencing cannabis under circumstances in which it was still a novelty, and they got frightened by symptoms which are now more familiar. It might be useful if we could separate out from the total reported cases those that reflect truly serious medical situations that warrant an emergency room call and require treatment, and to list those separately from the total statistics.

Fischman: I want to add to the concept of behavioural toxicity the idea of preoccupation with drug-seeking and drug-taking. These are important aspects of drug toxicity. They include lost productivity, or the lost time in which people can engage in more socially appropriate behaviour.

Anthony: I have to say that the epidemiologists have done a bad job of providing toxicologists and pharmacologists with the evidence required to assess cocaine's impact on public health consequences of the emergency room type, also the behavioural consequences, and also its impact on the aspects of life that might be impaired by too great a preoccupation with drug-seeking. I would urge extreme caution in the evaluation of the ratio of DAWN cocaine emergency room 'mentions' to the total number of active cocaine users as an index of the intrinsic toxicity of cocaine. If you had used data from 1982, or 1979, Dr Benowitz, the ratios would have been dramatically different, in that cocaine was accounting for many fewer emergency department episodes; yet that was the peak of the epidemic for 18- to 25-year-olds, who account for most of those emergency room visits.

Part of what we have to understand is the evolution that Dr Kalant described, namely that as different experiences with the drugs accumulate, a different profile of user presents itself to the emergency department. For this reason, the ratio of 'mentions' to users in any given year is not something constant (unlike, say, the plasma levels of cocaine taken by different routes, which I suspect could be replicated). If we look at the annual ratios of emergency room 'mentions' to users we shall find considerable variations even from one year to the next. This suggests to me that the epidemiological evidence available now is too flimsy to give us a picture of the intrinsic toxicity of cocaine.

Des Jarlais: Most people who work with the DAWN data treat it as trend, qualitative data rather than absolute, quantitative data, and would not calculate ratios. They would not use arithmetical operations like division or even addition.

Edwards: So you are warning us against over-confident interpretations?

Des Jarlais: Yes. In terms of medical examiner (coroner) data, there was a period of 4–5 years when New York City ceased to report, so for this time the national data were seriously incomplete. The DAWN system is now trying to make the emergency room visits a nationally representative sample; they were previously purely a convenience sample, so you could not generalize to the USA as a whole. Most people working with those data treat them as indicating trends that may reflect something happening in the real world, but comparisons and quantification ratios are considered to go beyond the quality of the data. The National Household Survey data for cocaine use are highly questionable also, because of suspected under-reporting.

Negrete: The point is worth noting that when the rate of cocaine use peaked, there were lower figures for cocaine in the DAWN data. But we should remember two things. First, chronic users have accumulated more years of use now; second, there are new patterns of use which became more prevalent after 1980, and are more hazardous. Smoking crack is worse than snorting cocaine, as far as the possibilities of health complications are concerned. The DAWN data are 'soft' data in many ways, as has been said, but with the same approach and the same method of collection, the profile has changed over the years. In 1980, heroin was the first cause of drug-related deaths, according to the medical examiners' data in the DAWN system. With the same way of registering things, the profile has changed over the years. Obviously cocaine has become the problem of most concern now.

Kleber: Our position at the Office of National Drug Control Policy on DAWN is that (as Dr Des Jarlais said) it should not be treated from a quantitative point of view, but viewed instead as an instrument that may have a 'constant error' built in. That is, the emergency rooms were making the same mistakes in 1988 or 1986, for example, so we should consider it as trend data rather than quantitatively exact data.

The reasons for cocaine deaths are partly the toxicity and partly the lack of appropriate treatment for overdose. With heroin we have naloxone, which is likely to save someone brought to the emergency room with a heroin overdose. But we don't have any comparable way to treat cocaine overdose and have to just give symptomatic treatment. This is another reason for the increased cocaine toxicity.

Benowitz: It's been my experience that most cocaine-intoxicated people who reach hospital alive will survive; very few die in the hospital as a result of the direct toxic effects of cocaine. I do not think an antagonist will really help. Most serious injury from cocaine, such as brain injury, occurs before victims reach the hospital. I don't think we have a problem in treating cocaine toxicity in the hospital.

Kleber: You referred to our paper on sudden death after cocaine in which we speculated that it was similar to a neuromalignant-like syndrome (Kosten & Kleber 1988). The classic case we were seeing was someone who had binged on cocaine, becoming very paranoid and hyperactive, and often behaving violently. The police would be called and had to wrestle the person down. Sudden death would occur in the vehicle going to the hospital or after arrival there and it would at times be attributed to 'police brutality'. Our belief was that this was in fact sudden death from cocaine, often accompanied by a fever of 104–106 °F. If subjects did live to get to the hospital they were sometimes treated inappropriately, by being given a neuroleptic, which makes that syndrome worse. I have not followed this since; what is the current thinking?

Benowitz: The largest number of cases of the hyperpyrexia and malignant hyperthermia type syndrome have come from Florida (Wetli & Fishbain 1985; A.J. Ruttenber, personal communication). A great many patients have been reported. Most look like the patient you describe. Whether the pathogenesis of hyperpyrexia is seizures or muscular hyperactivity because of agitation, or a central amphetamine-like effect, or a combination, is unclear. It has also been speculated that street cocaine may be contaminated with anticholinergic chemicals such as benzoyltropine and tropacocaine, which could inhibit sweating and further aggravate hyperpyrexia (Meyer et al 1990). The pathogenesis is unclear, but the phenomenon, since you reported it, has been well documented.

Strang: How far could one extend the experience of black market product refinement from cocaine to the amphetamines? The smokable methylamphetamine problem is very different from amphetamine snorting. Do you think the differences that you are seeing between amphetamines and cocaine are dose related or route related, and would you expect to see the same effects?

Benowitz: We see virtually all the same toxic effects with amphetamines and cocaine. But because amphetamine is so long-acting, people don't tend to take the huge amounts over a very short period of time that they do of cocaine. Differences in toxicity between amphetamine and cocaine I believe are related primarily to differences in the dose and route of dosing. Concerning smoked methamphetamine ('ice'), we haven't seen many cardiovascular complications; we mostly see neuropsychiatric disturbances. But in theory we could expect to see all of the same medical complications that one sees with cocaine.

Edwards: I argued at the beginning of the symposium that there are two perspectives—the experimental animal study, and the peasant woman arrested in Bolivia—and that it could be difficult to bring them together as the symposium unfolded. And of course it is difficult; there's no reason why the person talking about the forefront of molecular biology should try to talk about anthropology at the same time, or should genuflect towards social and cultural sensitivity and history; and there's no reason why the historians should try to reciprocate. I nevertheless was interested in your story of the young man who is brought in off the street with a plastic bag in his mouth and is found to be brain damaged. The one culture will of course debate what happened to his sympathetic storm, or what happened to his heart, what blew his brain. There is also the question of why he swallowed the cocaine, which is an entirely different issue. It was evidently because he knew that cocaine was illegal, and that he would be in trouble if the police got him; he preferred taking the risk of swallowing this bag (presumably not realizing the magnitude of the risk) to the risk of being arrested. There are researchable issues here, relating to the prevention of cocaine-induced harm.

References

Dow-Edwards DL, Freed LA, Fico TA 1990 Structural and functional effects of prenatal cocaine exposure in adult rat brain. Dev Brain Res 57:263–268

Finnell RH, Toloyan S, Van Waes M, Kalivas PW 1990 Preliminary evidence for a cocaine-induced embryopathy in mice. Toxicol Appl Pharmacol 103:228–237

Hogya PT, Wolfson AB 1990 Chronic cocaine abuse associated with dilated cardiomyopathy. Am J Emerg Med 8:203–204

Karch SB, Billingham ME 1988 The pathology and etiology of cocaine-induced heart disease. Arch Pathol Lab Med 112:225–230

Kosten TR, Kleber HD 1988 Rapid death during cocaine abuse: a variant of the neuroleptic malignant syndrome? Am J Drug Alcohol Abuse 14:335–346

Maillet M, Chiarasini D, Nahas G et al 1991 Altérations myocardiques expérimentales chez l'animal par intoxication à la cocaine. Proceedings of the I Internationales Symposium gegen Drogen in der Schweiz. Verlag Menschenkenntnis, Zurich, p 597–606

Meyer EM, Potter LT, DeVane CL et al 1990 Effects of benzoyltropine and tropacocaine on several cholinergic processes in the rat brain. J Pharmacol Exp Ther 254:584–590

Peng S, French WJ, Pelikan PCD 1989 Direct cocaine cardiotoxicity demonstrated by endomyocardial biopsy. Arch Pathol Lab Med 113:842–845

Ramoska E, Sacchetti AD 1985 Propranolol-induced hypertension in treatment of cocaine intoxication. Ann Emerg Med 14:1112–1113

Wetli CV, Fishbain DA 1985 Cocaine-induced psychosis and sudden death in recreational cocaine users. J Forensic Sci 30:873–880

Wiener RS, Lockhart JT, Schwartz RG 1986 Dilated cardiomyopathy and cocaine abuse. Am J Med 81:699–701

Woods JR Jr, Plessinger MA, Clark KE 1987 Effect of cocaine on uterine blood flow and fetal oxygenation. JAMA (J Am Med Assoc) 257:957–961

Determinants of cocaine self-administration by laboratory animals

William L. Woolverton

Department of Pharmacological and Physiological Sciences, The University of Chicago, 947 East 58th Street, Chicago, IL 60637, USA

Abstract. The reinforcing effect of a drug is that effect that increases the probability that the drug will be self-administered again. Like other drug effects, a reinforcing effect is the result of an interaction between organism, drug and environment. Laboratory research using animal subjects has helped elucidate the contribution of each of these factors to the self-administration of cocaine. A substantial amount of research indicates that increased dopamine neurotransmission in the brain, particularly in mesolimbic and mesocortical regions, plays a major role in cocaine self-administration. Both indirect and direct dopamine agonists can function as positive reinforcers in animals, whereas noradrenergic and serotonergic (5-HT, 5-hydroxytryptamine) agonists have not been found to do so. In addition, evidence suggests that dopamine but not noradrenaline (norepinephrine) or serotonin antagonists can attenuate the reinforcing effect of cocaine. Environmental factors have also been shown to be critical determinants of the reinforcing effect of cocaine. The schedule of reinforcement essentially determines the rate and pattern of drug-maintained behaviour. In addition, punishing self-administration, increasing the value of alternative reinforcers that are available, and increasing the cost of cocaine have all been shown to decrease the reinforcing effect of cocaine. With regard to organismic factors, recent research has suggested that there are significant genetic determinants of cocaine consumption. Taken together these research findings in animals imply that certain individuals may be more sensitive to the reinforcing effect of cocaine but that cocaine abuse can be decreased by pharmacological or behavioural means or by a combination of the two.

1992 Cocaine: scientific and social dimensions. Wiley, Chichester (Ciba Foundation Symposium 166) p 149–164

Among the pharmacological effects of drugs of abuse is the reinforcing effect, which is that effect that increases the probability that the drug will be self-administered again (i.e. it strengthens its self-administration). If not for its reinforcing effects, a drug like cocaine would be of little interest, save as a local anaesthetic. In a real sense, then, the reinforcing effect of cocaine also maintains the behaviour of many drug abuse researchers. Clearly, its influence is pervasive. Knowledge of the determinants of the reinforcing effect of cocaine can make a substantial contribution to our understanding and solution of the problems that cocaine presents. Therefore, although the title of my chapter is cocaine self-administration in animals, what I shall really be discussing are the determinants of the reinforcing effect of cocaine.

Methods for studying drug self-administration in animal subjects were originally developed in the early 1960s. Several investigators developed techniques that involved implantation of chronic intravenous catheters through which drug injections could be delivered as a consequence of some behavioural response, usually a lever press (see Weeks 1962, Thompson & Schuster 1964). The subsequent application of the theoretical framework of the experimental analysis of behaviour to this preparation has made significant contributions to our understanding of the variables that determine reinforcing effects of drugs. It has become clear that many drugs delivered by any of several routes of administration can function as positive reinforcers to maintain behaviour in animals in essentially the same way that other positive reinforcers, such as food, maintain behaviour. In addition, almost without exception animals will self-administer with similar rates and patterns the same drugs that humans abuse. That is, this is a valid and reliable animal model of drug self-administration in humans.

Research using this model has made it clear that the reinforcing effects of drugs are determined by both pharmacological and environmental factors. More recently, genetic determinants of the effects of cocaine have begun to be elucidated (see e.g. George 1991, George & Goldberg 1988). The purpose of this chapter is to review research on cocaine self-administration in animals from the point of view of the first two categories of independent variable: pharmacological and environmental. Pharmacological determinants are those related to the mechanism of action of the drug, such as neurotransmitters and receptor interactions in the central nervous system (CNS). Environmental determinants are those relating to the behaviour/environment and, generally, are initiated outside the organism. Organismic determinants—that is, those related to differences between organisms that existed before drug exposure—will not be discussed because of limitations on length (for review see Pickens & Svikis 1988). A comprehensive understanding of cocaine abuse will necessarily include a complete knowledge of each of these categories and, ultimately, of their interaction. It is important to emphasize that an enormous amount of research has been done with cocaine self-administration in animals and that this review is, of necessity, selective. I have chosen experimental results that I feel make major points about the determinants of cocaine self-administration in animals. For more detailed treatment of these topics the reader is referred to the cited references and any of a number of published reviews (e.g. Johanson & Fischman 1990, Spealman & Goldberg 1978).

Pharmacological determinants

A major neuropharmacological effect of cocaine is to block the uptake of the monoamine neurotransmitters dopamine, noradrenaline (norepinephrine) and serotonin (5-HT, 5-hydroxytryptamine). In addition, cocaine is a local anaesthetic. Much research has been directed at establishing which of these actions or combinations of actions mediates the reinforcing effect of cocaine. This question has been addressed in a number of ways. One involves the self-administration of selective agonists. If a compound shares a pharmacological action with cocaine and functions as a positive reinforcer under the same conditions that cocaine functions as a positive reinforcer, then there is reason to suspect that the pharmacological action that they share plays a role in the reinforcing effect of cocaine. Obviously, it does not demonstrate that the common mechanism determines the reinforcing effect of both compounds, but it does imply that the mechanism merits further investigation.

A number of compounds with indirect agonist actions that are more-or-less selective for the particular monoamine neurotransmitters have been evaluated for reinforcing effects in several self-administration paradigms (see Ritz et al 1987 for a summary). Compounds that increase dopaminergic neurotransmission, by either releasing or blocking the re-uptake of dopamine, have consistently been found to function as positive reinforcers. Moreover, drugs that directly stimulate dopamine receptors can function as positive reinforcers in animals (Gill et al 1978, Yokel & Wise 1978). In contrast, neither the noradrenaline uptake blocker nisoxetine (Woolverton 1987) nor the 5-HT (serotonin) uptake blocker fluoxetine (K. E. Vanover & W. L. Woolverton, unpublished data) has been to found to maintain self-administration. These data suggest that increased dopaminergic neurotransmission plays a primary role in the reinforcing effect of cocaine, whereas noradrenaline and 5-HT actions do not. Interestingly, several local anaesthetics have been found to function as positive reinforcers (Ford & Balster 1977, Hammerbeck & Mitchell 1978, Johanson 1980). This is not a general effect of local anaesthetics, however, but seems to be limited to those local anaesthetics that are esters (Woolverton & Balster 1979); amide local anaesthetics have not been found to function as positive reinforcers. Since not all local anaesthetics function as positive reinforcers under these conditions, it seems unlikely that local anaesthetic actions are responsible for the reinforcing effect of cocaine. Rather, it is probably the case that local anaesthetics and cocaine share some other mechanism (the blockade of dopamine re-uptake) that is responsible for the reinforcing effects of these compounds.

A second pharmacological approach that has been used involves the possibility of antagonizing the reinforcing effect of cocaine. It has been known for some time that, under simple schedules of reinforcement, pretreatment of animals with dopamine antagonists can alter the rate of cocaine self-administration in a manner that is consistent with antagonism of the reinforcing effect of cocaine (Wilson & Schuster 1972, deWit & Wise 1977). This effect is not seen with selective noradrenaline or 5-HT antagonists (Risner & Jones 1976, Woolverton 1987). Although there is significant ambiguity in the interpretation of these effects (see Herling & Woods 1980), the results are consistent with the notion that dopamine plays a primary role in the reinforcing effect of cocaine.

There is more than one type of dopamine receptor in the CNS. Although the number of types appears to be growing, pharmacological data are clear for two types, which have been termed D_1 and D_2. The role of these two receptors in the reinforcing effect of cocaine has been examined in studies of both agonist self-administration and antagonist pretreatment, using receptor-selective compounds. Dopamine agonists that function as positive reinforcers have in common action at D_2 receptors (Woolverton et al 1984). In contrast, the D_1 agonist, SKF 38393, was not self-administered by monkeys over a wide range of doses.

Studies with antagonists have suggested that either D_1 or D_2 antagonists can attenuate the reinforcing effect of cocaine in animals (Bergman et al 1990, Koob et al 1987, Woolverton 1986). In our recent research with dopamine antagonists (Kleven & Woolverton 1990), rhesus monkeys were trained to press a lever under a three-component, multiple schedule of food and drug reinforcement. In the first and third components, food pellets are available under a fixed-ratio (FR) 30 schedule (in which every 30th response is reinforced by food). Pellet delivery is followed by a brief time-out, in which no lights are illuminated and responding has no consequence. Cocaine is available in the second component under the same schedule of reinforcement (FR 30) but with a longer 'time-out' after each injection. Although the response rate is usually slightly lower for cocaine than for food pellets, the patterns of responding are similar for the two reinforcers. This equivalence helps to control for effects of drugs that may depend upon the rate or pattern of responding. To maintain a preparation that is at equilibrium, at least with respect to the test drug, we infused antagonists via a syringe pump, 24 hours per day. When the D_1 antagonist SCH 23390 was administered under these conditions, cocaine-maintained responding was decreased at doses that did not affect food-maintained behaviour in two of the four monkeys tested (Fig. 1). That is, the D_1 antagonist apparently decreased the reinforcing effect of cocaine without altering behaviour maintained by another positive reinforcer. Interestingly, the magnitude of the decrease in cocaine-maintained behaviour diminished over the two-week infusion period, as if tolerance to cocaine were developing. When we redetermined the cocaine dose–response function after the treatment with SCH 23390, the curve was shifted to the left in all monkeys, suggesting that the monkeys had been sensitized to the reinforcing effect of cocaine.

The results of these experiments support the not altogether surprising conclusion that CNS pharmacology plays an important role in cocaine self-administration.

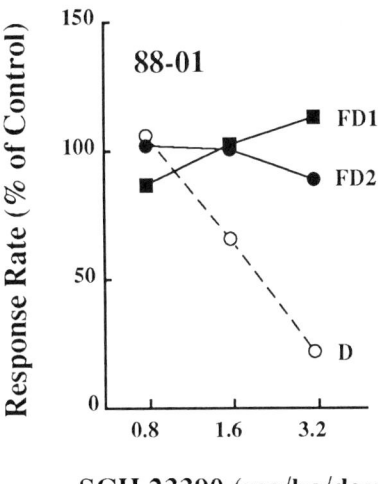

[Figure: Response Rate (% of Control) vs SCH 23390 (mg/kg/day) for monkey 88-01, showing FD1, FD2, and D curves at doses 0.8, 1.6, 3.2]

SCH 23390 (mg/kg/day)

FIG. 1. Effects of the D_1 dopamine antagonist SCH 23390 on responding maintained by cocaine or food in rhesus monkey 88-01. Response rate is expressed as a percentage of average rates of responding during control sessions ($n = 3$) which immediately preceded each dose of SCH 23390. The dose of cocaine maintaining responding was 0.1 mg/kg per injection. Doses of SCH 23390 were infused intravenously, 24 hours per day. FD1: first component in which food was available under an FR 30 schedule of reinforcement with a time-out after each reinforcer; D: the second component; cocaine was available under an FR 30 schedule of reinforcement with a time-out after each reinforcer; FD2: the third component; food was available under conditions identical to the FD1 component. For clarity, the variability is not shown, but in most cases it was less than 20% of control.

Specifically, blockade of dopamine re-uptake by cocaine appears to be the primary pharmacological action mediating its reinforcing effect. Across a relatively constant set of behavioural conditions, drugs that act primarily as agonists, either indirectly or directly, of dopaminergic systems in the brain, consistently functioned as positive reinforcers, while drugs that act primarily to block uptake of other monoamines, or are local anaesthetics, did not. Taken together with the self-administration data from direct agonists, the results of studies with antagonists suggest that stimulation of D_2 receptors is necessary for expression of the reinforcing effect of cocaine, whereas stimulation of D_1 receptors appears to be necessary but not sufficient for the expression of this effect. Such a role for D_1 receptors is consistent with their proposed role in other dopamine-mediated behaviours (Braun & Chase 1986, Walters et al 1987). Additional research has suggested that mesocortical and mesolimbic regions are the sites in the CNS where this effect of cocaine is initiated (Goeders & Smith 1983, Roberts & Koob 1982).

Environmental/behavioural determinants

Drug-seeking behaviour in humans is generally an extended sequence of behaviour that evolves over time and is ultimately maintained by the self-administration of a drug. The reinforcing effect of the drug is rarely the only consequence of drug-seeking and drug self-administration. Furthermore, drug-seeking and drug self-administration occur in the context of other behaviours that are maintained by consequences other than drug effects. Given these considerations, it is not surprising that cocaine self-administration is strongly determined by environmental factors. A number of these factors have begun to be elucidated in laboratory studies with animals. This research makes it clear that the rates and patterns of cocaine-maintained behaviour, indeed whether cocaine functions as a positive reinforcer at all, are strongly determined by the environmental circumstances under which it is made available.

The first environmental determinant to emphasize, and the one for which the most data are available, is the schedule of reinforcement. It is well established that cocaine can function as a positive reinforcer under a wide variety of schedules of reinforcement (for reviews see Spealman & Goldberg 1978, Johanson & Fischman 1990). Fixed-ratio schedules of cocaine injection maintain high rates of responding (Griffiths et al 1979, Winger & Woods 1985), fixed-interval schedules maintain positively accelerated rates of responding (Johanson 1982) and variable-interval schedules maintain moderate, steady rates of responding (Nader & Woolverton 1992, Spealman 1979). The brief presentation of stimuli that have been associated with a drug injection can greatly increase drug-seeking behaviour that is maintained by cocaine (Goldberg et al 1979). That is, the rate and pattern of cocaine-maintained behaviour are substantially determined by the environmental conditions of drug availability. In one study (Spealman 1979), the behaviour of squirrel monkeys was simultaneously maintained by cocaine injection and by the termination of cocaine availability—that is, cocaine was functioning as a positive and as a negative reinforcer simultaneously in the same monkey. Clearly, conditions of availability are major determinants of the behavioural effects of cocaine.

In human drug abusers, cocaine is rarely, if ever, the only reinforcer that is available to the organism. In addition, self-administration of cocaine has consequences for the user (such as punishment). Therefore, to more clearly understand the determinants of cocaine self-administration, we need to establish animal models in which cocaine is available under more complex environmental circumstances. To study the effects of punishment on cocaine self-administration, Johanson (1977) trained rhesus monkeys in a procedure (discrete-trials choice) that allowed the monkeys to choose between an injection of 0.1 mg/kg cocaine and an injection of an equivalent or higher dose of cocaine that also resulted in the simultaneous delivery of electric shock. That is, the

Cocaine self-administration by animals 155

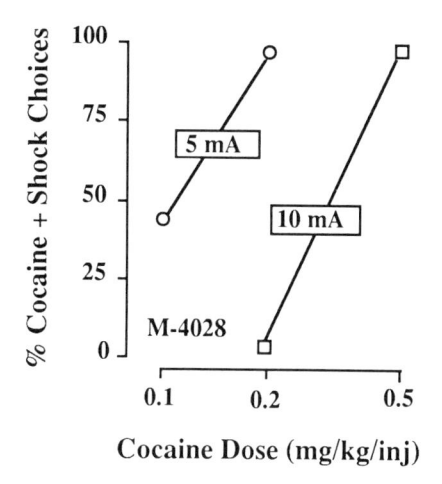

FIG. 2. Effects of punishment on cocaine self-administration in rhesus monkey M-4028. The graph represents the frequency of choice of the doses of cocaine indicated on the abscissa relative to 0.1 mg/kg per injection. The intensity of electric shock that was delivered with the injection of the high dose is indicated in the boxes. Redrawn from Johanson (1977).

choice was between two doses of cocaine, one of which was paired with the delivery of electric shock. When the shock was 5 mA (Fig. 2, 5 mA), there was little effect on preference: the 0.1 mg/kg cocaine injection was chosen as frequently when it was shocked as when it was unshocked. When the dose paired with 5 mA was increased to 0.2 mg/kg, preference for this dose increased to nearly 100%. However, when the shock intensity was increased to 10 mA, the preference for the 0.2 mg/kg injection was eliminated. Increasing the dose of cocaine again to 0.5 mg/kg per injection restored the preference for the shocked option. Thus, cocaine self-administration could be effectively punished by electric shock but, under these circumstances, suppression by punishment could be overcome by increasing the dose of cocaine that was available for self-administration.

Recently, we have begun a series of studies designed to examine the determinants of cocaine self-administration in an environment in which alternative non-drug positive reinforcers are available to the organism. We have utilized a 'discrete-trials choice' paradigm similar to that used by Johanson and Schuster (1975) and described in detail elsewhere (Woolverton & Balster 1981, Woolverton & Johanson 1984). Briefly, when a session begins, white lights are illuminated above the left lever and red or green lights are illuminated above the right lever. Red and green colours are each associated with one of the reinforcers, cocaine or food (one-gram banana-flavoured food pellets). Responding on the left lever changes the light colour above the right lever from red to green and from green to red. After a minimum of three colour changes, a monkey can choose between reinforcers by pressing the right lever when the light associated with that reinforcer is illuminated and completing the terminal link of the behavioural chain, an FR schedule on that lever. After the monkey has completed a choice, there is a 10 minute time-out, after which a new trial is initiated as before. Using this paradigm we have been investigating variables that influence the animals' choice between cocaine and a non-drug positive reinforcer, food.

The hypothesis of our first study (Nader & Woolverton 1991a) was that increasing the magnitude of the alternative reinforcer could decrease the frequency of cocaine choice. To test this hypothesis, we trained monkeys to choose between cocaine and food and varied the dose of cocaine that was available and the numbers of food pellets available as the alternative. The terminal link of the chain was an FR 30 for both reinforcers. When a given number of food pellets was available and the dose of cocaine was increased, the frequency of choice of cocaine increased (Fig. 3). On the other hand, when a given dose of cocaine was available and the number of food pellets available as the alternative to cocaine was increased from one to 16, the frequency of choice of cocaine decreased in all four monkeys that were studied. Put simply, the reinforcing effect of cocaine decreased as the magnitude of an alternative reinforcer that was simultaneously available increased. Carroll et al (1989) have also reported that the availability of an alternative positive reinforcer could decrease cocaine self-administration in rats.

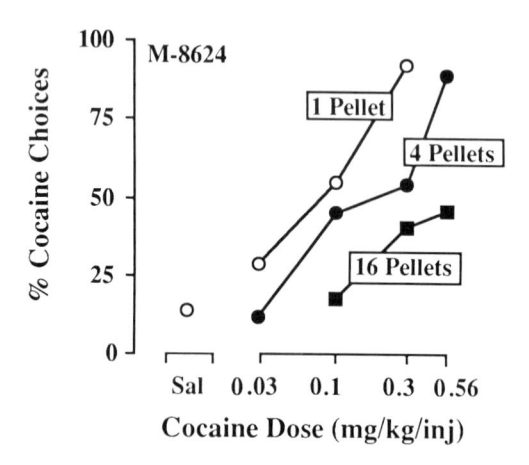

FIG. 3. Effects of increasing the magnitude of an alternative reinforcer on cocaine self-administration in rhesus monkey M-8624. The graph represents the frequency of choice of the doses of cocaine indicated on the abscissa relative to various numbers of food pellets available as the alternative. The numbers of food pellets are indicated in the boxes.

The hypothesis of our next study (Nader & Woolverton 1991b) was that increasing the *cost* of a cocaine injection relative to the cost of the alternative reinforcer would decrease the frequency of cocaine choice. To test this hypothesis, we trained monkeys in the same food–drug choice procedure and increased the number of lever presses (response cost) that were required in the terminal link of the chain for a cocaine injection while holding the response requirement for food (one or four food pellets) constant at 30. Under a given response cost, the frequency of cocaine choice increased as dose was increased (Fig. 4). However, at any given dose, the frequency of cocaine choice decreased as the response cost increased, again in all four monkeys studied. In fact, when the response cost was sufficiently high, the preference for cocaine could not be restored by increasing the cocaine dose up to 1.0 mg/kg per injection. As with the magnitude of the alternative reinforcer, increasing response cost for cocaine can dramatically decrease its reinforcing effect relative to that of an alternative positive reinforcer.

Conclusion

The basic conclusion of this review is one that has been made numerous times before, but of which we often seem to be in danger of losing sight: the reinforcing effect of cocaine is the result of an interaction between a drug, an organism and an environment. With regard to the pharmacological actions of cocaine,

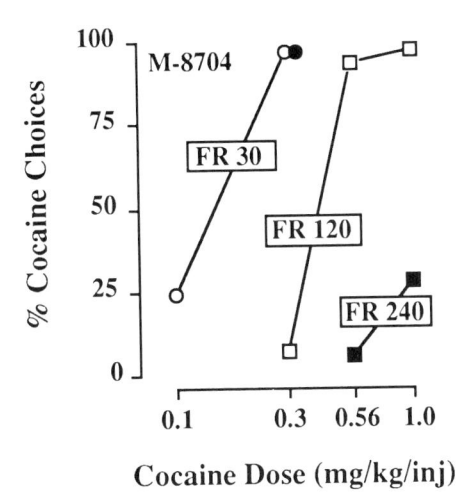

FIG. 4. Effects of increasing the response cost for cocaine on cocaine self-administration in rhesus monkey M-8704. The graph represents the frequency of choice of the doses of cocaine indicated on the abscissa relative to four food pellets available as the alternative. The number of responses required for an injection of cocaine is indicated in the boxes. The number of responses required for food was always 30.

the blockade of dopamine re-uptake, and the subsequent action of dopamine on its receptors of the D_2 type, appear to play a necessary role in the reinforcing effect of cocaine. In fact, direct stimulation of D_2 receptors is, apparently, sufficient to maintain self-administration in animals, at least under some conditions. However, the action of dopamine at D_1 receptors also seems to play an important role in the reinforcing effect of cocaine. The data on this point are at least consistent with the necessary-but-not-sufficient role that has been postulated for D_1 receptors in the expression of other dopamine-mediated behaviours. Although other monoamine neurotransmitters do not appear to mediate the reinforcing effect of cocaine directly, it is possible that they may play important modulatory roles in this effect of cocaine. For instance, it has been suggested that 5-HT may contribute an aversive component to the effects of cocaine (Loh & Roberts 1990). Moreover, little or nothing is known about the role that other neurotransmitters may play in the reinforcing effect of cocaine. Clearly, this is a fertile area for future research.

Although an increased concentration of dopamine in synapses in the CNS may be necessary, it is not sufficient for cocaine to exert its reinforcing effect. It is well to note that neuroleptics increase the concentration of dopamine in synapses in the CNS, but there is little concern about neuroleptic abuse. Reinforcing effects are determined by the environment as well. The schedule of reinforcement critically determines the rates and patterns of drug-maintained behaviour. Moreover, punishment, the availability of alternative reinforcers and response cost all determine whether or not cocaine has a reinforcing effect. In a sense, these are not surprising results. Recently, it has been argued that results such as these are consistent with well-established microeconomic theories of the consumption of any commodity (Bickel et al 1990). Although current rhetoric would often have one believe otherwise, these results emphasize that the self-administration of cocaine is governed by the same laws that govern behaviour maintained by other positive reinforcers.

One of the challenges of research on drug self-administration is the synthesis of the contributions of the drug, the organism and the environment to the self-administration of drugs. Clearly, self-administration research with animals has made substantial contributions to our understanding of this dynamic interaction. However, much remains to be learned. For instance, the possibility that the conditions of drug availability alter the neurobiology of cocaine—either the initiation of its effect or some downstream manifestation—should be investigated. Given the enormous number of environmental conditions that are known to modify drug effects, this is, at least for me, a sobering thought. Nevertheless, given technological advances such as *in vivo* microdialysis, it becomes increasingly possible to investigate these factors. From a more applied point of view, these data from animals imply that it should be possible to reduce human cocaine abuse pharmacologically with treatments that decrease the reinforcing effect of cocaine by modifying its basic neurobiological impact on the organism. At this point, at least, environmental changes appear to be effective as well. Given the interaction between the drug, the organism and the environment that determines the reinforcing effect of cocaine, one would predict that the combination of pharmacological and environmental changes might be the most effective strategy for reducing the reinforcing effect of cocaine. It is a challenge of future research to determine what those combinations might be.

Acknowledgements

Preparation of this manuscript was supported by grants DA 00250 and DA 00161 from the National Institute on Drug Abuse. I gratefully acknowledge the insightful comments of M. S. Kleven and M. A. Nader.

References

Bergman J, Kamien JB, Spealman RD 1990 Antagonism of cocaine self-administration by selective D_1 and D_2 antagonists. Behav Pharmacol 1:355–363

Bickel WK, DeGrandpre RJ, Higgins ST, Hughes JR 1990 Behavioral economics of drug self-administration. I. Functional equivalence of response requirement and drug dose. Life Sci 47:1501–1510

Braun AR, Chase TN 1986 Obligatory D-1/D-2 receptor interaction in the generation of dopamine agonist related behaviors. Eur J Pharmacol 131:301–306

Carroll ME, Lac ST, Nygaard SL 1989 A concurrently available non-drug reinforcer prevents the acquisition or decreases the maintenance of cocaine-reinforced behavior. Psychopharmacology 97:23–29

de Wit H, Wise RA 1977 Blockade of cocaine reinforcement in rats with the dopamine receptor blocker pimozide, but not with the noradrenergic blockers phentolamine or phenoxybenzamine. Can J Psychol Rev Can Psychol 31:195–203

Ford RD, Balster RL 1977 Reinforcing properties of intravenous procaine in rhesus monkeys. Pharmacol Biochem Behav 6:289–296

George FR 1991 Cocaine toxicity: genetic differences in cocaine-induced lethality in rats. Pharmacol Biochem Behav 38:893–895

George FR, Goldberg SR 1988 Genetic differences in responses to cocaine. In: Clouet D, Asghar K, Brown R (eds) Mechanisms of cocaine abuse and toxicity. (National Institute on Drug Abuse Research Monograph 88) US Government Printing Office, Washington, DC, p 239–249

Gill CA, Holz WC, Zirkle CL, Hill H 1978 Pharmacological modification of cocaine and apomorphine self-administration in the squirrel monkey. In: Deniker P, Radouco-Thomas C, Villeneuve A (eds) Proceedings of the Tenth Congress of Collegium International Neuro-Psychopharmacologicum. Pergamon Press, New York, p 1477–1484

Goeders NE, Smith JE 1983 Cortical dopaminergic involvement in cocaine reinforcement. Science (Wash DC) 221:773–775

Goldberg SR, Spealman RD, Kelleher RT 1979 Enhancement of drug-seeking behavior by environmental stimuli associated with cocaine or morphine injections. Neuropharmacology 18:1015–1017

Griffiths RR, Bradford LD, Brady JV 1979 Progressive ratio and fixed ratio schedules of cocaine-maintained responding in baboons. Psychopharmacology 65:125–136

Hammerbeck DM, Mitchell CL 1978 The reinforcing properties of procaine and d-amphetamine compared in rhesus monkeys. J Pharmacol Exp Ther 204:558–569

Herling S, Woods JH 1980 Chlorpromazine effects on cocaine-reinforced responding in rhesus monkeys: reciprocal modification of rate altering effects of the drugs. J Pharmacol Exp Ther 214:354–361

Johanson CE 1977 The effects of electric shock on responding maintained by cocaine injections in a choice procedure in the rhesus monkey. Psychopharmacology 53:277–282

Johanson CE 1980 The reinforcing properties of procaine, chloroprocaine and proparacaine in rhesus monkeys. Psychopharmacology 67:189–194

Johanson CE 1982 Behavior maintained under fixed-interval and second-order schedules of cocaine or pentobarbital in rhesus monkeys. J Pharmacol Exp Ther 221:384–393

Johanson CE, Fischman MW 1990 The pharmacology of cocaine related to its abuse. Pharmacol Rev 41:3–52

Johanson CE, Schuster CR 1975 A choice procedure for drug reinforcers: cocaine and methylphenidate in the rhesus monkey. J Pharmacol Exp Ther 193:676–688

Kleven MS, Woolverton WL 1990 Effects of continuous infusions of SCH 23390 on cocaine- or food-maintained behavior in rhesus monkeys. Behav Pharmacol 1:365–373

Koob GF, Le H, Creese I 1987 The D-1 dopamine receptor antagonist SCH 23390 increases cocaine self-administration in the rat. Neurosci Lett 79:315–320

Loh EA, Roberts DCS 1990 Break-points on a progressive ratio schedule reinforced by intravenous cocaine increase following depletion of forebrain serotonin. Psychopharmacology 101:262–266

Nader MA, Woolverton WL 1991a Effects of increasing the magnitude of an alternative reinforcer on drug choice in a discrete-trials choice procedure. Psychopharmacology 105:169–174

Nader MA, Woolverton WL 1991b Cocaine vs. food choice in rhesus monkeys: effects of increasing the response cost for cocaine. In: Harris LS (ed) Problems of drug dependence 1990. (National Institute on Drug Abuse Research Monograph 105) US Government Printing Office, Washington, DC, p 621

Nader MA, Woolverton WL 1992 Further characterization of adjunctive behavior generated by schedules of cocaine self-administration. Behav Pharmacol, in press

Pickens RW, Svikis DS 1988 (eds) Biological vulnerability to drug abuse. (National Institute on Drug Abuse Research Monograph 89) US Government Printing Office, Washington, DC

Risner ME, Jones BE 1976 Role of noradrenergic and dopaminergic processes in amphetamine self-administration. Pharmacol Biochem Behav 5:477–482

Ritz MC, Lamb RJ, Goldberg SR, Kuhar MJ 1987 Cocaine receptors on dopamine transporters are related to self-administration of cocaine. Science (Wash DC) 237:1219–1223

Roberts DCS, Koob GF 1982 Disruption of cocaine self-administration following 6-hydroxydopamine lesions of the ventral tegmental area in rats. Pharmacol Biochem Behav 17:901–904

Spealman RD 1979 Behavior maintained by termination of a schedule of self-administered cocaine. Science (Wash DC) 204:1231–1233

Spealman RD, Goldberg SR 1978 Drug self-administration by laboratory animals: control by schedules of reinforcement. Annu Rev Pharmacol Toxicol 18:313–339

Thompson T, Schuster CR 1964 Morphine self-administration, food-reinforced and avoidance behaviors in rhesus monkeys. Psychopharmacologia 5:87–94

Walters JR, Bergstrom DA, Carlson JH, Chase TN, Braun AR 1987 D1 dopamine receptor activation required for postsynaptic expression of D2 agonist effects. Science (Wash DC) 236:719–722

Weeks JR 1962 Experimental morphine addiction: method for automatic intravenous injections in unrestrained rats. Science (Wash DC) 138:143–144

Wilson MC, Schuster CR 1972 The effects of chlorpromazine on psychomotor stimulant self-administration in the rhesus monkey. Psychopharmacologia 26:115–126

Winger G, Woods JH 1985 Comparison of fixed-ratio and progressive-ratio schedules of maintenance of stimulant drug-reinforced responding. Drug Alcohol Depend 15:123–130

Woolverton WL 1986 Effects of a D_1 and a D_2 dopamine antagonist on the self-administration of cocaine and piribedil by rhesus monkeys. Pharmacol Biochem Behav 24:531–535

Woolverton WL 1987 Evaluation of the role of norepinephrine in the reinforcing effects of psychomotor stimulant in rhesus monkeys. Pharmacol Biochem Behav 26:835–839

Woolverton WL, Balster RL 1979 Reinforcing properties of some local anesthetics in rhesus monkeys. Pharmacol Biochem Behav 11:669–672

Woolverton WL, Balster RL 1981 The effects of antipsychotic compounds in rhesus monkeys given a choice between cocaine and food. Drug Alcohol Depend 8:69–78

Woolverton WL, Johanson CE 1984 Preference in rhesus monkeys given a choice between cocaine and d,l-cathinone. J Exp Anal Behav 41:35–43

Woolverton WL, Goldberg LL, Ginos JZ 1984 Intravenous self-administration of dopamine receptor agonists by rhesus monkeys. J Pharmacol Exp Ther 230:678–683

Yokel RA, Wise RA 1978 Amphetamine-type reinforcement by dopaminergic agonists in the rat. Psychopharmacology 58:289–296

DISCUSSION

Kalant: The concept of reinforcement, independently of any specific neurochemical mechanism, is strictly speaking an 'operant' term, which means that the consequence of a behaviour or action increases the probability of the repetition of the behaviour that produced that consequence. Given that food and cocaine in your studies were competing for, presumably, something that we measure by a single measure of reinforcement—the repetition of behaviour—can we draw any inferences of the existence of a *state*, as opposed to an observed behaviour, that can tell us what an effect on D_1 dopamine receptors does that makes people want to take cocaine? Does it enable us in any way to make projections or guesses as to what the change in the nervous system is that makes the animal or the human want to take this drug?

Woolverton: I think not. Part of the point of what I was saying is that, regardless of what is going on in the central nervous system as a result of the self-administration of cocaine, that self-administration is *not* simply determined by that effect. Does that answer your question?

Kalant: Strictly speaking it does, but the purpose behind my question is that there is a very common tendency to equate reinforcement with 'reward', and with human sensations of 'rush', or euphoria. I think your observations make the point very strongly that 'reinforcement', as observed behaviourally, tells us nothing about the subjective experience that leads to the repetition of drug taking. Therefore I am wondering whether it matters very much whether D_1 or D_2 receptors are acted on, in terms of intervention into human behaviour.

Woolverton: Certainly, pharmacology plays a role in the reinforcing effects of drugs—the effects that maintain self-administration. If one is interested in the possibility of developing therapeutic interventions for cocaine, then pharmacological blockade of those effects should be useful. I think it is a mistake to make assumptions about the subjective experience driving drug-taking.

Kalant: But could one develop a pharmacotherapeutic intervention that won't also decrease food intake, or water intake?

Woolverton: In fact, our data obtained with the D_1 antagonist argue that it is possible. Similar results have been found with opioid self-administration under antagonist treatment. But if the dopamine theory of reward is correct, and all behaviour maintained by dopamine-mediated reinforcement shares a final common pathway, we may be blocking reinforcement from all stimuli with neuroleptics.

Kuhar: Hasn't it been shown that food reward is in fact mediated through that dopamine system? If this is the case, then food competition with cocaine would be mediated through the same mechanism.

Fibiger: We have unpublished data showing that consumption of a palatable meal in rats causes a significant increase in dopamine release in the nucleus accumbens (in preparation). It is quite selective in that it does not occur in the caudate/putamen. So you could argue that when your monkeys are taking the food reward (banana-flavoured pellets), you are already elevating dopamine release to a certain extent. Under such circumstances, the animals might need less cocaine to achieve whatever desired level of dopamine release they are seeking to achieve. This could explain your behavioural data. I might also mention that we have found that sex also turns the meso-accumbens dopamine system on very dramatically! (Pfaus et al 1990.)

Balster: On the question of developing pharmacotherapies for cocaine use that interact with dopaminergic systems, it is premature to be too negative about this. If you were to consider methadone as an example of an effective therapeutic agent, and were to expect methadone to be effective as a treatment for opiate abuse at doses that didn't produce opiate-like effects, you would have a hard road to go. There is still a lot of work to be done to evaluate possible pharmacotherapies for cocaine. The animal models that Bill Woolverton discussed have merit in doing that. I personally am enthusiastic about developing *agonists* that could substitute for cocaine during treatment. It should be possible to develop drugs that have just the right agonistic efficacy, with a favourable onset and duration of action and with diminished abuse liability of their own, that could be useful at various stages of treatment.

My other point relates to the one that Dr Kalant was making, on the relevance of understanding the neurobiology of drug reinforcement to solving problems of drug abuse. In fact, the studies of Bill Woolverton, Mike Kuhar and Chris Fibiger, and my own studies, have supported the hypothesis that dopamine has a critical role in the reinforcing effects of cocaine. Clearly, this is at least one of the mechanisms of action of cocaine. What the 'dopamine hypothesis' doesn't explain is individual differences in the effects of cocaine. Why are some people abusers, and others not? Why do some people take cocaine today, and not tomorrow? Why do they take it now instead of 30 minutes from now? What are the bases for individual differences and the situational determinants of cocaine-taking behaviour? It is difficult to relate these to changes in the underlying neurobiology and the ebb and flow of dopamine neurotransmission. We have a long way to go towards explaining individual differences in those terms. Bill Woolverton is correct in pointing out that an understanding of the interplay of environmental factors with neurobiology is essential for understanding a complex phenomenon like cocaine abuse.

Kaplan: You specified three types of environmental factor, Dr Woolverton (schedule, response costs, and alternative reinforcers). Have you ranked their importance in determining drug-related behaviour?

Woolverton: It's hard to do this, because the factors are not directly comparable: what sort of increase in response cost is equivalent to adding one banana-flavoured food pellet as an alternative? To assess that quantitatively is a tricky undertaking. In the field of drug self-administration there is developing a method of analysis of these data that has been called 'behavioural economics', where people are looking at drug consumption in animals and humans in terms of economic concepts such as 'elasticity of demand'. If you analyse these data in those terms—to see which manipulation makes demand more elastic—then it looks as if 'response cost' is a more effective means of reducing cocaine self-administration than increasing the value of the alternative. But this sort of statement should be taken with a very large grain of salt.

Kalant: I was being deliberately negative in my initial question, even though I do in fact believe that there is value in examining the neurochemical basis of response mechanisms to different drugs and to other non-drug stimuli which act as reinforcers; but I also think it's necessary to do a lot more work in attempting to define what motivates human drug-taking behaviour in order to look for the appropriate animal model. So long as we look only at the linkage between dose and number of responses, we cannot have great confidence in the predictive value of any manipulations that are done on such a model, with respect to the consequence of the same manipulation of the human behaviour.

Anthony: I would like to try to link the images of Professor Edwards' photos of the rat in the cage and the woman being taken away by the police (p 4 and 5) with what Juan Carlos Negrete said about the array of alternative reinforcers for the peasants in Peru, who might choose to sell their coca leaf for $3600 per 1000 kg rather than for $600 on the legal market (p 42). The line of research that has been described by Dr Woolverton links those two images together with some clinical issues and with the issue of the array of alternative reinforcers.

I think we have to ask 'What *is* the array of alternative reinforcers?', whether the behaviour is growing coca leaf or taking cocaine, whether the animal will eat banana-flavoured pellets or take cocaine, or whether we have before us a cocaine user with a compulsive pattern of cocaine use needing intervention. This is an important question in these later stages of the American cocaine epidemic, because many of the cocaine users now presenting themselves for treatment have a very limited array of alternative reinforcers available to them. The rat in Professor Edwards' picture had very few options in that isolated environment. The woman growing coca had few options, too. Perhaps we now are finding in America that users very heavily involved in cocaine have very few alternative reinforcers.

Woolverton: This was a major consideration in the design of the experiment that I discussed. With several notable exceptions, much of intravenous self-administration research in animals has been done under conditions where the drug is the only reinforcer available to the animal, under some specified schedule of reinforcement. It is well established from these studies that the reinforcement schedule is a critical determinant of rates and patterns of drug-seeking, which is ultimately what we are interested in studying. Nevertheless, this is not an environment that mimics very closely the human situation, where there are concurrently available alternative reinforcers that are more or less effective in controlling behaviour. That is why we are evolving towards a more complex environmental situation for our experimental animals. The first stage for us has been to have two reinforcers available, namely food and cocaine.

Des Jarlais: This type of experimental situation does not seem to reflect the animal's natural environment, either; being isolated in a bare cage is not the environment in which monkeys have evolved, and it should also be thought of as a radical change in the environment for that animal. Thus the behaviour of a particular species, in its sensitivity to the reinforcing effects of a drug, may be very different in that highly constricted environment from its normal free-ranging and highly social behaviour.

Dr Woolverton, given the cost of these animals, I assume that most of the monkeys you work with have been previously exposed to cocaine, perhaps many times. Do you see any differences in sensitivity to cocaine between a relatively naive animal, and one with a lot of experience of this drug?

Woolverton: I have not looked at that specifically, and exposure to cocaine has not emerged as an obvious factor modifying self-administration. I am not aware of evidence that animals become sensitized to or tolerant to the reinforcing effects of cocaine as a function of length of exposure.

Reference

Pfaus JG, Damsma G, Nomikos GG et al 1990 Sexual behavior enhances central dopamine transmission in the male rat. Brain Res 530:345–348

Self-administration of cocaine by humans: a laboratory perspective

Marian W. Fischman and Richard W. Foltin

Department of Psychiatry and Behavioral Sciences, The Johns Hopkins University School of Medicine, 600 North Wolfe Street, Baltimore, MD 21205, USA

> *Abstract.* Laboratory research evaluating the behavioural and physiological effects of cocaine has produced important basic information relevant to the prediction and control of cocaine abuse. Adaptation for human subjects of laboratory procedures originally developed with non-humans has provided the methodology for assessing the relationship between cocaine-taking and the self-reported effects of cocaine. This laboratory model for evaluating drug-taking has been adapted to include all the routes of administration by which cocaine is abused. Data collected in cocaine choice/self-administration studies indicate that there is a generally good correlation between cocaine self-administration and its stimulant-like 'positive' effects. There are, however, areas in which these two measures clearly diverge, and drug self-administration procedures provide a sensitive measure of cocaine's effects when it is taken by the routes and in the patterns people use outside the laboratory. Combining these measures with other behavioural evaluations provides useful information for understanding cocaine use and abuse. In addition, and importantly, these laboratory procedures are useful tools in the development and assessment of treatment interventions which might be used effectively.
>
> *1992 Cocaine: scientific and social dimensions. Wiley, Chichester (Ciba Foundation Symposium 166) p 165–180*

A major reason for the present-day interest in the pharmacology of cocaine relates to its widespread abuse by humans. Laboratory models of drug abuse were originally developed to study drug self-administration behaviour (i.e. drug-taking) in non-humans (see Woolverton 1992: this volume), and have been shown to have substantial predictive power for drug-taking in humans (Schuster et al 1981). In contrast, the traditional laboratory approach to studying drug-taking and its consequences in humans has been to evaluate the subjective effects engendered by a drug dose administered by the experimenter (Fischman & Foltin 1991). It has generally been assumed that the effects of a drug which maintain drug-taking are related to drug-induced changes in subjective state and that what drug users say about the dose of drug they have just taken can be used to predict the likelihood that the drug will be used excessively and non-medically (Fischman 1989). However, this approach does not incorporate into the laboratory model the most salient feature of drug abuse, namely, the drug-taking *behaviour*. In addition, although the single dose paradigm, with drug administered by the experimenter, is a useful procedure for identifying an appropriate dose range to study as well as for evaluating profiles of action, including toxicity, administering a single dose of a drug within a laboratory context provides little information about the effects of that drug when it is relatively freely available and users can take it as they would outside the laboratory. For example, if we want to know the effects of a drug which is generally used (or abused) in repeated dosing patterns, that is the way we should study it in the laboratory.

Cocaine is commonly abused in multiple-dose cycles (known as binges), with users taking the drug repeatedly until their drug supply is exhausted. This pattern is similar to that demonstrated under controlled laboratory conditions when non-human primates were given access to intravenous cocaine (Johanson & Fischman 1989). Rhesus monkeys given continuous free access to cocaine readily self-administer it in erratic bursts, in marked contrast to the stable patterns of drug self-administration seen when the animals are allowed access to the drug for only a few hours each day. They also fail to eat and become severely debilitated. This compulsive behaviour may very well be comparable to the loss of control that some humans exhibit when using cocaine.

This chapter describes research on the effects of cocaine in humans in which experimental designs were applied that integrate laboratory models used with non-human and human research subjects. Volunteers for these studies were given the opportunity to take repeated doses of cocaine, with doses and patterning approximating those reported in the natural ecology. This work provides an important interface between laboratory research using non-human research subjects and the clinic, where various treatment interventions for individuals seeking drug-abuse treatment are being evaluated.

Studies of cocaine self-administration

Subjects

Normal healthy volunteers with histories of cocaine and other drug use (marijuana, alcohol, nicotine cigarettes etc.) participated in these studies (Fischman & Schuster 1982, Foltin et al 1988, Fischman et al 1990). Subjects resided on a hospital Clinical Research Unit for the duration of the 2–3 week studies, and were tested daily in experimental sessions lasting 2–4 hours, during which they received either drug or placebo.

Procedure

Each day subjects were allowed to choose between two unidentified intravenous injection solutions (saline or different doses of cocaine). They were told that these solutions could be active or inactive drug. On the first day of each 2–3 week study, each subject was told that the right-hand response button and light were associated with a specific drug solution and the left-hand response button and light were associated with a second drug solution. Subjects were allowed to choose repeatedly between solutions each day in experimental sessions that lasted 2–4 hours. Under these conditions, subjects generally selected cocaine over saline and higher doses of cocaine over lower doses. Similar dose relationships were observed when intranasally administered doses were available, indicating the dose-related nature of the reinforcing effects of this drug.

Results

In general, the initial few doses of cocaine exerted maximal effects, with subsequent doses exerting smaller, or no effects. This was true despite steadily increasing cocaine plasma levels, with peaks as high as 1200 ng/ml. Subjects exhibited no residual tolerance to the self-reported effects of cocaine 22 hours later, when the next test session was carried out. Although there was clear evidence of within-session tolerance (i.e. acute tolerance, defined as a decrease in responsiveness to cocaine within a single session) to many of the cardiovascular and subjective effects of cocaine, no change in self-administration behaviour was seen. In fact, in many of the self-administration sessions, subjects continued to choose to self-administer cocaine when we had to withhold the dose because of medical concerns (i.e. elevations in blood pressure or heart rate). These results provided a clear demonstration of why this drug is so harmful (see p 170 below).

This divergence of subjective and reinforcing effects no doubt occurs outside of the laboratory when people take the drug repeatedly. It is possible that the development of acute tolerance to the subjective effects of cocaine thus might be an important factor for those who 'binge' on this drug, leading them to escalate the dose when the initial drug effects are no longer achieved. The dissociation between changes in plasma concentration and the physiological measures was also evident, suggesting that users are getting minimal feedback from their bodies on the amount of drug that they have taken as tolerance develops, and provides information about a possible mechanism through which cocaine binges might occur.

The documented development of tolerance (Fischman et al 1985, Foltin & Fischman 1991) is supported by anecdotal reports from street users. Tolerance, measured in the laboratory, developed under conditions of repeated self-administration over 1–3 hours, and was not present 22 hours later. On subsequent sessions, each separated by a day, subjects did not need a larger dose to get the same effect. Nor were there any systematic changes that could be attributed to withdrawal after six or eight intravenous injections of cocaine within a 1–3 hour period. When cocaine users on the street stop taking cocaine after multiple doses, they describe a 'crash'. Gawin & Kleber (1986) have described the earliest stage of this crash as including anorexia, and high cocaine craving—subjective reports given by our research subjects as well. However, laboratory subjects do not report the depression, anhedonia (stated inability to experience pleasure) and lack of craving for cocaine that has been described by street users. Thus, while the development of acute tolerance to cocaine's cardiovascular and subjective effects has been documented, there are no laboratory indicators of a withdrawal syndrome following cocaine use, although clinical reports of the phenomenon are common.

Tolerance also develops to the subjective effects of cocaine when subjects smoke the drug (Foltin & Fischman 1991). Results, from a study in which the effects of experimenter-administered smoked or intravenously injected cocaine were compared (Foltin & Fischman 1991), were used to select doses of cocaine which would provide comparable venous blood levels for each route. Subjects were allowed to smoke pellets of the cocaine (i.e. 'freebase' or 'crack') as they would outside the laboratory (see Foltin & Fischman 1991 for a description of the procedure). Sixteen mg of intravenous cocaine and 25 mg smoked cocaine yielded similar venous blood levels which were approximately half those obtained after 32 mg intravenous cocaine and 50 mg smoked cocaine. The cardiovascular and subjective effects of these doses were not as readily differentiated. However, the subjects' ratings of the drugs they had received differentiated between the smoked and intravenous routes, with the smoked route being more favourably rated.

The reinforcing functions of cocaine when used via the intravenous or smoked routes are being compared in an ongoing study using the self-administration/choice procedure described above (Foltin & Fischman, unpublished), in which subjects choose between a smoked (placebo: hot air smoked through the pipe; 25 mg, 50 mg) and an intravenous (saline placebo, 16 mg, 32 mg) dose of cocaine. Preference favours smoked over intravenous cocaine when doses are matched for venous blood level. Epidemiological data also suggest that smoked cocaine is preferred, because declines in cocaine use via the smoked route have lagged behind the declines observed with other routes of cocaine administration (National Institute on Drug Abuse 1988).

Interestingly, verbal ratings of cocaine's effects via these two routes do not necessarily predict differences in preference. Although most subjects chose to self-administer smoked rather than intravenous cocaine, this is not always the case. Figure 1 demonstrates the choice behaviour of two subjects with different preferences. Subject 134, who chose both doses of intravenous cocaine over 25 mg smoked cocaine, and 32 mg intravenous over 50 mg smoked cocaine, rated himself as more 'stimulated' after smoked cocaine, while subject 120, who consistently chose smoked over intravenous cocaine, provided ratings of 'stimulated' after both routes of cocaine administration. Other self-reported effects of cocaine varied similarly.

Evaluation of pharmacological adjuncts to treatment

The self-administration model is also a useful tool for evaluating the mechanisms

Cocaine self-administration by humans

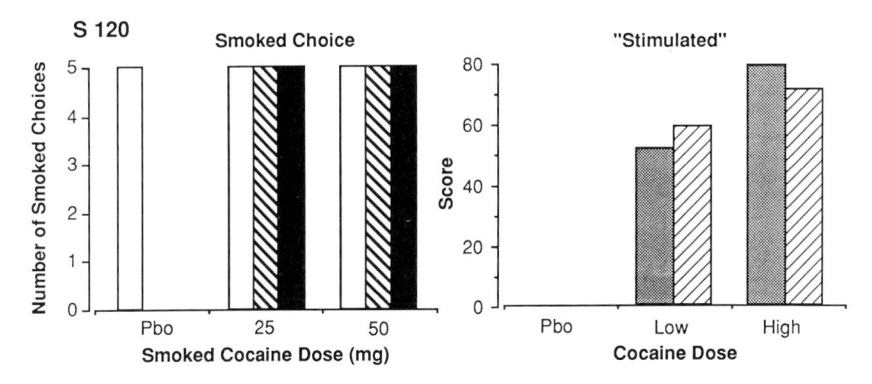

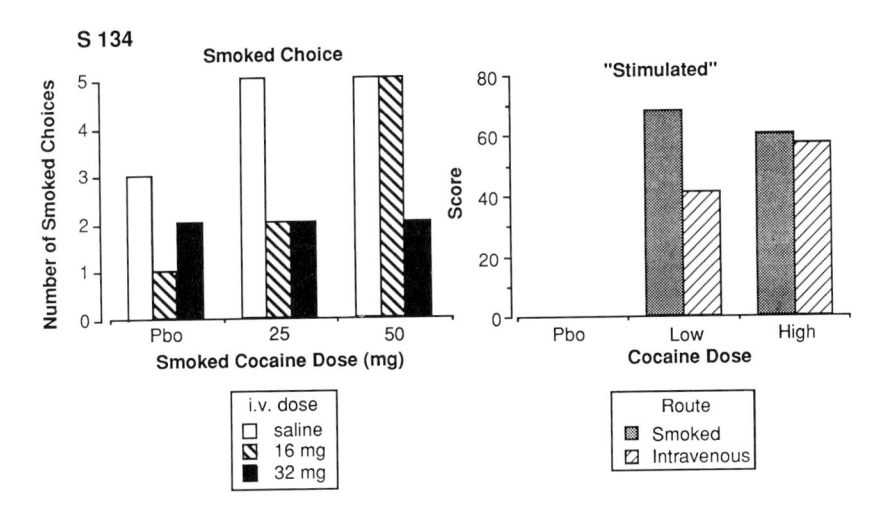

FIG. 1. Choice of smoked or intravenous cocaine doses by two subjects, S 120 and S 134. The left panel presents the number of times (maximum = 5) that the choice was of smoked cocaine. Comparisons were between placebo or 25 or 50 mg smoked cocaine and intravenously injected saline or 16 or 32 mg cocaine. The right panel presents scores on the 'stimulated' Visual Analog Scale after the initial dose of placebo by the two routes, low dose (16 mg intravenous or 25 mg smoked), or high dose (32 mg intravenous or 50 mg smoked) cocaine.

of action of pharmacological interventions in the treatment of cocaine abuse (Fischman et al 1990). Since separate measures can be made of drug-taking, cardiovascular effects, and subjective effects, it is theoretically possible to parcel out specific effects of a treatment medication, thereby eventually providing targeted treatment.

Procedure

Subjects were tested daily in three-hour sessions using the two-lever cocaine choice procedure. The lever associated with each dose (saline, or 8, 16 or 32 mg intravenous cocaine) remained constant within a day, but could change from day to day, and subjects could choose up to seven injections during the 90-minute period of each daily session.

A 3-4 week period of maintenance on the tricyclic antidepressant desipramine was inserted between two determinations of cocaine dose choice. The self-administration protocols were carried out while subjects resided on a hospital Clinical Research Unit. For the desipramine maintenance period the subjects were outpatients, reporting to the laboratory daily; blood samples were taken to monitor desipramine blood levels twice weekly. Blood levels of desipramine were maintained at approximately 125 ng/ml during the final determination of cocaine dose choice. This protocol allowed evaluation of desipramine's effects on drug-taking, dose preference, self-reported drug effects and cardiovascular effects under the conditions in which the drug was taken outside the laboratory (i.e. the opportunity for repeated dosing was available).

Results

Desipramine had no effect on cocaine-taking behaviour, with a mean of approximately six injections requested during sessions in which cocaine was available. Response rates and latency to first response were also unchanged. However, cocaine could not always be administered because of medical considerations (i.e. diastolic blood pressure about 100 mmHg or heart rate above 131 b.p.m.), which were generally related to the desipramine-induced elevations in baseline cardiovascular measures. The self-administration of cocaine in the face of detrimental cardiovascular effects shows clearly why this drug is so highly toxic.

Decreases in craving for cocaine have been reported anecdotally for cocaine abusers being treated with desipramine. In an effort to provide an operational definition for 'craving', a Visual Analog Scale labelled 'I want cocaine' was administered as part of the self-report questionnaires answered repeatedly during each session. Figure 2 indicates that before the period of maintenance on desipramine, subject's scores on this scale were close to the maximum of 100, while during desipramine maintenance, scores on this scale were substantially and significantly lower. Despite such shifts in reports of 'wanting' cocaine, however, the subjects' drug-taking behaviour remained unchanged.

Desipramine maintenance also resulted in a change in cocaine's profile of subjective effects. Desipramine had the effect of attenuating scores on many of the scales that are sensitive to stimulant drugs, including Arousal and Positive Mood of the Profile of Mood States (McNair et al 1971) and the Benzedrine

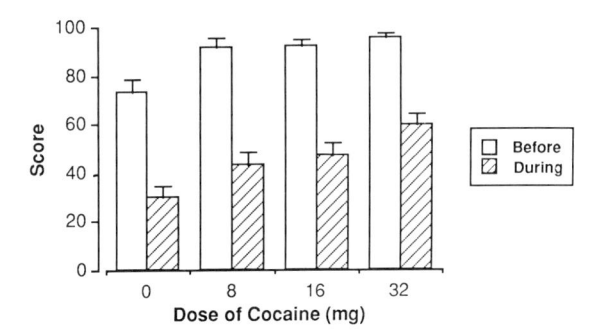

FIG. 2. Mean Visual Analog Scale ratings of 'I Want Cocaine' before and during maintenance on desipramine. Subjects were allowed to choose between intravenous injections (saline, or 8, 16 or 32 mg cocaine) up to six times daily, making ratings at the beginning of each session and after each choice. (Data taken from Fischman et al 1990.)

Group Scale of the Addiction Research Center Inventory (Haertzen 1966). Before desipramine maintenance, these scores were increased by the initial daily dose of cocaine in a dose-related fashion; during desipramine maintenance, cocaine engendered significantly lower scores on these scales.

A second pattern of interaction between cocaine and desipramine was observed on other self-report scales. Desipramine maintenance resulted in lower placebo scores and significantly higher scores in response to cocaine on the Confusion and Anger scales of the Profile of Mood States, and the Addiction Research Center Inventory LSD scale, a measure of dysphoric drug effects. Desipramine thus seemed to enhance cocaine's effects on these more 'negative' scales.

Desipramine maintenance was not always associated with changed effects of cocaine. In some cases, desipramine had no effect on reports of cocaine's effects. Most notable and consistent in this regard were the series of questions answered at the termination of each choice session, approximately 30 minutes after the last cocaine injection, when blood levels were considerably decreased. Subjects were asked to rate the overall effect of the cocaine administered during that session. Despite differential effects recorded during each session immediately after the drug was administered, and at approximately its time of peak effect, ratings made at the end of the session were related only to the cocaine dose level, regardless of the presence or absence of desipramine maintenance. Ratings of 'High', 'Liking', 'Potency' and 'How much would you pay for this drug?' all showed increases with increasing doses of cocaine. Thus, for example, subjects said they would pay an average of approximately 40 dollars for the drug administered in the 32 mg sessions. There are thus some properties of cocaine which do not appear to change when it is taken in conjunction with desipramine maintenance. And this unchanged retrospective rating of cocaine's effects when people are maintained on desipramine would also predict continued cocaine-taking when the desipramine is administered, at least in the absence of a treatment programme.

Although desipramine maintenance, under these controlled laboratory conditions, did not appear to affect the self-administration of cocaine, it did modify some of cocaine's subjective effects as reported by our subjects. What this dissociation suggests is that desipramine by itself is not an adequate pharmacological intervention for treating cocaine abusers: cocaine remains a potent reinforcer. The desipramine, however, may sufficiently alter cocaine's profile of effects so that users participating in a behavioural treatment intervention will learn to use other reinforcers in their environment rather than continuing to take cocaine.

Conclusion

This research demonstrates the way in which procedures developed in the laboratory for use with non-humans can be adapted for use with humans and combined with measures of verbal report. Such designs provide data with cross-species generality, thus increasing their utility. Self-reports do not substitute for measuring actual drug-taking behaviour, and in the absence of a good measure of such behaviour there is no way to be certain about whether a drug will maintain self-administration, or about the conditions that influence self-administration. For example, on the basis of verbal reports alone, the prediction would have been that our desipramine-maintained subjects, who showed minimal drug-induced 'euphoria-like' responses, would not self-administer cocaine. In addition, based on the decreases in the magnitude of verbal reports of stimulant effects and increases in the magnitude of 'dysphoric' drug effects during desipramine maintenance, the prediction would have been of a decrease in cocaine self-administration during desipramine maintenance. Neither outcome was observed. It is only by evaluating the most parsimonious measure of drug abuse—drug-taking behaviour—within a behavioural context, that we can fully understand and predict the likelihood that a drug will be abused. While it is frequently the case that drugs which readily serve as reinforcers in human and non-human research subjects also cause effects which lead to self-reports related to 'euphoria', or 'liking' or some combination of self-reported effects judged to be 'positive', the correspondence is far from perfect. Verbal reports of 'euphoria' or other 'positive' drug effects and drug self-administration dissociate from each other under a number of conditions. Therefore, it is important to measure both. Such divergence in these two measures provides interesting topics for future research.

Acknowledgements

The research described here was supported by grants DA-03818 and DA-06234 from the National Institute on Drug Abuse. Subjects resided on the Johns Hopkins Clinical

Research Unit supported by grant MO1-RR-00035 from the National Institutes of Health. We appreciate the thoughtful comments of Dr Thomas Kelly.

References

Fischman MW 1989 Relationship between self-reported drug effects and their reinforcing effects: stimulant drugs. In: Fischman MW, Mello NH (eds) Testing for abuse liability of drugs in humans. (National Institute on Drug Abuse Research Monograph 92) US Government Printing Office, Washington, DC, p 211–230

Fischman MW, Foltin RW 1991 Utility of subjective-effects measurements in assessing abuse liability of drugs in humans. Br J Addict 86:1563–1570

Fischman MW, Schuster CR 1982 Cocaine self-administration in humans. Fed Proc 41:241–246

Fischman MW, Schuster CR, Javaid JI, Hatano Y, Davis J 1985 Acute tolerance development to the cardiovascular and subjective effects of cocaine. J Pharmacol Exp Ther 235:677–682

Fischman MW, Foltin RW, Pearlson G, Nestadt G 1990 Effects of desipramine maintenance on cocaine self-administration. J Pharmacol Exp Ther 253:760–770

Foltin RW, Fischman MW 1991 Smoked and intravenous cocaine in humans: acute tolerance, cardiovascular and subjective effects. J Pharmacol Exp Ther 257:247–261

Foltin RW, Fischman MW, Pedroso JJ, Pearlson GD 1988 Repeated intranasal cocaine administration: lack of tolerance to pressor effects. Drug Alcohol Depend 22:169–177

Gawin FH, Kleber HD 1986 Abstinence symptomatology and psychiatric diagnosis in cocaine abusers. Arch Gen Psychiatry 43:107–113

Haertzen CA 1966 Development of scales based on patterns of drug effects using the addiction research center inventory (ARCI). Psychol Rep 18:163–194

Johanson CE, Fischman MW 1989 The pharmacology of cocaine related to its abuse. Pharmacol Rev 41:3–52

McNair DM, Lorr M, Droppleman LF 1970 Profile of mood states (manual). Education and Industrial Testing Service, San Diego

National Institute on Drug Abuse 1988 National Household Survey on drug abuse: main findings 1988. US Government Printing Office, Washington, DC

Schuster CR, Fischman MW, Johanson CE 1981 Internal stimulus control and subjective effects of drugs. In: Johanson CE, Thompson T (eds) Behavioral pharmacology of human drug dependence. (National Institute on Drug Abuse Research Monograph 37) US Government Printing Office, Washington, DC, p 116–129

Woolverton WL 1992 Self-administration of cocaine in animals. In: Cocaine: scientific and social dimensions. Wiley, Chichester (Ciba Foundation Symposium 166) p 149–164

DISCUSSION

Negrete: You noted that your subjects say they prefer the injection route to smoking. Was there any difference between those who were used to smoking and those who were not?

Fischman: Just as I don't give cocaine to people who haven't used it before, I don't expose them to a new route of cocaine administration. These are all people who have tried both routes. But you have to understand that smoking cocaine is a very wasteful way of using this drug, because you need a substantially larger initial dose to get the same amount to the brain. Much of the initial piece of cocaine is destroyed or lost before it reaches the lung.

Negrete: Smoking is also a more active process, perhaps, where they have to undertake more manoeuvres to get the drug?

Fischman: In my studies, after choosing a dose of smoked or intravenous cocaine, the subjects do very little. The nurse places the drug on the screens in the pipe, holds the lighter, etc. We try to keep the smoking procedure as standardized as possible. Likewise, for the injection route, the intravenous catheter is already in place.

Kalant: Could the actual preference for smoking, rather than the subjects' stated preference for intravenous injection, be that they didn't get the chance to inject themselves? With other drugs, it has been shown many times that the act of injecting is itself rewarding. One of my colleagues, studying the intravenous use of amphetamine, showed that subjects would actually get a 'rush' with a saline placebo, before they discovered that the follow-up effects of amphetamine weren't there (the late Dr R.J. Gibbins, unpublished studies). The act of injection is an important part of the ritual and of the pleasure.

Fischman: It is absolutely true that the stereotyped behaviour in which the drug taker engages comes to evoke a drug response. After a few days in the study, subjects show cocaine-like cardiovascular responses to the stimuli associated with an injection of cocaine, although these responses are extremely short lived. When we do cocaine research with humans, we do not always have the luxury of designing perfect studies, and, in this case, we need the permission of our institutional Clinical Investigations Committees. We are allowed to administer cocaine intravenously only if a nurse or physician puts the needle in the subject's vein. Therefore, subjects cannot engage in their regular intravenous drug-taking rituals. We have, in studies using intranasal cocaine, allowed subjects to do all of their ritual preparation. We give them the cocaine as 100 mg of white powder, placing it on a mirror and providing a single-edge razor blade. Subjects, under these conditions, chop the cocaine and place it in 'lines' before inhaling it. They would not, however, choose a dose of inhaled cocaine over an intravenous dose.

Kalant: Does that change your conclusions? Earlier, I thought you were saying that the subjects prefer smoking because the onset of the effects is faster. Maybe it is that they prefer an active process in which they administer the drug to themselves.

Fischman: It is possible that active involvement is important, but they would not choose to take a slower onset intranasal dose, which they actively administer, over an intravenous dose, which requires little behaviour on their part.

Benowitz: Your approach to looking at the effects of pharmacological interventions on the self-administration of cocaine as a screening test for potential medications for treating cocaine addiction may be a bit conservative. Take, for example, our experience in studying the self-administration of nicotine via cigarette smoking. When we gave intravenous nicotine, our subjects did not smoke fewer cigarettes; they smoked the same number (Benowitz & Jacob 1990).

They inhaled a little less nicotine, but as long as there was free access to cigarettes, they didn't change their smoking behaviour very much. However, if smokers are trying to stop smoking, it's much easier to stop when other sources of nicotine, such as nicotine chewing gum or transdermal nicotine, are provided. Thus, even if you don't find an effect of a medication on cocaine self-administration in your experimental paradigm, it does not mean that the medication would not be useful, if someone really wanted to stop using cocaine.

Fischman: You may well be right. However, clinicians who treat cocaine abusers will tell you that it is rare to find cocaine abusers who come into the clinic and say 'I really want to stop taking cocaine; I can't stand this euphoria'! It is more likely that the judge has told them they must either get into treatment or go to prison; or their employer has told them that they will lose their job if they do not stop using cocaine; or a family member has provided them with an ultimatum to stop using cocaine or lose their family. *Wanting* to stop cocaine use is not the issue; these are people who are being forced into treatment. We have to figure out how to make it work.

My research attempts to mimic some of the conditions present in a treatment programme, with recent experimental design changes moving towards providing a range of non-drug as well as drug options during choice sessions. The procedure we used to study the effects of desipramine (described in my paper) did not address the issue of what might happen if there were non-drug alternatives to cocaine-taking available during each test session. In our current design, subjects choose among three options—two intravenous cocaine solutions and one 'token' option. Tokens can be exchanged for luxury food items, candies, cigarettes, videotaped movies, cassette tapes, etc. The standard range of hospital-provided necessities are available, and subjects can choose to supplement these items using tokens obtained during experimental sessions, or they can use cocaine during these sessions. A basic aim of any treatment programme is to teach drug abusers to seek non-drug reinforcers in their environments. The idea in our research is that if a treatment medication works to make cocaine a less efficacious reinforcer, we might see a switch from drug-taking to token-taking under some conditions. We would like to understand how to shift behaviour from cocaine-taking to token-taking.

Kalant: I want to take up your point that animal models of drug-taking are good predictors of human drug-taking, and, secondly, that people on the street don't take cocaine once, they take it repeatedly; and that animals 'binge' as humans do. But isn't it true that the great majority of cocaine users do take it once, not repeatedly?

Fischman: They generally do not take it *once*; they may take it a number of times, but on one occasion. We consider this as one drug-taking occasion.

Kalant: I agree with that: a number of doses on a particular occasion. But I question the claim that the animal model is an excellent predictor; this is only partially true. Any drug that is self-administered in the animal model is also self-administered by humans, but there are many drugs that humans will take, but that the animal will not. For example, the animal model is poor for predicting alcohol use by humans, and even worse for hallucinogenic drugs such as cannabis and LSD. There is thus a range of psychoactive drugs that humans take which it is difficult or impossible to get experimental animals to self-administer. So I question the extrapolation from the animal model to the human.

Fischman: I actually think the animal model is quite a good model for predicting abuse liability. In general, those drugs that are taken by non-human research subjects in the laboratory are the same as those that are abused by humans on the street, and those that are not self-administered in the laboratory are generally not abused on the street. There are, of course, exceptions, but most of these can be explained with reference to route of administration, pattern of use, or similar mechanisms. For example, LSD is a drug of abuse, although it is only used occasionally by humans. If we make it available to non-human research subjects, it is taken at a rate as low as (or lower than) placebo. Since our definition of a drug of abuse requires that the drug be self-administered more than placebo, LSD would not qualify as a drug of abuse. However, this model cannot predict liability for abuse in drugs taken only occasionally. The model provides an excellent initial screening procedure for sorting through a range of drugs, and predicting their abuse liability. It cannot, however, predict abuse.

Kalant: I agree that animal experimentation is an excellent way, but in one direction only—a drug that is self-administered in the animal model works also in humans, but others work very effectively in humans that don't work in the animal. I think alcohol poses the biggest problem in this respect.

Woolverton: There are exceptions in the opposite direction as well. Procaine is a good example; it is readily self-administered by rhesus monkeys, but there's no evidence of a human abuse problem with procaine. There are, however, good reasons for that difference that have little to do with its reinforcing effects. Procaine is only one-tenth as potent as cocaine behaviourally, which means that self-administration by a human would require about 1 g of drug. Sniffing 1 g of procaine repeatedly would probably be quite challenging! Also, procaine is very short acting. Even if it were taken intravenously, one would have to inject it very frequently to stay intoxicated.

Fischman: In fact, I have compared lidocaine and procaine with cocaine (Fischman et al 1983a,b). Procaine engenders a number of subjective effects similar to those of cocaine and, when intravenous procaine is made available, humans will self-administer it. They do so repeatedly, even at doses that do not engender measurable subjective effects. However, when subjects are allowed to choose between intravenous injections of procaine or cocaine, they will choose extremely low doses of cocaine (e.g. 8 mg/injection) over procaine (48–96 mg/injection (Fischman 1989). We believe that this choice is related to the pharmacological properties of procaine that Dr Woolverton has just described.

Woolverton: There are clearly a variety of reasons why the animal self-administration model might not be a perfect predictor of the *abuse* of drugs by humans.

Jones: The procaine 'paradox' doesn't trouble me. Before our 'War on Drugs' in America made pure cocaine so readily available, cocaine was commonly adulterated with procaine and self-administered compulsively by some humans, even though they were probably taking far more procaine than cocaine. I am more concerned, as Harold Kalant is, about places where there is a divergence between animals and humans. Nicotine should be high on the list of drugs that don't fit animal-based models very well. I can't think of a drug which is more avidly and compulsively self-administered by humans, whereas animals only do so when tricked into taking it.

Woolverton: Dr Kalant also mentioned alcohol as a drug where the animal model is poor. But humans don't typically self-administer alcohol by the intravenous route either, whereas animals can readily be conditioned to drink alcohol. With regard to nicotine, animals self-administer nicotine by the intravenous route quite readily under appropriate schedules of reinforcement. If intravenous nicotine is made available under a fixed-interval schedule, animals self-inject it readily, probably because there is an enforced time between injections.

Strang: Are we confident that the animal model allows, at the human level, for the value judgements of drug use? We have asked heroin users who have used both routes why they choose smoking over injecting heroin. They comment on the intravenous route being very 'vulgar'. This is why, presumably, intravenous LSD never took off, and perhaps similarly for phencyclidine. Outbreaks of intravenous alcohol use do occur, but it never becomes established. There is something other than just getting the drug quickly.

Fischman: It is true that the rapidity with which cocaine is delivered via the smoked route is not the only variable controlling its use. Social and cultural variables clearly play a role in drug-taking. However, before we begin to study cocaine use under complex and uncontrolled conditions, it is useful to study it under more controlled conditions where these variables are somewhat less relevant. Once we have a baseline against which to compare the effects of more sophisticated manipulations, we can begin to approximate the natural ecology in trying to understand more of the controlling variables for cocaine self-administration. We have to start by eliminating some of the obvious variables first.

Anthony: I believe Marian Fischman's work has been under-appreciated, and I think in the laboratory it's great, but we should recall that about 70% of her subjects had been intravenous users of cocaine. And in Neal Benowitz's DAWN data, we saw that about 70% of the cocaine deaths were related to the intravenous use of cocaine. By comparison, in the general population of cocaine users in the USA, the fraction who have ever injected cocaine is well under 10%

(Anthony & Trinkoff 1989). So we must ask the degree to which we would find Dr Fischman's results replicated in users whose lives had not been substantially involved with cocaine. I am questioning whether the same results would be found if she had studied individuals who were more typical of cocaine users on the streets of America during the entire course of the cocaine epidemic—individuals for whom cocaine use was a more casual experience and who certainly did not inject cocaine.

Fischman: In 1985 we published data on the demographics of my population of research subjects at that time (Schuster & Fischman 1985). We found that a majority of those volunteering were intranasal users, a considerably smaller percentage were intravenous users, and none had smoked cocaine. My recent data, however, are comparable to the data collected on this slightly different population.

Des Jarlais: To me, the potential from the animal model hasn't been tapped yet. In the human use of drugs, the fundamental social problem is what it is about the drug history of some individuals that makes them insensitive to the increasing cost of maintaining their drug use. Why do some people continue to use drugs, even though the financial and interpersonal consequences are becoming increasingly negative? Bill Woolverton showed that some of his monkeys are sensitive to the increasing 'cost' of using drugs. We need an experiment that shows what type of animal with what type of drug history then becomes *insensitive* to the increasing cost of obtaining and using drugs—the addiction problem that causes our social problem. We should not just be showing that animals will take drugs, and that the patterns are similar to ours; we need a good animal model for addictive behaviour.

O'Brien: We have learned a great deal from animal models, but we could learn even more if behavioural pharmacologists would allow themselves to be more flexible and daring in the kinds of models that they develop. Everyone likes to study animals that have limited access to a drug like cocaine for, say, two hours a day, because this gives stable baselines and reproducible results. However, a study of animals with relatively unlimited access to cocaine would be more like the human condition. It would be more complicated to perform, but such a model may be more relevant. We then may ultimately get what I believe, as a clinician, is the most sorely needed animal model, which is a model of relapse—not a model that tells you that a certain medication will depress the self-administration rate of cocaine by a monkey that is continually working for it, during a two hours per day access. Rather, this model would involve a monkey that has learned to 'like cocaine', that will work hard for it, in an uncontrolled way, and then, after complete detoxification, that monkey will resume the avid pursuit of cocaine. It could be very interesting to see what medications or procedures will help us to prevent the *resumption* of that self-administration.

Fibiger: Dr Fischman, what effects do neuroleptics have on the paradigm that you are studying? I think this is a fundamental question with respect to the dopamine hypothesis of cocaine reinforcement.

Fischman: I have never pretreated subjects with a neuroleptic, prior to allowing them to self-administer cocaine. I have, however, administered chlorpromazine before a single dose of cocaine. Under those conditions, the cardiovascular toxicity was such that we could not complete the study. Chlorpromazine is a 'dirty' drug from a neurochemical perspective. By itself, cocaine causes increases in heart rate and blood pressure, and in combination with chlorpromazine these effects were exacerbated in an unpredictable fashion.

Fibiger: You haven't tried haloperidol, then?

Fischman: No.

Fibiger: That would be a fascinating thing to do. What, if any, effects did desipramine by itself have on these volunteers, who presumably were not depressed?

Fischman: The effects of desipramine on mood are minimal in our subjects. These are non-depressed research subjects. Probably the major effect is dry mouth.

Negrete: They do not become jittery?

Fischman: I have not seen that at all. They are not living in the hospital during the desipramine treatment, so we have to depend on their reports. They don't report being jittery.

Fibiger: Dr Fischman, if the euphoria-inducing effects of cocaine 'peak out', or show an acute tolerance effect, would you care to speculate on what it is that is maintaining the self-administration behaviour at that point?

Fischman: I think *cocaine* is maintaining their behaviour! If you want to know what the subjects *say* about their self-administration of these low doses, they tell me that they were not choosing cocaine over placebo. They often insist that they were sampling equally from each of the two choice options and both were placebo. On the other hand, if you look at the *data* from that session, you see that they were choosing the low dose (as low as 4 mg) or the dose with no measurable effect. Subjects will choose 4 mg intravenous cocaine over placebo repeatedly, despite the fact that I can measure no cardiovascular or subjective effects of that dose. I do not believe that measuring subjective effects provides us with the information about 'what' is maintaining their cocaine-taking. The best we can say at this point is that it is the cocaine that is maintaining cocaine-taking.

Musto: So there *is* an effect from a 4 mg dose!

References

Anthony JC, Trinkoff AM 1989 United States epidemiologic data on drug use and abuse: how are they relevant to testing abuse liability of drugs? In: Fischman MW, Mello NK (eds) Testing for abuse liability of drugs in humans. (National Institute on Drug Abuse Research Monograph 92) US Government Printing Office, Washington, DC, p 241–266 (especially Table 5)

Benowitz NL, Jacob P III 1990 Intravenous nicotine replacement suppresses nicotine intake from cigarette smoking. J Pharmacol Exp Ther 154:1000-1005

Fischman MW 1989 Relationship between self-reported drug effects and their reinforcing effects: stimulant drugs. In: Fischman MW, Mello NK (eds) Testing for abuse liability of drugs in humans. (National Institute on Drug Abuse Research Monograph 92) US Government Printing Office, Washington, DC, p 211-230

Fischman MW, Schuster CR, Hatano Y 1983a A comparison of the subjective and cardiovascular effects of cocaine and lidocaine in humans. Pharmacol Biochem Behav 18:123-127

Fischman MW, Schuster CR, Raifer S 1983b A comparison of the subjective and cardiovascular effects of procaine and cocaine in humans. Pharmacol Biochem Behav 18:711-716

Schuster CR, Fischman MW 1985 Characteristics of humans volunteering for a cocaine research project. In: Kozel NJ, Adams EH (eds) Cocaine use in America: epidemiologic and clinical perspectives. (National Institute on Drug Abuse Research Monograph 61) US Government Printing Office, Washington, DC, p 158-170

General discussion

AIDS and HIV infection in cocaine users

Des Jarlais: In the United States, where almost all persons who inject heroin also inject cocaine, there have been a large number of studies indicating that, of the two drugs, cocaine injection is more strongly associated with exposure to the human immunodeficiency virus (HIV) (see Table 1). The exact reasons for this stronger association are not well-understood. Because it is the sharing of injection equipment while injecting, and not the drug being injected, that transmits HIV, this difference requires explanation.

First of all, there clearly is measurement error in the self-reporting of injection behaviour. For a heroin 'addict', heroin injection tends to be fairly regular, with injections on the great majority of days and a moderate number of injections per day. A cocaine 'addict', in contrast, will often engage in 'binge' injecting, with a large number of injections per day for one or two days, followed by days with no injection at all. To the extent that the cocaine injector reports fewer injections than actually occurred (partly due to unreliable memory of one's own behaviour during binges)—and to the extent that a research questionnaire which classifies the highest frequency of injection as 'daily' is insufficiently precise to account for binge behaviour—the resulting undermeasurement of cocaine injections may lead to an artificially stronger association between cocaine injection and HIV exposure.

Nonetheless, the preponderance of studies in which this stronger association with cocaine injection has been found suggests that there may be real behavioural differences between cocaine and heroin injection that are relevant to HIV exposure. We have conducted one study in New York where a researcher went into cocaine 'shooting galleries' to actually observe the injections (Friedman et al 1989a). The researcher reported that cocaine injectors usually try, at first, to practise 'safer' injection; they intend to avoid sharing equipment or to clean it if the equipment is to be shared. They actually maintain this good injection hygiene for the first five to 10 injections. But, by that time, they are pretty stoned. For the next 10 to 15 injections, their ability to maintain good needle hygiene breaks down. They may get confused about whose needle is whose; one or more of the needles may jam, points may get dull, or they may run out of the bleach used for disinfecting the injection equipment. So it may be an inability to maintain good hygiene during binging that is one cause of the stronger association between cocaine injection and HIV exposure. We clearly need more non-participant observation research to determine what is happening during cocaine injection. The evidence is surprisingly consistent that, for people

TABLE 1 (*Des Jarlais*) Cocaine injection and HIV in the United States

Location	Period of study	Reference
New York	1978–1983	Novick et al 1989
New York	1984–1989	Schoenbaum et al 1989
New York	1987–1988	Friedman et al 1989b
San Francisco	1986	Chaisson et al 1989
San Francisco	1987–1988	Moss et al 1989
Baltimore	1980–1988	Vlahov et al 1990

who inject both drugs, their reported cocaine injection correlates much more strongly with HIV exposure than does their cocaine injection.

Cocaine, of course, is injected not only in the United States but also in South America. Indeed, cocaine is the dominant drug injected there, with very little heroin injection. There is some injection of pharmaceutical drugs, but cocaine is by far the most frequently injected drug in South America. Moreover, studies from Brazil and Argentina are showing disturbingly high rates of HIV seroprevalence among people injecting drugs (see Table 2). Thus, HIV infection among drug injectors is not just a problem of North America, Europe, or Southeast Asia; it is already well-established in South America.

However, the number of people injecting drugs in South American countries is not clear. The sampling procedures for the studies in Table 2 involved recruiting drug injectors off the street, or drug injectors coming into cocaine treatment programmes, or drug injectors from general hospitals, but lacked even the simplest capture–recapture estimations of the total population of injecting drug users. Still, it is clear that we must consider the HIV epidemic among drug injectors to be well under way in South America, and we have to start planning how to get clean needles to injecting drug users and how to get azidothymidine (AZT) to drug injectors who have already been exposed to HIV. These will not be easy tasks. We also must consider how to change the sexual behaviour of these cocaine injectors so that they do not spread HIV to their sexual partners and to their potential children.

TABLE 2 (*Des Jarlais*) HIV infection among cocaine injectors in South America

Location	Seroprevalence rate	Reference
Rio de Janiero	36% HIV+	Lima et al 1991
Santos (Brazil)	57% HIV+	Mesquita et al 1991
Buenos Aires	44% HIV+	Calello et al 1991
Rosario (Argentina)	40% HIV+	Fay et al 1991

HIV infection and crack use

The other particular concern about cocaine use and HIV infection has been the dramatic increase in sexually transmitted diseases that we have seen in the United States, associated with the smoking of 'crack' (the free base form of cocaine). Crack use has been frequently, although not yet conclusively, associated with increases in syphilis, gonorrhea and chancroid (Marx et al 1991). Clearly, the unsafe sexual behaviour that transmits these diseases can also transmit HIV. Ulcerative genital diseases, such as syphilis and chancroid, may also increase the infectivity of HIV, adding a further risk for HIV transmission associated with crack use.

Having outlined this scenario, I should emphasize that in regard to the heterosexual transmission of HIV, only a few studies to date (and all of those from New York City) have shown an association of crack use and HIV among persons without a history of injecting illicit drugs (Marx et al 1991, Ratner et al 1991).

There is also a substantial overlap between smoking crack and injecting drugs; our street-recruited samples of intravenous drug injectors in New York show that 60% also smoke crack. This overlap creates methodological problems in disentangling HIV exposure due to crack use from that due to the sharing of drug injection equipment. We may find that it is also necessary to have large numbers of HIV-positive drug injectors engaging in crack-related sexual activities before HIV becomes widespread among crack users in general. The studies from places other than New York show very high levels of 'unsafe' sexual activity, but these samples include very few HIV-positive people who smoke crack without also injecting drugs. Another factor to consider is that much of crack-related sexual activity is oral sex, which is probably much less efficient for transferring the virus than vaginal sex, and certainly much less efficient than anal sex.

Research has advanced to the point where the ethnographic studies of the crack houses are starting to differentiate between different types of crack-related sexual behaviour (Ratner et al 1991). There are basically three major types. One is a simple casual exchange of crack for sex, very similar to the exchange in the 1970s and 1980s of inhaled cocaine for sex. Somebody is giving a party, there is a 'have-a-good-time' atmosphere, and there is an implicit trade-off whereby the male provides drugs and the woman will then agree to have sex in return for the good time. This type of 'exchange' typically occurs among friends or acquaintances, and should be considered as a variation on longstanding patterns of using various drugs, including alcohol, as aids to seduction. This type of exchange is not considered to be prostitution behaviour by either the man or the woman involved, although both usually understand that providing the drug will lead to sexual activity.

In the second type of exchange of sex for crack, women will exchange sex for money in order to buy crack. These women do have something of a professional prostitute orientation. They seem, more than any other crack-using group, to be willing to use condoms, and to take a health-conscious, professional occupational-risk attitude towards the exchange of sex for money to buy crack. They are perhaps analogous to the traditional female prostitute who engages in prostitution as a way of obtaining money to buy heroin.

The third type of crack-related sexual behaviour is a direct exchange of sex for crack, occurring particularly in the crack houses. This occurs mainly among young women who do not have a professional prostitute belief system, and so the chances for the use of condoms and safe sex are minimal (Williams et al 1988). This type of exchange of sex for crack is not simply drug-taking behaviour; it involves what sociologists would call 'degradation rituals' (Garfinkel 1956). The men are involved not just in having sex, but in exerting power over and often humiliating the women. The sexual activity will often be performed publicly, adding to the real humiliation and degradation of the women in these situations. Hamid has described this type of sexual activity as an evolution from a crack house to a 'freak' house (A.H., personal communication).

The findings from our current New York studies of women who have engaged in crack-related sexual activity are quite depressing. In investigating the background of women who get involved in this situation, we find that about 50% report that they had been raped prior to their 'crack for sex' activity. About half of these rapes were committed by a family member or a family friend, and occurred when the women were relatively young. Clearly, these women are not psychologically healthy people who somehow got involved in crack use and crack for sex. They are women who were already psychologically vulnerable.

In considering the direct exchange of crack for sex, we need to be careful that we do not demonize the addictive potential of crack. Rather than presuming that these women are willing to perform these humiliating activities simply to obtain crack, we should consider whether an amplifying positive feedback loop may be occurring. The prior psychological vulnerability, particularly low self-esteem, may create an increased reinforcement effect for crack, since cocaine has long been reported to alleviate feelings of low self-esteem. Engaging in humiliating behaviour to obtain crack may further damage self-esteem, such that the immediate positive drug effect is actually increased. In this 'crack for sex' situation, there may be mutual causation, with the activities you have to do to get crack first reducing your self-esteem, which the crack use then temporarily medicates. When the crack effect wears off, self-esteem has been further reduced, resistance to additional humiliation has been reduced, and the effect of the next use of crack will be still further enhanced.

We do not have a good understanding of the behaviour of the men in these direct crack-for-sex situations. It is clear that crack is 'advertised' as an enhancement to male sexual pleasure; in New York there is the 'master blaster', which involves having an orgasm as one is inhaling crack from the crack pipe.

This has been advertised on the street as the ultimate sexual experience. Yet we also know that high levels of cocaine use can impair sexual performance. It may be that some of the humiliation of the women in the crack-for-sex exchanges—particularly men requiring that the women perform sex with the man's friends—may stem from projected anger that the man himself has used cocaine to the point of sexual impairment.

Areas for future research

First, we need better treatment for cocaine dependency. Indeed, if we are to stop a major HIV epidemic among drug injectors in South America, we need to develop and implement treatments for cocaine dependency on a public-health scale. Treatments of the kind that are very labour-intensive, will take two years, and cost $30 000 to $50 000 per person, may help individuals, but will not affect the spread of HIV among cocaine injectors in South American cities. Given the medical costs of AIDS treatment in the United States, such treatments would be comparatively cost-effective there, but it is unlikely that they would be made available to the hundreds of thousands of people who are injecting cocaine in the United States.

We also need to know much more about the specifics of cocaine injection behaviour. We have done very few studies to explain the strong relationships between cocaine injection and HIV exposure in the United States. We do not know how effectively people can use bleach while they are injecting cocaine. We do not know how the dynamics of very frequent injection (i.e. every 10 or 15 minutes) would work with over-the-counter sales of syringes or syringe exchanges. Clearly, large stockpiles of sterile injection equipment would be needed to prevent the sharing of equipment if groups binge on injected cocaine.

We shall also have to examine changing the sexual behaviour of cocaine users—particularly those who are injecting cocaine and thus are at high risk for transmitting the virus to their sexual partners and their children. We also need to change the sexual behaviour of crack users, both those who use crack as a part of seduction and those who directly exchange sex for crack. I am afraid that, in regard to the direct exchange of sex for crack, AIDS prevention will require much more than just AIDS 'education' and giving out condoms. There are indications of severe psychological and social problems that will also need to be addressed.

In the interim, while we are conducting this needed research, the best short-term strategy may be to focus on preventing the initial HIV infection from occurring among drug injectors. Sharing of injection remains the predominant known source of HIV infection among cocaine users in both North and South America. It is drug injectors who not only transmit HIV to their 'regular' sexual partners, but who also appear to be the source through which HIV enters the crack-for-sex situations.

Edwards: At this stage in the symposium we are being asked to move our focus from the D_2 dopamine receptor site to the crack house. Thus the particular fascination of this meeting.

Moore: Can you amplify this—for what purpose is it necessary to keep these two different images in mind?

Edwards: I think we are conducting our science not simply for its intrinsic and elegant pleasure. It is quite legitimate to be selfish, and I hope to be able to go on doing things because they interest me! But if our science in its totality is to serve our society, it will be necessary to keep both these images in mind. The totality of our science is greatly impoverished if we don't make that attempt. Tell me I am wrong!

Moore: It seems to me that you suggest two slightly different strands of thought. One is the importance of integrating the scientific community so that the totality of knowledge about the effects of cocaine use and their causes could be maximally developed, so that the scientific community could have a more coherent picture of the problem, and where its solution might lie.

The second idea is that, somehow or other, this scientific enterprise ought to be able to serve the broader society, and that the accumulated insight that would come from the scientific community unifying itself would make available a different set of social responses than would be characteristic of a smaller science community, or a disintegrated science community. Those are two slightly different ideas, and I wasn't sure which should be our aspiration.

Almond: I would suggest that the idea of value-free science has been largely discredited, or at least challenged, since the Second World War, with the examples of Nazi medicine and then the work of scientists in connection with the production of the atomic bomb. I would therefore certainly support Professor Edwards' remarks about taking one's vision out from the laboratory and into the community. Going back to what Don Des Jarlais has told us, I am struck again by the fact that the people he is reporting on are very young people when they get into these situations. So, in a way, the solutions generally proposed are rather like putting sticking plaster on serious cuts. One subject we haven't put on our agenda, which seems to be in fact the only one which is really relevant, is education. It is relevant in that some drug education projects may convey to the young people concerned the idea that drug-taking is a natural part of growing up. The point is, though, that the kind of lifestyles that we have just been hearing about are the kind of lifestyles which can lead to an abrupt and premature termination of life. In other words, some of these young people do not get as far as growing up—whether directly, through complications associated with drugs, or indirectly, through HIV/AIDS.

Kleber: Let me try to tie together some of what Don Des Jarlais said with what we shall hear about later, on treatment, on prevention, and also on behavioural aspects.

When I began my job as Deputy Director at the Office of National Drug Control Policy, I had just completed an elegant treatment study which took three years and about three hundred thousand dollars to do. It showed that desipramine might be significantly helpful in decreasing cocaine use. Since then there have been about five studies, three showing that it does work, two showing that it doesn't. But we really can't afford that luxury—if it takes us that kind of time to show some effect, we can't (given what's going on in the epidemic) afford this pace of work.

Major thrusts that we therefore encouraged at the National Institute on Drug Abuse included the development of animal models that could quickly screen possible compounds that might be of use; studies like Marian Fischman's, that perhaps in a few months could show which drugs might be promising and then one could carry out the longer-term studies on only the most promising compounds. Clearly, these animal and human laboratory studies are absolutely essential if we are to do much faster work in developing better treatments.

A major problem with the 'harm reduction' approach to HIV infection as it relates to drug use is, as Don pointed out, that the drug use interferes with putting into action the less dangerous behaviour. This is especially true with stimulants; as people get into heavy use of stimulants, they don't carry out what they were supposed to do to be safe. They become confused or intoxicated, or they remember perfectly and just don't care. Ultimately, the best way to prevent the spread of AIDS among drug abusers is to develop effective treatments, get people into them, and get them to stop the drug use behaviour, rather than to continue it in a 'safer' way.

Finally, we have to address prevention, because ultimately the answer has to be prevention. You will never *treat* your way out of a drug epidemic, from what I see historically, unless you have treatments that are 100% successful. We have to *prevent* our way out of an epidemic. But, ironically, those kinds of stories that Don tells aren't very effective in prevention. If you tell them to adolescents, in some ways they sound more exciting than degrading to many of them. The 'focus' groups where that has been tried show that it does not prevent this kind of behaviour; they know it 'won't happen to them' and, if it did, maybe they would be able to stop. There are some more or less effective prevention techniques, but they are not as good as we would like, and we need more research on that too.

Negrete: Dr Des Jarlais is telling us that there is a difference between cocaine and heroin users in their risk of becoming infected with HIV. I had not heard this before. I knew that cocaine users tend to inject more times than heroin users, and therefore the risk is higher, but very clearly the sexual behaviour is also different. Heroin users in general have a decreased sexual drive and lose sexual interest more rapidly than cocaine users.

In a study of HIV seropositivity prevalence in injecting drug users in Canada it was observed that Montreal presented higher rates than Toronto (unpublished personal communication from Drs F. Lamothe & J. Bruneau). Sexual patterns seemed likely to be the cause! In fact, one of the strongest associations found was that prostitution, sex for money, and sex for drugs, were more common among drug users in Montreal than in Toronto.

Des Jarlais: I hope that I didn't imply that injecting heroin is safe, in terms of HIV. The three fastest HIV epidemics, in Edinburgh, in Bangkok and in Manipur in India, were all epidemics where it was almost exclusively heroin use. But in situations where people are injecting both drugs, it does appear to be cocaine injection that is associated with the greatest risk of exposure.

Maynard: I would like to turn to the issue of the effectiveness of interventions. When I hear the idea that we should be looking at alternative policies in relation to their effectiveness, I have two questions. Firstly, what is the measure of effectiveness? There have been hints that we should be looking at length of life and additional life-years. You might also look at the quality of life. How would you choose between treating me after swallowing my cocaine, and getting severe brain damage, giving me another 20 years of very poor quality of life, as opposed to spending the money on a heart transplant for somebody? It might give that person a much better quality of life and the same number of years. The question of measuring the effectiveness of interventions is crucial and shouldn't be avoided.

The second question is: effectiveness at what cost? Which of two alternative interventions gives you your desired measure of outcome—length and quality of life, perhaps—at what cost? You are not going to make choices purely with regard to their effectiveness; you are going to make them on the basis of cost-effectiveness.

Jones: Our government's ultimate goal in the USA, and the endpoint for which we are urged to aim, for cocaine and all drugs of abuse, is zero use of drugs—at least, from what I read, from government sources and what I see on television, this goal is part of national drug abuse strategy. In most treatment trials of desipramine and other medications for treating cocaine addictions, although it has never been clearly stated, there is implicit a therapeutic goal of complete cessation of cocaine use. That goal is suggested in the way we commonly measure treatment outcome in the USA; if a patient has a urine with 300 ng/ml or more of cocaine metabolites, that's a positive urine and a treatment failure; if the patient has a urine with 299 ng/ml, that is reported as cocaine negative and this is considered evidence for a treatment success. A simplistic goal of 'negative' urines does not address issues of quality of life, or treatment effects on possible or concurrent diseases. The treatment goal is of stopping drug use. Not given as much attention are the merits of a new treatment that might change a patient's urine cocaine level from 30 000 ng/ml to 3000 ng/ml—that is, continuing but more controlled cocaine use.

Kleber: The goal of the national strategy is certainly a sharp *diminution* of illicit drug use in the United States. Ideally we would like to eliminate it altogether, but that may not be totally realistic. I would be happy if we could reduce it to the very low level of the early 1950s. In our first strategy, probably for the first time, numerical goals were expressed: every two years, we hope to reduce *this* amount of drug use by *this* percentage.

Edwards: And you knew that the curve was already coming down?

Kleber: Interestingly, those goals were designed before we knew that that this fall had occurred! We believed they were rather ambitious goals when we first set them and saw no need to revise them to be even faster. We are now saying publicly that we expect to reach our goals faster than we stated originally. Zero tolerance has not been widely talked about since 1989, as I described earlier. Diminished drug use is the critical goal. Even if drug seizures are up, or spending on drug education has risen, if drug use is not going down, then we are not being successful. This should lead to an improved quality of life. We believe that poverty, unemployment and racism are all very desirable goals as well, but they are the responsibility of the rest of the US government. Our goal at the Office of National Drug Control Policy, as clearly defined by Congress, is diminishing the use of drugs. We know that drug use makes poverty and unemployment worse, and harder to escape from.

Edwards: Don Des Jarlais has given us a different and very threatening perspective. We have been able to comfort ourselves with the elegance of science, and then he has pulled back the curtain and shown us the frightening world outside the laboratory. I would like to know whether Don believes that the things he has been telling us about are effectively and adequately addressed by research.

Des Jarlais: As a scientist myself, I have to believe in the unpredictability of scientific research, and that things being done in the lab. at some point will be directly relevant to the immediate field situation. I would not want to see the laboratory work discontinued or constrained by political imperatives. It is vital for people working in the lab. to let their imaginations run, in terms of choosing interesting topics to investigate. My concern is much more that the epidemiological research, and particularly the ethnographic research, because it is often coming up with bad news, is more likely to be underfunded. Ethnographic work is labour intensive. To talk your way into a crack house or a shooting gallery requires much preparation, so that you know it will be safe to go in, before you even start collecting data. There is the tendency for that work not to get the same continuing support as the laboratory experiments. I would also recommend that people doing lab. work occasionally talk with drug users, both as a source of ideas and as a source of a moral perspective on their own work.

Woolverton: On this point about the continued funding of animal research, I personally don't have any difficulty in translating the relevance of what we already know through animal research to the human situation. For example, it's been well demonstrated in the animal laboratory that punishment is an effective way to suppress cocaine-maintained behaviour but that the punishment has to be strong and has to be delivered immediately to be effective. Some of the research that I presented (p 149) has demonstrated, at least to my mind, that the monetary cost of cocaine, relative to other reinforcers in the environment, is an important determinant of cocaine self-administration. Alternatives that are available to the organism are vital determinants of self-administration. If anything, the idea that we should continue to fund animal research because it might at some point turn up something that is directly relevant to what's going on in the human may be arrogance in the reverse direction. What I would say is that we already know from behavioural work, with and without drugs, that given control of the contingencies of reinforcement, one can control behaviour. What has to be decided is how much control of those contingencies you want to give, and to whom. This is obviously not a simple issue. But in my mind, animal research is already telling us relevant things. Perhaps there is a failure on our part to communicate effectively to you what that animal research really means.

Moore: We have all come to this meeting with different agendas. My particular point of view is to be interested in things that I didn't know that have some bearing on future policy choices. It might interest you to know what thoughts might now be rattling through the head of a reasonably well-informed, occasionally thoughtful policy maker, based on what I have heard so far.

One thought is that cocaine is a vastly more complicated drug than many of the other drugs of abuse. I think this has to do with the intrinsic properties of cocaine and not just our close-up focus. It has a variety of different forms and it is astonishing to find out how complicated this all turns out to be.

A second thought, that perhaps we haven't underlined enough, is that the position of the scientific community on cocaine as a dangerous drug has changed radically since 1974. In the 1975 White Paper on Drug Abuse in the USA, I wrote that cocaine was not an addictive drug, and deserved less attention than heroin. I did that at least partly on instructions from the scientific community. (The epidemiological evidence at that time also made it clear that heroin was then the more serious problem.) I am now embarrassed by that view. What is interesting is to think about all the dimensions of danger and hazard that this group (as a representative group of drug researchers) is now depicting as important problems associated with cocaine. Through all the complicated mechanisms by which drugs produce damage, this drug seems to be producing lots of damage. If this is true, it is a significant and radical change.

As a further comment on that aspect, it's interesting that many of the adverse effects of cocaine that have been discovered have come out of human experience, as measured by epidemiology, which science then tries to understand, rather than as predictions of science. So it is *experience* that has taught us that this drug is dangerous, rather than science. Then science tries to help us understand in what ways and through what mechanisms cocaine might be dangerous.

AIDS/HIV in cocaine users

The third point that has come up is that it looks as though it will be difficult to develop a pharmacological treatment for cocaine abuse, given the complexity of the drug's actions.

We have also referred to science policy, and the balance between basic and applied research, without reaching any resolution—although Don Des Jarlais has suggested that the balance ought to shift a little bit, towards the applied end, given the uncertainty about what kind of science is going to produce what result, either in basic science or in applications.

These points appeal to me as important lessons that could be drawn at this stage. I am not sure that they are correct or appropriate ones, but you can feel the weight of science in their conclusions. Interestingly, they are not the conclusions of an *independent* science, but of a science that is alive with the experience of the societies.

I was interested by the Chairman's challenge in his Introduction that we should identify the things we are now saying about cocaine that will sound odd and quaint, a hundred years from now. When I listen to Don Des Jarlais, I think of Dr Benjamin Ward Richardson complaining about nervous women drinking tea in the afternoon; here we are now, talking about crack dens infested with AIDS and syphilis. We now think of the first example as an odd comment. Will this view sound odd too, or is the crack den the thing that is going to end the drug epidemic, because it will result in the death of a large number of drug users? I have no way of knowing, at this stage, whether in those powerful images we are seeing an important truth that we have to respond to, and round which our policy ought to turn, or whether we are allowing ourselves to become victims of horrible images for which we have receptor sites in our brains just because they are so compelling.

Musto: First of all, I am glad to know to whom to attribute that remark in the 1975 White Paper! I also had an interesting experience at about that time; two years after 1975, I was on the White House Strategy Council on Drug Abuse Policy. It was only by a very narrow margin that we did not recommend the decriminalization of cocaine in the 1979 strategy. I was one of those opposed, but many observers thought that cocaine was harmless. When one mentioned history, it was dismissed on the grounds that the earlier rejection of cocaine had been in an era of ignorance and fanaticism, whereas modern scientists were now demonstrating cocaine's safety.

I was struck by how powerful this conviction was. The trend against drugs in this declining phase of the current wave of drug use is as profound as the initial tolerant attitude. Even though we still hear comments that small amounts of cocaine use are possible without problems being created, my impression from a study of the American experience is that the antagonism and intolerance toward cocaine will only become more powerful in the next 10 years. 'Zero tolerance' is increasingly the attitude of the public that will fuel legislation and the provision of punishment. So I agree with Professor Moore that these large trends, which extend beyond the question of cocaine, are enormously powerful, and their roots are very curious. It also brings home to me how weak in affecting policy are references to history and past experience, when a contrary conviction grips a large number of a society's policy makers.

Kalant: I think the need is not only, as David Musto stated, to put together the views and knowledge and approaches of different sciences, but also to recognize that scientific skill is often accompanied by a certain arrogance that leads us to ignore past history on the grounds that it doesn't count because it wasn't studied with modern methodology. This can lead us to ignore the fact that, as Mark Moore said, we recognize problems from human experience, not from laboratory hypothesis. Human experience showed that cocaine created problems which were well recognized and described abundantly in the clinical literature, and no one has shown that modern scientific methodology invalidates the clinical observations of 50–100 years ago. We would do well to keep that in mind.

Anthony: As an undergraduate in 1967, I first encountered a discussion of cocaine in a biology class, and the drug was *not* then portrayed as a harmless drug. I took my first pharmacology course in 1972; again the drug was not depicted as harmless, although the extent of cocaine abuse in the USA was said to be small compared with that of marijuana or LSD. Can anyone else reflect back on this span of the past two to three decades and say whether the view that cocaine was harmless might have been held by a relatively small segment of the scientific community, or whether this was the general consensus?

Negrete: What was being said then in psychiatry or the social sciences, though? That was not a time in which the neurosciences were as important as they are now. We are in the 'decade of the brain' at present, whereas at that time the social sciences influenced the thinking of the day very strongly.

O'Brien: Jim Anthony's point is absolutely accurate that 'establishment' behavioural pharmacologists had developed techniques through the 1960s and 1970s which showed that cocaine was a very powerful reinforcer, and students in most pharmacology courses were being taught the same things that he was taught; we were also seeing rare cases of what you might call cocaine addiction among very wealthy people. But this was in a social environment where people were more likely to perceive that drugs were not harmful, and there were certain policy makers and people more on the fringe of science saying that cocaine was harmless. However, students in our courses didn't hear that cocaine was harmless, and I think that other establishment pharmacologists were not saying such things either.

Strang: I am concerned that we move between being scientists and politicians, because the fact is that the conclusions we reach will change over time. It may well be that scientists reported what they did in the mid 1970s because that was to a large extent correct; and if you looked at low dose snorting of cocaine, the conclusions of Robert Byck and his colleagues might not have been far off the mark (Van Dyke & Byck 1982). We keep trying to satisfy politicians by talking about cocaine as a whole. Presumably none of us would actually regard the topical local anaesthetic application of cocaine as being a major health or social hazard!

Kleber: The situation in the late 1970s was that part of the scientific community knew the danger of cocaine, but connected to the White House at that time were people with a different point of view. A key White House drug abuse adviser was a member of the board of NORML (National Organization for the Reform of Marijuana Laws) which wanted to legalize marijuana. In one textbook of psychiatry with a chapter describing cocaine to be safe in 1980, the author had not changed his views by 1985, in spite of the dangers that had become evident and the deaths from cocaine overdose. Some people just don't want to be beholden to experience!

Kuhar: One factor that may have been important in leading people to think that cocaine was not a serious problem was the lack of a physiological abstinence syndrome, such as you see with alcohol and heroin. In many people's minds, cocaine was 'only' psychologically addictive. One of the achievements of our era has been the demonstration that even though cocaine is 'only' psychologically addictive, the fact that it takes over your behaviour is just as bad, and just as damaging to society.

Edwards: The relationship between the objective evidence which may be to hand on a drug's harmfulness and society's subjective appraisal of that threat certainly raises general questions that go beyond cocaine. The history of America's prohibition experiment points to exactly that issue. At the outset of the experiment, the 'evidence' was read as suggesting that getting rid of alcohol would cure violence, empty the jails, and make the sun shine for ever. Prohibition was then repealed because by bringing alcohol back you would create employment, get rid of crime, and fulfil the American dream. History is replete with examples which should warn us that governments and society often experience great difficulty in distinguishing between fact and fiction, so far as the dangers resulting from drug use are concerned. Anyone listening to Don's presentation is likely to be persuaded that the widespread use of cocaine by the injected route constitutes a significant and growing public health threat because of the potential association with HIV. He puts these facts squarely before us. At the same time, some of us may feel that the dangers of crack, though real, have at times been exaggerated. It is getting the balance of concern right which is so difficult in the face of cocaine or other drug problems.

References

Calello M, Libonatti O, Boxaca M, Weissenbacher M 1991 Increasing risk of heterosexual HIV-1 spreading due to intravenous drug use in Argentina. Presented at the Seventh International Conference on AIDS, Florence (abstr W.C.3326)

Chaisson RE, Baccheti P, Osmond D, Brodie B, Sande MA, Moss AR 1989 Cocaine use and HIV infection in intravenous drug users in San Francisco. JAMA (J Am Med Assoc) 261:561–565

Fay O, Taborda M, Fernandez A, Fernandez E, Rodenas L, Rubio L 1991 HIV seroprevalence among different communities in Argentina after four years of surveillance. Presented at the Seventh International Conference on AIDS, Florence (abstr M.C.3263)

Friedman SR, Sterk CE, Sufian M, Des Jarlais DC 1989a Drug using environments, drugs injected, and risk among IV drug users. Presented at the Fifth International Conference on AIDS, Montreal (abstr Th.D.O.3)

Friedman SR, Rosenblum A, Goldsmith D, Des Jarlais DC, Sufian M 1989b Risk factors for HIV-1 infection among street-recruited intravenous drug users in New York City. Presented at the Fifth International Conference on AIDS, Montreal (abstr T.A.O.12)

Garfinkel H 1956 Conditions of successful degradation ceremonies. Am J Sociol 61:420–424

Lima ES, Bastos FIPM, Friedman SR 1991 HIV-1 epidemiology among IVDUs in Rio de Janeiro, Brazil. Presented at the Seventh International Conference on AIDS, Florence (abstr W.C.3287)

Marx R, Aral SO, Rolfs RT, Sterk CE, Kahn JG 1991 Crack, sex and STD. Sex Transm Dis 18:92–101

Mesquita F, Moss AR, Reingold AL, Ruiz M, Bueno RC, Paes GT 1991 Pilot study of HIV antibody seroprevalence among IVDUs in the city of Santos, Sao Paulo State, Brazil. Presented at the Seventh International Conference on AIDS, Florence (abstr M.C.3008)

Moss AR, Bachetti P, Osmond D, Meakin R, Kefelew A, Gorter R 1989 Seroconversion for HIV in intravenous drug users in San Francisco. Presented at the Fifth International Conference on AIDS, Montreal (abstr T.A.O.11)

Novick DM, Trigg HL, Des Jarlais DC, Friedman SR, Vlahov D, Kreek MJ 1989 Cocaine injection and ethnicity in parenteral drug users during the early years of the human immunodeficiency virus (HIV) epidemic in New York City. J Med Virol 29:181–185

Ratner M, Inciardi J, Bourgois P et al 1991 Crack pipe as pimp: an eight-city ethnographic study of the sex-for-crack phenomenon. Draft final report. National Institute on Drug Abuse, Rockville, MD

Schoenbaum EE, Hartel D, Selwyn PA et al 1989 Risk factors for human immunodeficiency virus infection in intravenous drug users. N Engl J Med 321:874–879

Van Dyke C, Byck R 1982 Cocaine. Sci Am 246(3):108–119 (p 128–134, US edn)

Vlahov D, Munoz A, Anthony JC, Cohn S, Celentano DD, Nelson KE 1990 Association of drug injection patterns with antibody to human immunodeficiency virus type 1 among intravenous drug users in Baltimore, Maryland. Am J Epidemiol 132:847–856

Williams TM, Sterk CE, Friedman SR, Dozier CE, Sotheran JL, Des Jarlais DC 1988 Crack use puts women at risk for heterosexual transmission of HIV. Presented at the Fourth International Conference on AIDs, Stockholm (abstr 8550)

Treatment of cocaine abuse: pharmacotherapy

Herbert D. Kleber*

Office of National Drug Control Policy, Executive Office of the President, Washington, DC 20500, USA

Abstract. Until recently the treatment of cocaine addicts was limited to non-pharmacological methods because cocaine abuse was viewed as a psychological addiction to the drug's euphoriant effects. Chronic stimulant abuse is now known to lead to neurophysiological adaptation. This physiological evidence, and the failure of many patients to respond adequately to psychological treatment, prompted clinicians and researchers to explore numerous pharmacological agents in the early 1980s. Promising medications that may affect the euphoria, the craving, withdrawal, or the toxic effects associated with cocaine are under development. Potential pharmacological agents being studied include tricyclic antidepressants, anticonvulsants, neurotransmitter precursors, stimulants and dopamine agonists, serotonin re-uptake blockers and agonists, neuroleptics and opioid agonists/antagonists. Most of the research to date is on anti-craving agents. While many positive clinical reports exist, most reports are anecdotal and uncontrolled. The available data are reviewed. Potential pharmacotherapies require further research to elucidate the differences between treatments, the target populations, the optimal dosages and duration, and the interaction with behavioural and psychotherapeutic approaches.

1992 Cocaine: scientific and social dimensions. Wiley, Chichester (Ciba Foundation Symposium 166) p 195–206

Many approaches have been developed to help addicts stop their drug use, but these methods do not work equally well for each type of addict. Unfortunately, the type of treatment a patient currently receives is frequently determined by the first door on which he happens to knock, when most addicts would stand a much better chance of success in treatment if aspects such as personality, background, psychiatric state, duration, extent and type of drug use were initially evaluated. The pre-admission screening process would then place an addict in a treatment programme most likely to meet his needs and produce the best outcome. Some patients need rehabilitation, but others need 'habilitation'— they lack the appropriate vocational, educational, or social skills to cope in

---

*Present address: Professor Herbert D. Kleber, Department of Psychiatry, Columbia University College of Physicians & Surgeons, 722 W 168th Street, Box 66, New York, NY 10032, USA.

society and, unless these needs are recognized and dealt with as part of therapy, relapse is almost inevitable.

For many years, both cocaine users and scientists viewed cocaine abuse as a psychological addiction to the very pleasant euphoriant effects of the drug. Evidence from the mid 1970s onwards makes it increasingly clear, however, that chronic stimulant abuse leads to neurophysiological adaptation (Fischman et al 1985, Gawin & Kleber 1986). This is not, however, the classic drug abstinence syndrome of the opiate or sedative variety. Instead, chronic high dose use of cocaine may generate sustained neurophysiological changes in brain systems regulating psychological processes. Changes in these neurophysiological systems could produce physiological addiction with a withdrawal syndrome whose clinical expression would be psychological (Gawin & Kleber 1984).

Cocaine withdrawal

The first 24–48 hours after cessation of prolonged cocaine use lead to a barrage of unpleasant symptoms that has been called 'the crash' (Gawin & Kleber 1984). After resolution of the crash symptoms, there are a few days of apparent normalcy. This is followed by a prolonged period of chronic dysphoria and limited pleasurable responses to the environment which has been called anergia, depression, anhedonia or psychasthenia. Such symptoms are usually not severe enough nor accompanied by sufficient additional impairment to meet criteria for a formal psychiatric diagnosis, but may be severe enough to contribute to an empty, subjective existence against which the memory of stimulant-induced euphoria is compellingly seductive. The cycle of stimulant binges may thus occur. Stimulant abusers describe the amelioration of such anhedonic symptoms after two to 10 weeks of sustained abstinence (Gawin & Kleber 1984).

Cocaine craving

Intermittent stimulant craving usually recurs even after initial abstinence has been achieved. This craving may or may not be accompanied by dysphoria, anhedonia, or other symptoms characteristic of the earlier withdrawal phase, and can be understood as a memory of the stimulant euphoria which contrasts with the less pleasant present. Unfortunately, there is a remarkable *lack* of memory of the crash or the adverse psychosocial consequences of abuse during this craving, but such negative memories may re-emerge after the episode of craving has passed. The craving tends to be episodic, lasting only minutes or hours with long free periods. It can re-emerge, however, months or even years after the last episode of stimulant use. Although abstinence from other drugs of abuse is also marked by episodic craving, craving in former stimulant abusers appears to have a particularly rapid onset and marked intensity. It can occur in association with a variety of factors, including mood states (positive as well as negative), geographic locations, specific persons or events, and intoxication with other substances, or in the presence of various objects directly or indirectly connected with cocaine use, such as money, white powder which looks like cocaine, or mirrors (which are commonly used to cut cocaine upon and separate it into lines to be snorted).

Pharmacological approaches to treatment

Because of the failure of many patients to respond adequately to psychological treatment approaches, clinicians and researchers began in the early 1980s to explore a number of pharmacological agents. These include lithium, tricyclic antidepressants, stimulants and dopamine agonists, and neurotransmitter precursors.

Lithium has been tried because of animal studies suggesting that it might block the effects of amphetamine and cocaine, but human studies so far have not achieved such results and there appears to be no blocking effect or general usefulness of the drug in these patients. A subgroup of patients, however (those with bipolar or cyclothymic disorders along with their cocaine abuse), do appear to benefit from lithium therapy (Gawin & Kleber 1984).

Tricyclic antidepressants such as desipramine were tried with a very different rationale. Because dopamine appears to mediate the acute cocaine euphoria, the anhedonia or dysphoria after long-term cocaine abuse could be based on homeostatic adaptation to cocaine in the dopaminergic system and might be reversed by pharmacological intervention. Desipramine was chosen because of its effect on both catecholamine and dopamine receptors and because it had fewer anticholinergic side effects than drugs with similar receptor effects. Both open (non-blind) and double-blind trials (Gawin et al 1989a) have now shown that a majority of patients demonstrated prolonged abstinence from cocaine and decreased craving for it after being treated with high doses of desipramine. The time course was a delayed one, consistent with desipramine's time course for neuroreceptor changes, and the drug did not usually take full effect until the second to third week. A majority of the subjects did not have a diagnosis of depressive disorder, and yet displayed desipramine-associated decreases in craving and abstinence-facilitating effects. The final dose of desipramine being used in this ongoing trial is higher than in many treatments for depression and is achieved faster. The starting dose is 50 mg a day, and the dose is increased rapidly, so that by the fourth day the patient may be receiving 200 mg per day. Patients who have not responded by the third week and whose blood level of desipramine is not in the 100–200 ng/ml range are given higher doses of the drug. Ongoing studies with desipramine, imipramine and similar drugs are being carried out by a number of centres in the USA. These drugs should not be given until a few days have elapsed after the crash, and blood pressure and cardiac rhythm should be regularly monitored. It is clear that desipramine is no panacea, however, because studies of its efficacy have yielded mixed results (Kosten 1991). It is probable that different populations of cocaine abusers will respond to different agents.

Since cocaine euphoria is presumed to be mediated by dopamine and since some neuroleptic agents are dopamine antagonists, animal studies have been tried to see whether neuroleptics would block cocaine euphoria, with variable results. Human trials are missing and, because of the frequent production of dysphoric reactions in non-psychotic individuals by these drugs and their potential in the development of tardive dyskinesia, it is unlikely that they will have a significant role in the treatment of cocaine abuse. One agent, however, appears somewhat promising. Flupenthixol, a xanthine derivative, has been tried at low doses with crack abusers in the Bahamas and has produced promising results (Gawin et al 1989b). Double-blind trials are needed.

The possibility that cocaine craving may be related to the depletion of dopamine, as well as the delayed onset of the effects of desipramine, have led to a search for agents that might have an earlier onset, such as dopamine agonists. The two that have been tried are amantadine and bromocriptine. Amantadine, a presynaptic dopamine agonist, has been tried alone and in combination with the neurotransmitter precursors tyrosine and tryptophan, and shown to ameliorate cocaine use and craving (Tenant & Sagherian 1987). Bromocriptine, a postsynaptic dopamine agonist, has also been shown to decrease craving on acute administration (Dackis et al 1987). Adequate double-blind trials are needed for both agonists. Preliminary data suggest that such agents may act quickly to decrease use and craving (i.e. within one week), but that their effects wear off within three weeks. Thus, their combination with drugs such as desipramine may be clinically useful. Methylphenidate has been tried as a treatment for cocaine abuse but appears to make the situation worse (Gawin et al 1985). This drug may be useful in cocaine-abusing patients with a clear history of attention deficit disorder (Khantzian et al 1984).

Cocaine blocks the re-uptake of serotonin at nerve terminals, so agents that act on the serotonin system are being tried as well as those that affect the dopamine system. Serotonin re-uptake blockers have been reported to be of use in treating depression and as general anti-appetitive agents of possible use in alcoholism, gambling, and obesity. As yet, no adequate controlled study of their use in cocaine abusers has been described. Kosten recently presented a review of studies on serotonergic agents for cocaine treatment (Kosten 1991). Sertraline, in an open (non-blind) trial at Yale University, decreased cocaine craving but not use, by comparison with historical placebo controls. 'Open label' fluoxetine in one San Francisco study decreased cocaine craving and self-reported use, but these decreases were not matched by an equivalent decrease in actual positive urine tests. Another study on fluoxetine, conducted at the Addiction Research Center in Baltimore, using cocaine abusers not addicted to other substances, showed no effect on the number of positive urine tests. A mazindol study conducted at Yale University also showed no effect. Thus, at this time, trials of serotonergic agents have yielded no significant results.

Neurotransmitter precursors such as tyrosine, the precursor of dopamine, and tryptophan, the precursor of serotonin, are generally safe agents which can be purchased without prescription. It has been suggested that they may be helpful in ameliorating cocaine crash symptoms (Gold et al 1983), but adequate double-blind trials have not been done. Moreover, the recent finding of eosinophilia-myalgia syndrome secondary to tryptophan ingestion (Kaufman et al 1991) requires that tryptophan not be used clinically to treat cocaine abuse until the aetiology of this potentially fatal disorder is clarified.

One can sum up the status of the pharmacotherapy of cocaine abuse by noting that a number of positive clinical reports exist, but most reports are anecdotal and uncontrolled. Systematic controlled clinical trials demonstrating efficacy appear to be present only for certain of the tricyclic antidepressants so far. Potential pharmacotherapies require further research designed to elucidate the differences between treatments, the target populations, and the optimal dosages and duration of treatment. It is also important to recognize that the nature of addiction requires that pharmacotherapy be combined with appropriate psychological and behavioural therapy. It is unlikely that any 'magic bullet' will stop drug addiction in and of itself.

Completing treatment

Addicts never emerge from a treatment programme completely 'cured'. In fact, it is only after they leave the relatively protective environment of a treatment programme that they face the greatest challenges to their ability to stay off drugs. Unfortunately, former addicts tend to yearn for the days when they could control their use of drugs, and most believe that they can go back to that 'honeymoon' period, despite numerous warnings from counsellors and former addicts. The experience of many recovering addicts shows that they cannot. For psychological, social, and perhaps even biological reasons, attempts at moderate drug use after the completion of treatment often rapidly lead addicts back to their former patterns of compulsive drug use. As a result, most patients relapse at least once or twice. For some, relapse is temporary—a 'slip' rather than a 'fall'—and it serves as a hard lesson that they cannot go back to controlled use. But, for others, relapse leads back to ongoing, compulsive drug use and the need for additional treatment.

Specific training in relapse prevention, regular contact with out-patient treatment, and involvement in self-help and support groups like Narcotics Anonymous, all become very important in both preventing and surviving relapse. Pharmacotherapy may be an important part of that overall treatment. Addicts with strong support from family, friends and counsellors are better able to resist the temptation to go back to drug use. And drug testing as a regular part of a follow-up out-patient programme provides recovering addicts with the added incentive to resist their craving for drugs.

References

Dackis C, Gold MS, Sweeney D et al 1987 Single dose bromocriptine reverses cocaine craving. Psychiatry Res 20:261-264

Fischman MW, Schuster CR, Javaid JI, Hatano Y, Davis J 1985 Acute tolerance development to the cardiovascular and subjective effects of cocaine. J Pharmacol Exp Ther 235:677-682

Gawin FH, Kleber HD 1984 Cocaine abuse treatment: an open pilot trial with desipramine and lithium. Arch Gen Psychiatry 41:903-909

Gawin FH, Kleber HD 1986 Abstinence symptomatology and psychiatric diagnosis in cocaine abusers. Arch Gen Psychiatry 43:107-113

Gawin FH, Riordan CE, Kleber HD 1985 Methylphenidate treatment of cocaine abusers without attention deficit disorder: a negative report. Am J Drug Alcohol Abuse 2:193-197

Gawin FH, Kleber HD, Byck R et al 1989a Desipramine facilitation of initial cocaine abstinence. Arch Gen Psychiatry 46:117-121

Gawin FH, Allen D, Humblestone B 1989b Outpatient treatment of 'crack' cocaine smoking with flupenthixol decanoate. Arch Gen Psychiatry 46:322-325

Gold MS, Pottash ALC, Annitto WD et al 1983 Cocaine withdrawal: efficacy of tyrosine. Soc Neurosci Abstr (B157; 13th Annual Meeting, Boston)

Kaufman LD, Gruber BL, Gregersen PK 1991 Clinical follow-up and immunogenetic studies of 32 patients with eosinophilia-myalgia syndrome. Lancet 337:1071-1074

Khantzian EH, Gawin FH, Riordan C et al 1984 Methylphenidate treatment of cocaine dependence: a preliminary report. J Subst Abuse Treat 1:107-112

Kosten TR 1991 Pharmacotherapy of substance abuse with serotonergic drugs. In: National Institute on Drug Abuse Research Monograph. US Government Printing Office, Washington, DC, in press

Tenant FS Jr, Sagherian AA 1987 Double blind comparison of amantadine and bromocriptine for ambulatory withdrawal for cocaine dependence. Arch Intern Med 147:109-112

DISCUSSION

Negrete: Dr Halikas has completed a double-blind, random-assignment, placebo-controlled trial of carbamazepine (Halikas et al 1991). This was done on an out-patient population of male crack smokers, over 20 days, with the first 10 days on placebo and then the active drug for half the sample, and vice versa for the other half. He finds that this drug, at doses sufficient to reach blood concentrations of 4 µg/ml or higher, reduced significantly the number of urines positive for cocaine (urines were checked every day during those 20 days). There were 7.5 positives out of nine while on placebo, compared to 6.1 while on carbamazepine. These subjects continued to have complete access to cocaine, they were not seeking treatment, and they were paid for participating in this trial. Although modest, the reduction in daily use while on carbamazepine is significant, given the double-blind conditions of the experiment.

On the use of desipramine, studied by Dr Kleber and others, it was found that there were beneficial results in the reduction of craving, but some other cocaine experiences were not modified. Are there any dangers of potentiation of the effects of cocaine—is there any increase in toxicity?

Fischman: When we looked at the cardiovascular responses of our subjects, we could not give as much cocaine under desipramine maintenance, because of persistent elevations of blood pressure. However, the elevation of blood pressure in response to cocaine of subjects maintained on desipramine was somewhat smaller than before they were maintained on desipramine. Although desipramine maintenance pushed blood pressure up into the range where we felt it was inappropriate to give more cocaine, in fact desipramine didn't increase blood pressure to toxic levels. There was, therefore, potentiation of blood pressure effects under desipramine, but it was not believed to be toxic. It is something that physicians should monitor in desipramine-maintained drug users.

Anthony: I am concerned about the ramifications of the effects of alcohol consumption, in relation to the prognosis for pharmacotherapy and cocaine. My question is stimulated in part by the observation that many of the individuals who are intensively involved in cocaine also are, or have been, intensively involved with alcohol, qualifying as alcohol dependent or as problem drinkers, or with some degree of alcohol dependence (Anthony 1991). So one might suspect that a history of alcohol dependence would modify the response to treatment.

Kleber: One reason it took so long to do our desipramine study was that under the terms of our grant we had to exclude anyone who had serious alcohol problems. This is part of the problem of doing research in the real world, where most patients are dually dependent, and trying to do as narrowly focused research as possible. The people in our desipramine study were not alcohol-dependent individuals. The recent finding that cocaine plus alcohol leads to the formation of a new toxic byproduct, cocaethylene (see p 89), should intensify research on the interaction between these drugs.

Edwards: I have two questions that may perhaps help to clarify the issues which we need to address in relation to pharmacological treatment. First, do we think that something is already available that we can recommend to physicians? And, second, and more difficult, where do we believe the future lies, in the sense of making a link between the laboratory research and the job of the clinician?

Jones: Of the psychopharmacological treatments that have been proposed, I don't think any treatment so far has been shown to be different enough from placebo to justify its use in routine clinical practice. That is not to say that a physician can't use clinical judgement and suggest something as innovative treatment, but we should not mislead ourselves or our patients. I share Juan Carlos Negrete's concern about the likely toxicity of our treatments. It strikes me as unlikely that we shall come up with a powerful medication affecting the dopaminergic system, be it an agonist or an antagonist, that would not have some kind of associated acute or chronic toxicity—alterations in seizure threshold, or in temperature regulation, or something else. There will be a price to pay for the treatments. As yet, not enough patients have been treated long enough with any of the currently popular research treatments for perhaps subtle toxicity to appear, if it exists. Even with the 'worst case' interpretation of the toxicity figures that Neal Benowitz presented, for example, hyperthermia is a relatively rare event among cocaine users—even though it can lead to a disaster when it occurs. So, in answer to your first question, I don't think there's a proven treatment yet, and I suspect there will be a price to be paid for any yet to be established treatment.

Jaffe: I would agree with this. At present, researchers are happy to see even statistical significance, and even if it turns out to be only the difference between 7.5 urine specimens out of nine positive for cocaine, versus 6.1, with a large enough group of subjects you can show statistical significance. This usually allows you to publish the results. In contrast, if you work with smaller groups and show dramatic results, it may still be said by those anonymous referees that because the results didn't reach statistical significance (your group wasn't big enough), the finding should not be published. This discourages people from undertaking the search for promising agents unless they have enough funding to get a big enough n value (size of group) not only to see differences, but to be able to show that the differences are statistically significant. I conclude that I have yet to see any pharmacological intervention for cocaine that has clinically robust effects comparable to methadone's effect in the heroin user.

Kleber: I don't disagree with either of your replies to Dr Edwards' first question. At this point, my conclusion would have to be that if I have a cocaine-dependent patient, I would first use non-pharmacological means to treat him or her: supportive psychotherapy plus relapse prevention plus referral to a self-help group. If that patient was not responding adequately, however, I would want to try pharmacotherapy. On the basis of current research, the best-studied drug is desipramine. It is clearly not a magic bullet; none of the drugs is. We don't have any methadone or naltrexone equivalent. It is simply a question of one drug being a little more promising than another. It is also important to recognize that these medications may be more effective than the research currently suggests if one does a better job of separating groups. For example, taking out the patients diagnosed as having anti-social personalities may yield much better results.

Jaffe: Nevertheless, it is useful to have a study such as yours that shows a statistically significant decrease in cocaine use in subjects treated with desipramine, and perhaps the recent study on carbamazepine referred to by Dr Negrete will, if confirmed, suggest still another clinically useful tool. The patients we deal with (drug users) have developed a kind of 'magical' relationship to something that you ingest. The physician who begins by saying that he is going to help using purely psychological means therefore works at a disadvantage. If you can in good conscience offer a medicine, you can sometimes get people to return often enough so that you can build the psychological link that gives you the opportunity to do something helpful for that patient. But our drug-using patients typically have a scepticism about the power of interpersonal relationships that must be bridged. Whatever you use that helps you to build that bridge increases your chance of helping the patient. This is my clinician's intuition; I have no evidence for it.

Negrete: But pharmacotherapy must be tested through double-blind placebo-controlled studies.

Jaffe: I would never use a double-blind procedure in a non-research clinical situation, however. I would ask the patient to try the medication in question and say 'This works for some people! Maybe it will help you!' I would use all the tools at my disposal, because my task is to help somebody in trouble, and I know that these tools are useful.

Gerstein: Dr Jaffe's statement that these patients as a rule have a scepticism about the power of the human relationship should be emphasized. On a clinical level, this is generally the most fundamental problem that needs to be treated! Drug-dependent patients have a faith in pharmacological relationships, and this undercuts their interest in and ability to successfully carry on regular interpersonal activity that is not based on or sealed with a drug exchange. In most cases, this behavioural and psychological disability is the primary clinical issue. In some cases, it is not a matter of restoring faith in interpersonal relationships—this was never there to begin with—but of socializing or internalizing that ability from scratch.

Moore: Are we in danger of romanticizing the development of methadone? My recollection is that we kept looking for three different effects that became more and more difficult to estimate. One was that methadone could block the effects of heroin; the second was that it could suppress the use of heroin in people who were prescribed methadone; the third was that it would produce attractive behavioural consequences for addicts who stayed on the regime. But my recollection of the pharmacology is that it turned out that methadone could not block heroin; large doses of opiates would override the blocking effect of any dose of methadone.

Kleber: In theory that is so, but in average clinical practice, it is unlikely; it is easy to give enough methadone that the subject is not going to get high on heroin, on any expectable heroin dose that he can afford.

Moore: And that was also the dose of methadone that didn't produce any euphoria?

Kleber: Absolutely. The euphorigenic effect of methadone is primarily based not on the dose, but how long it took you to get there—that is, what is the individual's current tolerance. Methadone blocks heroin euphoria via a cross-tolerance mechanism, not by the antagonistic effect of a drug like naltrexone.

Moore: So the principle of the blocking of euphoria did survive 10 years of experience with methadone?

Kleber: You can treat people on 70 mg of methadone for 10 years; it's a high enough dose not to be overriden by heroin, in the majority of cases. Nor will you be able to tell, except occasionally by some drowsiness, that the subject is taking methadone.

Des Jarlais: It's important to point out that much of the blockade treatment did not survive the ideology of 'just a substitute for heroin'. Low doses were prescribed in many methadone treatment programmes, whereby the least methadone was considered the best methadone dose. In the majority of methadone clinics in the USA, they are not giving large enough doses of methadone to produce a blockade effect.

Jaffe: That is the triumph of ideology over science! There's no evidence that the lower dose of methadone did anything but lower the efficacy of methadone treatment, yet such doses became popular and have been accepted even by clinicians who should know better.

Moore: I wonder if we were ever able to distinguish what was producing the reduction in heroin use? We did observe a reduction in the illicit use of heroin in association with oral methadone treatment, and we could attribute part of that to the blockading effect, and the fact that heroin was no longer producing euphoria. But another possible explanation for reduced opiate use was that the regime of daily urine testing, with the prospect of loss of continued supplies, discouraged patients from using it.

Des Jarlais: A double-blind, random-assignment controlled study was done in Hong Kong (Newman & Whitehill 1979). It showed that it was giving the medication that made a difference; it was not an effect of turning up at the clinic every day.

Moore: Do we know for sure whether the reduction of heroin use was producing the observed changes in unemployment and crime?

Des Jarlais: Reducing the use of heroin was a necessary but not sufficient condition for those social improvements.

Jaffe: On this question of what factors make the drug-using behaviour change, you have to look at studies designed to assess that issue systematically. A study at the University of Pennsylvania has modified the clinical treatment, other than the dose of methadone, which was held constant for all the three groups at an adequate (60 mg) dose. The study showed that systematic changes decreased illicit drug use and social problems as the level of psychological, social and medical services was increased (A. T. McLellan et al, unpublished work).

O'Brien: When methadone was held constant (approximately 60 mg/day), there was a dose–response curve for psychological interventions (counselling or psychotherapy): the more counselling you give, the less opiate in the urine, and also the less the risk behaviours for AIDS (which is another outcome measure). Thus we verified the increased efficacy of adding counselling by preventing increases in the numbers of HIV-positive patients. Thus methadone by itself, while adequate for some opiate-dependent patients, requires the addition of counselling or psychotherapy for optimal results.

Moore: So the example of methadone continues to be an alluring model for the effective treatment of cocaine!

Edwards: Would the laboratory scientists here, having heard this discussion of the clinical research issues, like to give us their sense of where future leads lie?

Balster: I think it's likely that the medications for cocaine abuse that we may be using in 10–15 years are already on the shelves of pharmaceutical companies or in the minds of pharmaceutical chemists, and that the likelihood of finding the ideal pharmacotherapy among drugs developed for other indications is relatively small. Thus we need policies and strategies that support the development of new medications designed specifically for the purpose of treating cocaine abuse. This requires a basic pharmaceutical development activity which should be done within the industry itself, perhaps with the support of government agencies, utilizing the general strategies of drug development for treatments for other disorders. Until that kind of programme is mounted we won't have any new medications specifically designed for the treatment of cocaine abuse.

Kleber: At present, the US government is funding a 35–40 million dollar medication development initiative, trying to do just what Bob Balster says—to work with the pharmaceutical companies to get the drugs that they may have on the shelf into trials where we can see whether they have any effect on cocaine euphoria or craving.

Fibiger: The opioid drug, buprenorphine, is one candidate for the treatment of cocaine abuse that may raise interesting political questions. There is evidence that buprenorphine decreases the rate of cocaine self-administration in animals. I don't know its present clinical status, but even if it is also found to be useful in decreasing cocaine intake in humans, there is reason to believe that it may not prove to be acceptable for use in the clinic. Specifically, we have obtained evidence that buprenorphine may improve cocaine's efficacy and that it doesn't reduce cocaine intake by blocking the stimulant's reinforcing effects. Rather, our data suggest that it may simply decrease the amount of cocaine required to produce a desired effect (Brown et al 1991). The political question is whether such a mechanism of action would be acceptable for the treatment of cocaine abuse.

Kalant: We should note that all the drugs that are being used now to try to treat cocaine abuse or dependence are based on attempts to interfere, one way or another, with various presumed mechanisms of action of cocaine. The availability of the cloned gene for the receptor (if the dopamine transporter is the receptor) should make it possible to find something which, for cocaine, would be more analogous to naloxone for opiates, in the sense of blocking whatever cocaine does, at the point at which the whole sequence of reinforcing action begins. This might be a better approach to specific therapy.

References

Anthony JC 1991 The epidemiology of drug addiction. In: Miller NS (ed) Comprehensive handbook of drug and alcohol addiction. Marcel Dekker, New York, p 55–86 (especially Table 2)

Brown EE, Finlay JM, Wong JT, Damsma G, Fibiger HC 1991 Behavioral and neurochemical interactions between cocaine and buprenorphine: implications for the pharmacotherapy of cocaine abuse. J Pharmacol Exp Ther 256:119–126

Halikas J, Crosby R, Carlson G et al 1991 Cocaine reduction in unmotivated crack users using carbamazepine versus placebo in a short-term double blind crossover design. J Clin Pharmacol Ther 50:81–95

Newman RG, Whitehill WB 1979 Double-blind comparison of methadone and placebo maintenance treatments of narcotic addicts in Hong Kong. Lancet 2:485–488

Psychotherapy for cocaine dependence

Charles P. O'Brien, A. Thomas McLellan, Arthur Alterman and Anna Rose Childress

Department of Psychiatry, University of Pennsylvania/Veterans Affairs Medical Center, 3900 Chestnut Street, Philadelphia, PA 19104/6178, USA

Abstract. Dependence on cocaine is a new disorder for contemporary US clinicians. Until the 1980s sufficient quantities of the drug were not available to produce a true dependence. Thus far the only models for pharmacological intervention involve an interaction between medication and psychotherapy; that is, medication may be able to facilitate a drug-free interval during which time the patient can be engaged in psychotherapy. Psychotherapy programmes for cocaine dependence have generally been modelled on group-oriented treatments of the type used by Alcoholics Anonymous. Controlled studies of therapy programmes for cocaine dependence are currently being conducted and one prospective random-assignment study comparing day hospital and in-patient rehabilitation shows generally good results. Behavioural treatments aimed at reducing or extinguishing conditioned responses in cocaine addicts have also shown efficacy in a controlled study. More general relapse prevention procedures including rehearsal and role-playing are also used in the treatment of cocaine dependence. Combinations of psychotherapy and pharmacotherapy have so far shown the most promise in the treatment of this disorder.

1992 Cocaine: scientific and social dimensions. Wiley, Chichester (Ciba Foundation Symposium 166) p 207–223

Cocaine dependence, as it is known in the 1990s, is a new disorder for the current generation of US clinicians. Until the 1980s, cocaine was not available in quantity, so compulsive use and other complications that force the user to seek treatment were not commonly seen. Use was limited by high price and scarce supplies. Now, cocaine dependence is the most common presenting problem in American urban substance abuse treatment programmes and we have had to develop new treatments, evaluating them as we go along. Early in the cocaine epidemic we noted that most alcoholics were also using cocaine. Accordingly, we integrated our cocaine-abusing patients into day hospital rehabilitation treatment, using the 12-step Alcoholics Anonymous model, an approach that had functioned successfully for many years in the treatment of alcoholism.

Day hospital treatment (partial hospitalization) enables patients to come to the clinic daily for several hours of treatment, but to return to their homes in the evening. Our impression was that the cocaine-dependent patients generally became engaged in this treatment programme and appeared to do well. To test this impression, we decided to conduct a prospective, random-assignment trial, comparing the results of day hospital treatment with those of the standard in-patient treatment for cocaine abuse/dependence.

In-patient versus day hospital treatment of cocaine dependence

The research subjects were 96 men seeking treatment for cocaine dependence at the Philadelphia VA (Veterans Affairs) Medical Center. Prospective candidates had to be less than 60 years of age, willing to accept either in-patient or day hospital treatment for one month, have a relatively stable residence for follow-up contact, have no present evidence or history of a psychotic disorder, have no indication of dementia and have no major medical problems. All met the study criterion of cocaine dependence by DSM-III-R (Diagnostic and Statistical Manual III, Revised) criteria. Those with mixed cocaine dependence and alcohol dependence were included in the cocaine category. Forty-eight subjects were randomized into each of the two rehabilitation programmes. The groups did not differ from each other on socio-demographic and substance abuse history, except that subjects assigned to the in-patient group were more likely to have had previous treatment for drug-taking (54% versus 31%) than those assigned to the day hospital group. As a group, the subjects were about 33 years of age, had about 12 years of education, and were almost all African-Americans. They averaged fewer than three years of cocaine use, although they had been drinking alcohol to intoxication for over seven years. There was little evidence of use of drugs other than cocaine, alcohol or marijuana. On the average, these patients were using cocaine about 13 times a month and were spending about $600 monthly on drugs. Relatively few of the subjects had not consumed alcohol in the past 30 days. Both groups had worked about 10 days in the past month and reported having psychological problems on 10 days out of the past 30. On the substance-use characteristics, the day hospital and in-patient groups did not differ significantly at baseline.

Despite the difference in settings, the two programmes were quite similar in terms of actual treatments rendered. The day hospital programme is in operation for 27 hours during weekdays, while in-patient treatment is obviously residential. Both programmes are 28 days in duration. The major therapeutic modality in both programmes takes the form of group meetings that focus on overcoming denial and helping the patient to learn to cope with everyday problems and stresses. Individual counselling and ancillary psychotropic medication are available when needed in both programmes. Both programmes provide education about the effects of addiction; both provide recreational therapy and encourage participation in a self-help group. The latter is provided on the campus of the in-patient programme, while attendance in community meetings is required and monitored during out-patient treatment. Both programmes offer medical care,

Treatment outcome

In this chapter we shall present programme completion data, Addiction Severity Index (ASI) (McLellan et al 1980) data (i.e. patients' self-reports), and results of urine drug screening comparing baseline data and follow-up at seven months. A complete data analysis is in progress and will be presented in another publication when all follow-ups are complete. In-patients (40 of 46, or 87%) were significantly more likely ($\chi^2 = 11.81$, 1 df, $P = 0.0006$) to complete their treatment than were day hospital patients (25 of 48, or 52%). The four and seven month follow-up results include all patients assigned to a given treatment, whether or not they completed the 28 day rehabilitation programme. Outcome findings at four months are based on 76 subjects (41 attending day hospital, 35 as in-patients); seven month outcomes (Table 1) are based on 56 subjects

TABLE 1 A comparison of in-patient and day hospital treatment of cocaine-dependent patients

ASI variables	Day hospital (n = 28) Intake	7 months	In-patient (n = 28) Intake	7 months	Significant differences Between groups at 7 months	Within groups over time
Abstinent from alcohol (%)	19	56	7	44	NS	0.05
Days intoxicated (of past 30)	6.11	2.19	5.67	2.7	NS	0.012
Days of cocaine use (of past 30)	12.8	3.22	11.6	3.27	NS	0.001
Did not use cocaine (%)	0	59	0	46	NS	0.05
Days of marijuana use (of past 30)	3.63	2.52	3.89	1.26	NS	NS
Amount spent on drugs (in past 30 days) ($)	521	79	476	358	NS	0.012
Drug factor score[a]	0.25	0.1	0.24	0.09	NS	0.001

All variables reflect the 30 days prior to interview.
[a]Factor scores vary from 0 to 1, with larger values indicating more serious problems.
NS, not significant.

(28 in each group). The follow-up rates at both time periods are over 90% for each group. The n values (group sizes) available for this report reflect delays in both data entry and data analysis, and follow-up time lags. The outcomes reveal considerable self-reported (ASI) improvement in virtually all drug- and alcohol-related behaviours at both four and seven months after entry into treatment. An example of these improvements is the change in cocaine use. Virtually none of the subjects had been abstinent from cocaine at entry, but over 60% reported abstinence at the four month follow-up and 59% (day hospital) and 46% (in-patient) reported no use at seven months. The two groups did not differ significantly on any substance abuse variable at either the four month or the seven month follow-up. The reductions reported at four months generally appear to have been maintained at seven months, with one exception. The amount of money spent on drugs appears to have increased between four and seven months for the subjects who had received in-patient treatment; however, this effect did not achieve statistical significance.

Results of screening urine samples for cocaine, opiates and benzodiazepines were available for about two-thirds of the subjects at each of the follow-up evaluations. Forty-nine urine drug screens (out of 76, or 64.5%) were available at the four month follow-up evaluation. Seventeen out of 27 (63.0%) of screens obtained for day hospital patients were negative for cocaine, as contrasted with 12 out of 22 (54.5%) of those obtained from the in-patient subjects. The two groups did not differ significantly in this respect. Thirty-nine urine drug screens (out of 56, or 69.6%) were available at the seven month follow-up evaluation. Eleven of 19 urine drug screens (57.9%) obtained for the day hospital group were negative for cocaine, as contrasted with 13 out of 20 (65%) of those for the in-patient group. Again, the groups did not differ significantly. Thus, the ASI (self-report) findings with respect to abstinence from cocaine are generally supported by the urine cocaine levels. Additionally, the urine data support the ASI finding of little regression in the level of improvement between the four and seven month follow-up evaluations.

With respect to the patients' level of functioning in areas unrelated to substance abuse, the ASI (self-assessment) data indicate significant improvements for both groups at both follow-up periods with respect to family/social, psychological and employment problems. The two treatment groups did not differ in the degree of improvement. There was little indication of improvement in medical problems at either follow-up point. There was some indication at the seven month follow-up of greater success in the area of employment for the in-patient subjects, as shown in the significant statistical interaction effects for employment income and for the employment composite score on the ASI.

Conclusions from the study

In this study of day hospital versus in-patient rehabilitation for cocaine dependence, our interim findings are that those allocated to in-patient treatment were more likely to complete the initial one month of rehabilitation (87% compared to 52%). However, when all patients entering treatment were re-examined four and seven months after beginning treatment, significant reductions in levels of *substance-related problems* were found for both groups at both follow-up evaluations. Over 60% reported no cocaine use during the 30 days before follow-up. There were no significant differences between treatment groups. Improvements shown at four months were generally maintained at seven months. These conclusions were supported by the results of urine drug screening. Furthermore, significant reductions in legal, family/social and psychological problem levels were revealed for both groups at both follow-up periods. There was no reported improvement in medical problems. At the seven month evaluation there was some indication of a better functioning in terms of employment in those who had received in-patient treatment.

This study shows that the majority of the cocaine-dependent patients did well in both treatment programmes, as measured by self-reports of improvement at the two follow-up points. There were no significant differences in efficacy between day hospital and in-patient rehabilitation programmes. Thus the day hospital approach appears to be a cost-effective alternative to in-patient rehabilitation programmes. Further research is needed to determine whether a subpopulation of patients can be identified who would not respond to the day hospital approach and thus require an in-patient rehabilitation programme.

Addressing the conditioned aspects of dependence

Researchers investigating treatment for drug dependence are constantly striving to develop new ways to prevent relapse to drug use in former addicts. This is a particular problem with cocaine dependence, where a return to compulsive cocaine use may occur shortly after a subject leaves a treatment programme. Both psychosocial and biological factors probably contribute to the phenomenon of relapse (O'Brien et al 1986). A critical part of the treatment programme, therefore, is analysing those factors that increase the likelihood of relapse after a period of abstinence. One of these relapse factors may be the presence of Pavlovian conditioned responses, produced by repeated drug administration in the presence of specific environmental cues. Such conditioned responses have been well-documented in the literature when humans or animals have repeatedly received psychoactive substances (O'Brien et al 1991). Cocaine among all drugs of abuse appears to be very potent in producing conditioned responses, which have been noted by numerous clinicians and studied systematically (Childress et al 1988, O'Brien et al 1990).

Former cocaine users report 'craving' when they are in situations where cocaine has been used or when they encounter stimuli (such as sights, sounds or odours) previously associated with the use of cocaine. It is true that the concept of craving is difficult to define and that it refers to a subjective phenomenon, but the concept has operational value in talking to patients, and studies using 'craving' as a measure have produced consistent results. Craving evoked by conditioned stimuli is puzzling to the former user, because it conflicts with his or her previous decision to avoid cocaine. Despite their expressed and apparently genuine intention to refrain from returning to cocaine use, these patients find themselves wanting the very substance that had recently got them into so much trouble. Some report intense craving, arousal and palpitations when they encounter a white powder such as talcum or sugar, or when they see a friend with whom they had used cocaine or when they encounter drug-buying locations, or experience a pharmaceutical odour—almost anything that has been repeatedly associated with obtaining and using cocaine. Thus a patient leaving a treatment programme is likely to encounter numerous stimuli that may increase the risk of relapse. Though many different factors probably contribute to the high rate of relapse among users of cocaine, the responses provoked by drug-related stimuli, presumably by way of a conditioning mechanism, are thought to play a role.

Preventing relapse in former cocaine addicts

We have done a series of studies attempting to understand and treat the causes of relapse after treatment for cocaine dependence. Several of these studies investigated the possibility that reducing or eliminating conditioned responses—by a process of systematic exposure to cocaine-related cues with no drug reinforcement (extinction)—may reduce the rate of relapse in abstinent patients who formerly were cocaine dependent. This procedure may be useful when integrated with traditional abstinence-oriented treatment programmes. Traditional treatment approaches have intuitively recognized the power of cocaine-related cues. Thus, abstinent patients are warned to avoid 'people, places and things' associated with previous cocaine use. In reality, even when well-motivated patients try to avoid stimuli connected with cocaine use, such avoidance is almost impossible. Patients need additional tools for coping with or reducing their drug craving.

Our approach to treatment complements attempts to avoid cocaine 'reminders' in the natural environment. We expose patients repeatedly to cocaine-associated cues while they are in a safe environment, in an attempt to reduce the craving and arousal often triggered by these stimuli. By repeated exposure of the patient to cocaine cues without cocaine being available, the power of these cues to produce conditioned responses (such as arousal and craving) which could lead to drug use and relapse should be gradually diminished.

Integration of cue exposure within a comprehensive treatment programme

A comprehensive treatment programme should address all categories of relapse-producing factors, including pharmacological, social, occupational, medical, legal, family, and additional psychiatric disorders, when they are present. Conditioning factors may play an important role in the tendency for some patients to relapse, but it is unlikely that conditioning factors would override all others. The influence of conditioning probably varies with the individual patient, depending on the relative importance of other relapse-producing factors in his or her life. Thus we have investigated the extinction procedure within the context of a treatment programme that addresses a wide range of issues thought to be important to the recovering addict.

A complete report of this treatment study is being published elsewhere (Childress et al 1992). In brief, the 37 patients were male, ranging in age from 28 to 53, with slightly less than two years of cocaine use. Though several of these patients also had histories of alcohol and marijuana use, those with a significant history of opiate dependence were specifically excluded. In general these relatively 'pure' cocaine-abusing patients tended to have significantly shorter addiction histories, and fewer previous episodes of treatment, than recently admitted patients presenting for the treatment of opiate dependence, or for dependence on more than one drug.

Assignment to treatment

After pre-treatment testing for the presence of conditioned responses, the patients in the study were randomly assigned to one of four treatment conditions: (1) supportive-expressive psychotherapy + extinction (SE-X); (2) supportive-expressive psychotherapy + activities to control for the extra attention received by patients assigned to the extinction condition (SE-C); (3) standard drug counselling + extinction (DC-X); and (4) standard drug counselling + control activities (DC-C). 'Control activities' consisted of sessions (equal in length and number to the extinction sessions) with self-help videotapes featuring suggestions for developing a healthy lifestyle, better relationships, and so on. Drug counselling was given by experienced counsellors according to a treatment manual developed in our treatment programme and represented good standard treatment for substance abuse. 'Supportive-expressive' psychotherapy (a psychoanalytically oriented form of psychotherapy) was administered by experienced doctoral-level psychologists and has been found to be significantly more effective than drug counselling for opiate-dependent patients (Woody et al 1983). The efficacy of psychotherapy for cocaine dependence has not been previously examined in a controlled study.

In-patients assigned to the 'extinction' groups (1 and 3) received 15, hour-long sessions of repeated, non-reinforced exposure to cocaine 'reminders' during the two-week period of hospitalization following their initial detoxification from cocaine. Therapy or counselling sessions were administered three times per week during this two-week period according to our manual. This in-patient treatment was followed by a two-month out-patient phase offering eight additional weekly sessions of extinction or control activities (with continued psychotherapy or counselling, according to group assignment). All these treatment sessions were additional to *standard* treatment for cocaine dependence at our clinic. Each hour-long cocaine extinction session contained three five-minute audiotape segments, three five-minute exposures to a cocaine-related videotape, and three simulated cocaine administration rituals.

Though most in-patient 'extinction' sessions were conducted on the treatment ward, sessions 1, 8 and 15 were conducted in the laboratory, to allow us to monitor physiological responses over the course of extinction. During all extinction sessions, the patient is first asked to rate the overall intensity of 'high', 'craving' and 'crash' (withdrawal), using a 1-10 scale for each. The type and intensity of symptoms are then probed through an accompanying list of 50 responses associated with early 'high' (euphoria), toxic (e.g. paranoia) and 'crash' phases of cocaine use. The entire rating scale developed in our programme is administered at the beginning and again at the end of each hour-long extinction session. These subjective responses were then analysed as described below.

Effects of the extinction sessions

Subjective responses. A one-way analysis of variance (ANOVA) was performed for each of the subjective variables of 'craving', 'high' and withdrawal/'crash', using number of sessions as the repeated measure. These analyses revealed a significant progressive effect of this treatment on all three subjective variables: craving ($P<0.0001$), high ($P<0.0001$), and withdrawal 'crash' ($P<0.0001$). Of these responses, craving was the most prevalent and persistent, reducing gradually over the course of 15 extinction sessions. Reports of 'high' and withdrawal/'crash' were less common, and were largely extinguished by the sixth hour of extinction.

Cocaine craving was the most intense and most frequently reported subjective response in the extinction setting. Extinction was effective in significantly reducing conditioned cocaine craving, 'high' and withdrawal over the course of 15 extinction sessions ($P<0.001$ for all three variables, on a one-way ANOVA with number of sessions as the repeated measure: Childress et al 1992). Figure 1 illustrates the reduction in reports of subjective 'high', craving and withdrawal as a function of extinction sessions in the first 25 patients. The results for the total sample were similar.

Physiological responses. With repeated exposure to the drug-related stimuli, psychophysiological evidence of arousal decreased (skin temperature, skin conductance), but these responses did not disappear even after 15 hours of exposure to the same stimuli. Heart rate responses were particularly resistant to extinction. As a whole, there were no significant differences in the heart rate responses to the cocaine-related stimuli from session 1 to session 15.

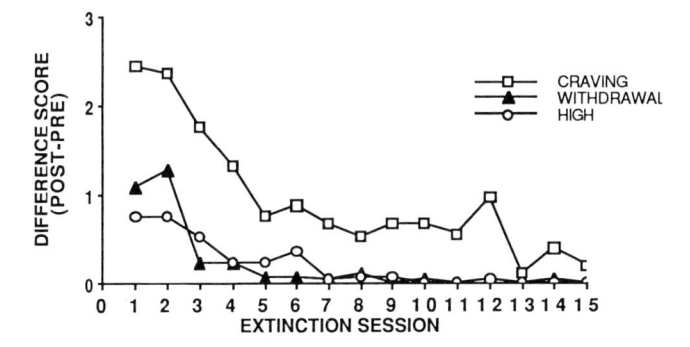

FIG. 1. Reduction in subjective responding to cocaine-related stimuli as a function of extinction ($n = 25$).

Outcome of treatment

The results of this randomized clinical trial of passive cue exposure or extinction are being reported in detail elsewhere (Childress et al 1992). Briefly, both groups exposed to extinction showed better 'retention' in out-patient treatment (i.e. remaining in treatment rather than dropping out) and a higher proportion of clean, cocaine-free urine samples than the two control groups. It was noteworthy that the group receiving counselling plus extinction did better than the group receiving supportive-expressive therapy from a doctoral-level therapist plus the non-extinction 'control' condition. When the two 'extinction' groups were combined, the differences between the groups on 'retention' and 'clean' urines were significant at the 0.05 level. These results were encouraging, because the extinction sessions were well accepted by the patients and the technique can be applied by non-professional drug counsellors. Our current work suggests that the beneficial effects can be enhanced still further by training the patient in active techniques (such as relaxation, covert sensitization and role playing) and then practising them in the clinic, to combat craving and arousal induced in response to drug-related cues.

The effects of this extinction procedure on retention in treatment and on cocaine use were roughly comparable in magnitude to the effects of available medication in promoting abstinence from cocaine (Gawin et al 1989). Combinations of medication and behavioural therapy may produce additive or even synergistic effects, and this combined approach should be examined in controlled studies.

Acknowledgements

This work was supported by US Public Health Service grants RO1 DA 000586 and P50 DA 5186 and by the Medical Research Service of the Department of Veterans Affairs. Parts of this review were presented at the 1990 meeting of the Association for Research on Nervous and Mental Disease.

References

Childress AR, McLellan AT, Ehrman R, O'Brien CP 1988 Classically conditioned responses in cocaine and opioid dependence: a role in relapse? In: Ray BA (ed) Learning factors in drug dependence. (National Institute on Drug Abuse Research Monograph 84) US Government Printing Office, Washington, DC, p 25-43

Childress AR, McLellan AT, Ehrman R, O'Brien CP 1992 Treatment effects produced by adding repeated cocaine cue exposure to a comprehensive cocaine outpatient treatment program. Am J Addict, under review

Gawin F, Kleber H, Byck R et al 1989 Desipramine facilitation of initial cocaine abstinence. Arch Gen Psychiatry 46:117-121

McLellan AT, Luborsky L, O'Brien CP, Woody CE 1980 An improved diagnostic evaluation instrument for substance abuse patients: the Addiction Severity Index. J Nerv Ment Dis 168:26-33

O'Brien CP, Ehrman R, Ternes J 1986 Classical conditioning in human opioid dependence. In: Goldberg S, Stolerman I (eds) Behavioral analysis of drug dependence. Academic Press, San Diego, p 329-356

O'Brien CP, Childress AR, McLellan T, Ehrman R 1990 Integrating systematic cue exposure with standard treatment in recovering drug dependent patients. Addict Behav 15:355-365

O'Brien CP, Childress AR, Ehrman R 1991 Conditioning models of drug dependence. In: O'Brien CP, Jaffe J (eds) Advances in understanding the addictive states. Raven Press, New York, p 157-177

Woody GE, Luborsky L, McLellan AT et al 1983 Psychotherapy for opiate addiction: does it help? Arch Gen Psychiatry 40:639-645

DISCUSSION

Edwards: The results you report of 59% abstinence from cocaine at seven months follow-up seem to be significantly better than one would be seeing with nicotine dependence. They are also better than one would generally see with alcohol problems. If I am right, then with what is considered to be an extraordinarily reinforcing drug, you are going against the tide and achieving amazing results. Can you give us some more information on your treatment sample, and how these people compare with the generality of cocaine users?

O'Brien: This question of whom we are treating is certainly important. I believe that it's a mistake to focus too much on the drug-taking behaviour and not to pay enough attention to the social dysfunctional syndrome that our patients tend to have.

Those whom we treat for heroin addiction and alcoholism have been using their drug for an average of 10 years before they come into treatment. They have lost many of their social support systems and their employment opportunities; they have a higher frequency of chronic psychiatric disorders than the cocaine-using patients, who tend to have more acute problems. So cocaine brings patients into treatment more rapidly. I accept that some never come into treatment for their cocaine use, but those cocaine users who get into trouble, and therefore whom we see in our clinic, tend to have a shorter history than opiate or alcohol cases. Since their course of illness is shorter, they have not broken their social support systems; therefore, they still have something to fall back on, and they respond better to psychological treatments than I initially predicted that they would.

Benowitz: To go back to the smoking analogy, your good results may be because your main focus has been on a long-term change of lifestyle. With cigarette smoking, it's relatively easy to get people to stop smoking for four or six weeks, or even three months, using pharmacological means (such as nicotine chewing gum). Because nicotine is not being used to maintain smokers in the way one uses methadone for heroin addicts, the toughest therapeutic problem is not short-term cessation but rather the prevention of relapse, or maintenance of abstinence. To me, considering treatment in two phases—initial cessation and maintenance of abstinence—is a much more helpful way to think about potential interventions. A pharmacological intervention is likely to be of use only for short-term cessation, unless we discover a maintenance agent like methadone, which seems doubtful for cocaine.

O'Brien: I agree, and this is why I feel so strongly that this is where animal models need to be focused, for the reasons you give.

Des Jarlais: Having monitored data on treatment for cocaine in New York State, over a sample of maybe 400 programmes, including more than 100 'drug-free' programmes that treat cocaine as well as heroin, I consider yours to be extraordinarily good results, Dr O'Brien.

Gerstein: In comparing the results of treatment across different programmes, it is crucial to notice that a sample of army veterans, such as Dr O'Brien is reporting on, is nothing like the sample of patients that would typically be found in a publicly funded treatment programme not specifically directed at veterans. The age, criminal history, and vocational and educational status would all be quite different. If we are hearing about honourably discharged veterans (and if they were not, I assume they would not be eligible for a Veterans Affairs [VA] programme), they have had a minimum of four years of successful military experience, which alone would greatly differentiate them from the undisciplined lives that so many public clients have led. In fact, these results don't look so different from the results that the Comprehensive Care Corporation's chain of treatment units reports in its follow-up of patients, and that programme does not have the reputation of being a research-quality programme, as the Philadelphia VA treatment programme does. The nature of the sample is critical in terms of predicting what would be a good or bad result, and one cannot compare programmes without reflecting on what their treatment samples are.

Des Jarlais: Certainly, many people going into publicly funded treatment programmes in New York City would never have entered the army, because their drug use was already at a level to exclude them, so Dr O'Brien may be working with a group that is particularly responsive to treatment because of factors originating prior to their drug use.

Jaffe: To underscore Dean Gerstein's point, let's think back to our experiences with the kind of chronic heroin users that we admitted to in-patient services, as we developed community hospital programmes in the late 1960s, where we found 80–90% relapse at the end of 90 days. And then let us recall our surprise when Lee Robins and her coworkers did the follow-up of heroin-dependent army veterans returning from Viet Nam in 1971 and found only a 5% relapse rate at the end of one year with minimal treatment (Robins 1974). We have to remind ourselves continually that it's not just the drug, or the individual; it's the interaction.

Nevertheless, the very fact that a programme like Dr O'Brien's can produce results of this kind is powerful evidence that treatment can play a major role in a nation's response to the drug problem. We need not assume that it's hopeless. These are large effects, and they are effects compared with a group without access to treatment; any calculus of cost–benefit analysis has to take that into consideration.

Negrete: I think your treatment service must also be commended for its continuing efforts to evaluate what it is doing, which adds to the therapists' burden! As regards the subjects dropped out of treatment, for whom you have data at four and seven months, were they paid to come back to give urine samples then?

O'Brien: Yes, they were.

Negrete: Concerning arousal reactions to cues, and your attempts to extinguish such responses, I have tried to establish who will be the more eligible candidates for undergoing cue desensitization therapy. However, their responsiveness to cocaine cues did not tell me much about the outcome of treatment; those who reacted strongly to cues were not necessarily those who did poorest, twelve months later; there was no statistical correlation with outcome. Are you happy with your desensitization efforts? Do they really add something to your programme?

O'Brien: There was an additive effect of desensitization with the general rehabilitation programme. Those who were randomly assigned to 'extinction' did somewhat better than those who received standard treatment. But we weren't satisfied with the results because the improvements over standard treatment, though statistically significant, were not large. The approach you have taken, Dr Negrete, to see if there is any predictive value from conditioned responses, is a good one, and we have been looking at our own data with prediction in mind. We would like to know if this cue-extinction is worth the effort. We need to know if the conditioned responses represent an epiphenomenon that is associated with drug use but does not necessarily have an important role in relapse, or if they are central.

Negrete: I have found that cue reactivity is more strongly associated with psychological distress at the time of exposure than with measures of cocaine addiction, such as duration of use, quantity/frequency index of use, or days of abstinence prior to the test (unpublished results).

Strang: Of those who were still using cocaine at the four month follow-up, I gather that the average frequency of use had become substantially less? Is that correct?

O'Brien: That's correct. The entire group was using cocaine on average on 13 days per month before treatment; the group as a whole was using cocaine for an average of two days per month at both follow-up points (four and seven months). This includes those who were using zero cocaine at follow-up and those who were using it for much more than two days.

Strang: So, in addition to the evidence of individuals who became drug free, you have impressive evidence of a moderation of the continued drug use in many of the others.

Secondly, two different interpretations have been suggested for your encouraging results. You yourself are suggesting that the nature of the drug and its use by the population means that you happen to have picked up early cocaine users. The other suggestion is that there is a stoical quality to army veterans that makes them better candidates for treatment than the average cohort. The nature of the interpretation has very different implications for the place of pharmacotherapies in treatment. If the good results you obtained are just to do with the chronicity of the condition, then one would need different strategies from those needed if the results are to do with the populations from which subjects are drawn.

O'Brien: There is a wide spectrum of different types of patients out there. Dean Gerstein is quite right, that these US military veterans have a better prognosis than people who are in public (free) treatment programmes. Our subjects had an average education of 12 years; they were high school graduates. This contrasts with a community clinic in a low socioeconomic community, where the average education may be only six years. But remember also that our group was 98% Black; about half were using cocaine intravenously; the other half were smoking crack. There were very few taking it intranasally. Moreover, the alcoholics and the heroin addicts in this population of military veterans do not generally do as well as this group of cocaine-dependent patients. So military veterans can have poor prognoses as well; they certainly are not as healthy as, for example, a population from an employee assistance programme, where the cocaine use has been detected even earlier. I would say that ours is an average population, better than some in its prognostic indicators, and not as good as others.

Kleber: Dr O'Brien has obtained excellent and important results. What I find especially interesting is that they fit into the numbers that I, as a policy maker, have been asked to give before Congress. I have based these on my clinical experience of many years, because the hard data are not as available as we would like. If you treat business executives, lawyers, or other upper-middle-class individuals with a cocaine problem, a success rate of about 65% is not unreasonable. Whereas with blue collar workers (people who are employed, are high school graduates, have vocational skills, and often have families) the success rate with good treatment can be in the 40–60% range. But if we treat crack addicts with no vocational and limited interpersonal skills, we are lucky to get 20–25% success. My guess is that these veterans fall into the middle group, so I am delighted to see the result.

Is cocaine addiction harder to treat than, say, heroin addiction? Cocaine is an extraordinarily addictive drug, but, like many stimulants, it 'burns you out', so users tend to come to treatment quicker. The group in the desipramine study came to treatment on average 3.5 years after first using cocaine, whereas yours had 2.9 years of use. This is one 'advantage' of cocaine, that because it 'burns you out' quicker, and gets you into trouble earlier, it may enable you to do better in treatment than a heroin user. People can continue for 10 or 20 years on heroin before stopping. If the patient is coming to us relatively healthier, he may be easier to treat.

Jaffe: I have another concern. If this treatment approach to cocaine dependence works well in other groups of cocaine users, in 3–4 years there won't be enough patients to provide clinical justification for the treatment capacity we are now trying to set up! In other words, if the cocaine epidemic is winding down, and there are fewer and fewer cocaine-addicted people coming to seek treatment, we need to give more thought to the nature of the structure that the United States is setting up to respond to the people who now need treatment. If the response to treatment can be so good, should we perhaps be looking for a more transient type of treatment system that will respond to a *crisis*, rather than to a chronic, endemic problem where we would expect that there will always be people seeking treatment?

Moore: I am interested in the question of what constitutes success in treatment, from both a policy and a clinical point of view. The imagery in people's minds is of drug abuse as an acute illness that we treat with a single intervention, and it works if we manage to suppress drug use to zero, and if there's some relapse, that's a failure. That image is reinforced by the way we keep track of the results of drug treatment. But we all know that drug use is a chronic condition, where the interesting question really is of how much effort we need to put in to maintain certain increments of improvement, both in drug-taking and in terms of other social and behavioural evidence. To my mind, the method of reporting the results, that shows a continuing failure of treatment at some level, tends to emphasize the instability of the effects that we are able to produce with the single-intervention type of treatment. The negative picture, of constantly losing patients because they are relapsing, continues to reinforce in the public's mind the image that the right result to seek is that 100% of subjects remain drug free for ever, after the treatment, and that things keep getting worse as users relapse, the longer the treatment goes on. This is a terrible image to leave with people.

The alternative way to represent the goal of drug treatment would be to keep reminding the public that cocaine addiction is a chronic illness, and to show them not the relapse from abstinence, but, instead, the improvement relative to what the individuals would have done if they had remained on the waiting list for treatment. The question of how to make this result vivid for people in general is a key to building the political support and understanding for treatment.

O'Brien: That is an important point that I had wanted to bring up myself. I am surprised that until now no one has attacked me for my definition of 'success'! In fact, when I present our detailed results I do make it clear that there is still drug use by our subjects, even while they are in treatment. Our staff wanted to kick some people out of treatment during the day hospital period (28 days) because they were showing some drug use, yet it was declining. It typically stopped during the course of treatment for those who continued to come in daily. The after-care was very important. There was clearly some drug use, but we defined success as being drug free during the prior 30 days and having clean urines at follow-up interview. We are saying that the treatment needs to be continuing. We need to educate policy makers about the nature of this chronic disorder, where you need to continue treatment. There are clinicians working in our field who could look at our data and say that we had a 90% failure rate, because most of our patients use drugs at least once after they enter treatment despite our best efforts keep them 100% abstinent.

Kalant: If you are down to 59% and 46% patients who are abstinent at seven months while continuing the same schedule of out-patient visits for both groups, and presumably the percentages who remain abstinent would fall further if you carry on to a year or 18 months, what can you do to keep improving the results? Do you put the subjects into hospital for a period? But the group that did better (day hospital attenders) had not been in hospital as in-patients. Do they receive an intensive group therapy again? I can see the value of maintaining a group under chronic treatment with periodic jacking-up of some kind, but what does it consist of?

O'Brien: We did precisely that. We have a programme of after-care whereby, when subjects get into trouble by using cocaine, they are taught that this is not something to be embarrassed about, and to come back and get help. We then try to work out with them why they relapsed. We shall continue to follow these people and see if the abstinence rate remains in the same range. We felt that seven months was probably the maximum time that we could follow them and be able to attribute changes to the effects of the one initial course of treatment.

Kalant: Is the attenuation of abstinence more or less continuous during that seven month period?

O'Brien: We have only the two 'slices' there, of cross-sectional follow-up times (four and seven months), so I can't tell you what it's like at any other point. Not all of these subjects are in after-care; the number there tends to fall. But if they become acutely ill again, so that they are willing to come back into treatment, we accept them back for treatment, either day hospital treatment or more of the intensive out-patient care.

Edwards: What is treatment really for? Is it to do with the greatest good for the greatest number? Is its worth to be judged in terms of its objective efficacy as a society-wide response, or do we also value and promote it because it carries some kind of symbolic power and humanizes society, even if in the harsh objective sense it often reaches only the minority of people in need, too late, and with questionable efficacy? Is it an attempt to avoid worse solutions?

Jones: The current aim of much of our drug abuse treatment in the USA is to lead or push people to the proper moral state! Dr O'Brien's study, where some of the people had been employed before treatment, and then with a good treatment outcome, seems to me as a physician to be more than adequate—at least as good as when we treat many other medical disorders. Most of his patients would be unemployable for any federal government job, or for large numbers of companies that do periodic testing for the presence of illicit drugs in a worker's urine. Although much improved by many criteria and (relative to their pretreatment state) seemingly more in control of drug use, they still occasionally use illicit drugs. These occasional slips will be picked up eventually, and Dr O'Brien's patients will lose their jobs, or get recycled back into another treatment programme. The dilemma is that judged on the basis that we judge outcome for most medical treatment, your result is good. But in terms of the morality-based judgements of some policy makers in government in America, your treatment has failed: you still have a group of unemployable veterans, since they occasionally have evidence of having used cocaine in their urine even though otherwise they are doing well.

Kleber: The purpose of treatment is to reduce the social and individual pathology that drug abuse carries with it. Chuck O'Brien would be the first to point out that the majority of his patients came there because of some external pressure. Without that pressure, many of them would not have come for treatment at 2.9 years of use—perhaps not till five or seven years, if they hadn't been pushed. They needed the incentive of knowing that something unpleasant would happen if they continued using drugs. There has to be some competing reinforcer or punisher; if you don't have that, drugs are too pleasurable for most users to want to give up.

Edwards: Nicotine substitution has been introduced as an effective treatment for cigarette smoking, and yet the number of deaths per year in the UK from smoking-related diseases has been revised upwards from 100 000 to 150 000. I really do want to know what people at policy level believe treatment is for. In reality, most smokers are never going to turn themselves in for treatment. Is it the controlled trial that carries persuasion with the policy makers, even if the results may not generalize beyond the exceptional research centre from which the report emanates? Is it enough to show that a treatment is effective for those self-selected people who walk through the treatment door, while failing to address the health service questions relating to help-seeking, barriers to help-seeking, the acceptability of the treatment to the mass of drug users in the community, and the 'market penetration' of the treatment you are purveying?

Kleber: When I testify before Congress, the committees break down to roughly half saying 'you are not spending enough on treatment; we need to do much more because of AIDS and crime', while the other half are saying that we have a lot of nerve to be asking for so much money for the treatment of addicts when it is clear that it doesn't work and that most of the time people relapse; treatment is a failure, they say, so we should put the money into building more prisons. Any evidence that treatment works helps us in justifying wanting to maintain and expand the treatment system, improving it, and doing better research. But if it's a question of discretionary dollars—you have 10 dollars; how much are you going to put into prevention, how much into prisons, and how much into treatment?—there is a feeling that since we are not going to treat our way out of an epidemic, only a certain percentage of those discretionary dollars for drug abuse should go into treatment. In the USA it has been decided that of $10 from federal sources, a little less than $2 will go into treatment, $1.50 into prevention, and $6.50 into a variety of international and domestic supply reduction activities. If everyone had Dr O'Brien's results, we might be able to increase it to $3 for treatment (and with poor results, it may get reduced to $1 out of $10).

O'Brien: I empathize with Herb Kleber's position, because the people he speaks with in government do not understand that for the most part, in dealing with cocaine dependence, we are not dealing with a specific medical disorder, as most physicians are. Cocaine dependence is a very complex syndrome, and the doctors who are giving treatment are given responsibility for everything that goes along with addiction. But in order to understand this problem properly you have to look at all the other social factors: the poverty, the lack of education, the unemployment, and so forth. It is a mistake to let ourselves, as physicians, accept all of this responsibility, when we can only be expected to focus, because of our training, on a small part of it.

Reference

Robins L 1974 The Viet Nam Drug User Returns: Final Report, September 1973. Special Action Office Monograph, Ser A, No. 2. US Government Printing Office, Washington, DC

Alternative strategies

Reese T. Jones

Department of Psychiatry, Langley Porter Psychiatric Institute, University of California, San Francisco, CA 94143, USA

> *Abstract.* Drug treatment alternatives in the United States are constrained by what is politically correct and expedient and by a federal policy of 'zero tolerance' for any illicit psychoactive drug use. A war on drugs will not solve all the problems posed by cocaine. Alternative strategies must address fundamental problems in ghetto life: violence, poverty, poor health, no education, no jobs, and few reasons for not taking drugs. Despite warnings of pharmacological determinism, cocaine is like other psychoactive drugs. Even with cocaine, when alternative behaviours are possible most people avoid out-of-control use. Public health strategies promoting a harm-reduction policy offer advantages. Recent reductions in cocaine use are a consequence of education, awareness of good health practices, and interest in other activities. Alternatives could include cocaine in a safer, non-lethal and controllable form but are unlikely in a political climate where politics and law prevail rather than medicine and humanity.
>
> *1992 Cocaine: scientific and social dimensions. Wiley, Chichester (Ciba Foundation Symposium 166) p 224–241*

Alternative strategies for what? After chapters on the pharmacotherapy and psychotherapy of cocaine addiction (Kleber 1992, O'Brien et al 1992), I might logically consider alternatives like acupuncture, self-help groups, prayer, electroconvulsive therapy or lobotomy. However, a focus on the treatment of individuals would not do justice to our understanding of the major cocaine problems. I shall instead consider some of the other strategies used in the United States in what has been termed a 'War on Drugs'. We are in the third year of what has been mostly a war on cocaine, though as drug wars evolve the drugs targeted for special attention vary (Musto 1991, Cahalan 1991). Critics have argued that strategies for fighting the drug war have consequences perhaps as devastating as does cocaine use itself (see Cahalan 1991, Alexander 1990). Suggestions for or even discussions of alternative strategies sometimes lead to questions of the patriotism or the sanity of the person mentioning the alternatives. People who question 'war on drug' strategies are 'the fellow travelers of the 1990's' (Zimring & Hawkins 1992). But that is sometimes the nature of war.

What about current strategies in the war against cocaine?

America's war plan is described in a paper called the National Drug Control Strategy (NDCS) (Office of National Drug Control Policy 1989). It must be read to be believed—easy to do, since it is only 90 pages long and presents strategic rather than tactical proposals. The NDCS document mentions the 'evil of drugs', the 'scourge of drugs', and defines drug use as a moral problem—insofar as it offers any definitions of the term 'drug problem'. An essay and critical analysis considers the NDCS in the context of contrasting approaches to drug control and argues that its legalistic position, among other things, exploits drug problems 'as a rallying point for authoritarian sentiments in America' (Zimring & Hawkins 1992). The NDCS offers a simple theme: drug abuse is a moral problem and can be best overcome by punishing illicit drug users through the law.

Federal spending designed to combat trafficking and drug abuse has gone from $6.3 billion in 1989 to $9.5 billion in 1990 and an estimated $10.4 billion in 1991. About 70% goes to law enforcement and supply reduction, the rest for prevention, treatment and education. For those concerned about cocaine, supporters of the government's policy point out that cocaine use has dropped by 72% in the past five years, the numbers of deaths and emergency room visits are down, and the cocaine epidemic is becoming localized. Critics of the policy point out that about 500 tonnes of cocaine still enter the United States each year (Treaster 1991). In Colombia alone, cocaine traffickers last year brought back an estimated $3.5 billion from their cocaine trade—roughly triple the amount Colombia earns from the sale of coffee, that country's largest legal export (Brooke 1991). The critics say that the optimistic government survey figures miss most of the real cocaine addicts. Critics of the current strategies also argue that it's clear we have already lost the war on drugs (Alexander 1990), or that it is now mainly a war on young African-American males and a war where the constitutional rights of all citizens are being constrained to fight what is falsely presented as a domestic threat to national security (Alexander & Holborn 1990, Nadelmann et al 1990). In recent years, severe limits on due process of law, removal of certain guarantees of freedom from unreasonable search and seizure, and justifications for excessive punishment, have all been justified by citing the threats posed by cocaine and other drug use.

Body counts and other consequences of drug wars

The NDCS concedes that 'locking up millions of drug users will not by itself make them healthy and responsible citizens' but suggests that 'the short-term reduction in the number of American casual and regular users will be a good in itself . . . because it is their kind of drug use that is most contagious' (Office of National Drug Control Policy 1989). Over one million Americans are now in prison—about 400 out of every 100 000 people, but about 3000 out of every 100 000 Black men. Thirty-eight per cent of people arrested for drug abuse charges are Black. About 80% of people in prison have drug abuse problems. In New York, one in four Black males in their twenties are in prison, on probation, or on parole, the majority because of drug-related offences. In 1990, the United States spent $1.5 billion for new prisons, increasing capacity by 100%. Currently, about 50% of all federal prisoners are in prison for drug-related offences. By the year 2000, if the current rate continues, almost three million people will be in prison. Since 1980, the overall crime rate in the United States decreased by 3.5%.

Cocaine is important in the current drug war and has to a great extent replaced marijuana, LSD, amphetamines and heroin as the drug most used by 'the enemy', separating society into the good and righteous who don't use and the bad, immoral, dangerous and damned who do. At this time, a war against cocaine is particularly attractive and makes for morally and politically accepted battles of good versus evil with overall success less important. The terrible cost to individual freedoms and the neglect of other social problems is presented as a necessity in a time of limited resources. Political and economic considerations take precedence over health interests. The drug war mentality fosters criminal justice bureaucracies and diverts attention, resources and energy away from issues like the serious economic and productivity problems in the United States.

Besides its $10 billion a year costs, the war has seriously damaged some of the guarantees of the Bill of Rights. Whether the aim of reinterpreting and weakening the protection offered to citizens by the Fourth, Fifth, Sixth and Eighth Amendments to the US Constitution is mostly to 'denormalize' cocaine and other drug use, or to decrease both supply and demand, is unclear. Life becomes more difficult and complicated for both the cocaine user and the cocaine seller, but at what cost to non-drug users and sellers?

For example, by a recent Supreme Court decision, police may now board any bus, train or aeroplane and without reasons to suspect any particular passenger engage in dragnet-style searches of passengers' luggage, seeking cocaine.

Or, if a person is to keep a job or to be hired into any job in about half of our major businesses in the USA, their urine can be tested. Twenty million people will have tests for cocaine in their urine in 1991 at a cost of about $350 million. If any cocaine metabolites are found, even though a result of a few doses of cocaine taken some days before the test, the job is refused or, if the subject is already an employee, treatment is mandated until that employee is cured of the propensity to use cocaine. This is all voluntary, of course, but the alternative, if testing or treatment is refused, is loss of employment.

People arrested for possession of cocaine can have their financial assets and material goods seized before they are tried and found guilty in court. With their money all gone, this sometimes makes it difficult for the accused to acquire their first choice of legal counsel.

In some areas in the USA where cocaine selling is rampant, automobiles are stopped at random and searched by police. Someone who has in their possession (in the car) unexplained amounts of money may have that money immediately seized by the policeman. The money is released only when an adequate explanation is later given to the court. If an explanation is not offered or considered adequate, the policeman seizing the money is able to keep it and use it for law enforcement purposes.

In Michigan a person arrested for possessing about $20 000 worth of cocaine (673 grams) was given a lifetime prison sentence without any possibility of parole, even though it was a first offence. The Supreme Court recently ruled that this lifetime penalty should not be considered excessive punishment because 'It was false to the point of absurdity to suggest possessing enough cocaine to yield 32 500 to 65 000 doses was a nonviolent and victimless crime'.

Anyone convicted of simple drug possession can have about 300 or so federal benefits withdrawn for up to five years—such as student loans, research grants, or media licences. If a drug rehabilitation programme is completed successfully (six months of negative urine tests), benefits may be restored.

Maybe cocaine is special and justifies a war?

In the usual 'war on drugs' rhetoric, rarely is smoked cocaine (crack) ever mentioned without it being referred to as highly addictive. Crack cocaine 'is, in fact, the most dangerous and quickly addictive drug known to man' (Office of National Drug Control Policy 1989). This is despite very little pharmacological evidence suggesting that smoked cocaine is any more or less addictive than other forms of cocaine or routes of use or, for that matter, more or less addictive than a number of other licit and illicit psychoactive drugs. In fact, whenever the data are examined objectively, they suggest that the intense interest in crack among some communities is as much driven by economic, capitalistic factors as by alterations in crack users' neurotransmitter systems (Cheung et al 1991, Fagan & Chin 1991).

Recall that in other times alcohol was depicted as being highly addictive ('the fatal glass of beer' metaphor) and, a little later, marijuana was presented as highly addictive in movies like 'Reefer Madness'; and, of course, heroin for many years was the prototype of the ultimate addictive drug (Musto 1991). Some observers have even suggested that perhaps nicotine deserves that label (Jones 1987, US Department of Health and Human Services 1988, Kozlowski et al 1989).

Cocaine seems to have some of the attributes of these 'most addictive' drugs. For example, it appears that, although many millions of people try, and use, cocaine, only relatively few appear to go on to use it more than a few times or to use it compulsively (National Institute on Drug Abuse 1989). Current estimates of 200 000 to 300 000 daily cocaine users amount to fewer than 4% of the people who may have used cocaine at some time in the past year and no more than 10% or so of those using cocaine currently (Goldstein & Kalant 1990). Thus, a small group of very atypical people who become compulsive cocaine users are the prototype.

One consequence of failing to distinguish between compulsive cocaine use (addiction) and cocaine 'experimentation' or, more accurately, occasional use, is that this diverts attention from the positive values that distinguish achievement-oriented, goal-directed occasional or past cocaine users from the smaller number of cocaine users who go on to become compulsive users and addicts. To ignore the distinction between the occasional and the compulsive user is to contribute to the wrongly assumed associations between crime, misbehaviour and the use of illicit drugs. As much attention should be given to those people who *don't* use cocaine, if we are to figure out why others do. For good reason, the best predictor of a good outcome in the treatment of cocaine addiction, be it pharmacotherapy or psychotherapy, is having a job or being able to get one, and having a family or other similar social structures in place (Gawin 1991). Cocaine users most likely to come to pharmacotherapy or psychotherapy are unlikely to give up the pleasures offered by cocaine unless they have available better choices as part of the bargain. Jobs, homes, and the promise of a better life for some people do not necessarily result from their simply stopping cocaine use. Alternative strategies are needed besides psychopharmacological drugs that might block desire, arousal, and the other consequences of cocaine use.

What about some alternative strategies?

Instead of presenting drug abuse as a moral and legal problem, many people have suggested a public health approach to demand reduction (Erickson 1990, Alexander 1990, Morgan 1991). Public health strategies also rely on law, but in a different and more humane way than does the more simplistic, legalistic prohibition policy. The criminal prohibition of cocaine use forbids the behaviour absolutely. Infractions must be subject to punishment. Its objective is absolute suppression consistent with a 'zero tolerance' for any philosophy that condones illicit drug use. From a public health perspective, however, some level of perhaps non-healthy cocaine possession and use may be tolerated, but legal regulations and policy focus more on enforcing standards of safety and, most importantly, they attempt to minimize harm (Erickson 1990). As an example, tobacco smokers are not arrested, yet legal controls on where and when they may smoke are regularly imposed. Yet tobacco addiction, at least in some countries, has been decreasing without a more draconian punishment-oriented public policy (Fiore et al 1990). A policy of something other than 'zero tolerance' for the use of psychoactive drugs is not so revolutionary (US Department of Health and

Human Services 1988). Most psychoactive drugs (the legal ones, that is) are regulated by law rather than prohibited—including, of course, cocaine. Even cocaine can be legally prescribed and can be used in the course of medical treatment, though practitioners who prescribe it, except in very limited circumstances, may well find themselves harassed by the law.

Punishment or threat of punishment by itself has not been demonstrated to be an effective deterrent of illicit drug use except in somewhat unusual, closely regulated groups; for example, among people in the army or navy. Judging from reports of possible and previous illicit drug users, the perceived likelihood of punishment has never been a significant factor in deterring drug use. In the United States, a strong correlate of the dramatically decreasing level of cocaine use in recent years has been the reports from cocaine users, or former users, of the increased perceived harmfulness of cocaine, and increased social disapproval of cocaine use. Cocaine is no longer in style. The few well-publicized deaths of public figures and exaggerated descriptions of cocaine's possible toxicity have probably accomplished more than the billions of dollars spent to cut cocaine supplies from South America. Perhaps, as seems to be happening with tobacco smoking, increased awareness of health hazards and restrictions on where smoking is acceptable is in itself enough to 'denormalize' drug use.

What about making cocaine available by a legal scheme?

Am I hinting at legalization in the sense of the unrestricted availability of cocaine? Of course not—at least, not in the sense that some libertarians might suggest. However, with a public health approach that emphasizes harm reduction, some of our now very constrained research strategies may change. For example, rather than search, probably unrealistically, for drugs that eliminate craving for cocaine or block the cocaine effects that a user seeks, we might consider a scheme of cocaine prescribing for some addicts, as is now done with opiates (methadone) and nicotine. A controlled-release, controlled-delivery, less abusable form of cocaine, analogous to the nicotine formulations used for treating nicotine addiction, seems technologically feasible. But, in a political climate where the use of cocaine represents as much a moral weakness as merely a pharmacologically unwise behaviour, this treatment strategy is not likely to receive serious consideration—not so much for purely scientific reasons, as for being politically incorrect. However, not too many years ago, some would have said the same about giving opiates to opiate addicts (Melkin 1973); but now, rightly or wrongly, that technological 'quick fix' for a complex social problem is accepted—a good example of the public health strategy of harm reduction. But, for now, the goal of the US National Drug Control Strategy is the zero use of cocaine and other illicit drugs, even though the health problems posed by some of the alternative drug replacements may not be trivial.

What is a better strategy?

Useful strategies are well described in the public health literature on alcohol and tobacco (Cahalan 1991). Important are efforts designed to make for a normative climate favouring non-drug use, as is happening with tobacco and alcohol, but in the context of more positive alternatives—health-related, increased well-being—rather than the loss of civil liberties and privileges. Even if a fraction of the government funds currently spent on the US Criminal Justice response to cocaine use were directed to prevention efforts, including proper education (without excess propaganda), effective rehabilitation offered in the context where it is attractive enough that people need not be forced into it, together with proper evaluation providing adequate data to make future policy adjustments, it would make it a better world. For most of the US population, demand reduction for cocaine has already been so very effective that for literally millions of former cocaine users, cocaine legalization is probably a non-issue. Survey data suggest that former users of this drug would not necessarily resume cocaine use, just because it was somehow more available.

The problem populations of cocaine users remain those whose health-related behaviours are most difficult to change (Cahalan 1991). What is really their primary problem? As scientists, do we really think that some of our inner city Black communities are so very vulnerable to compulsive crack use because the residents have a different serotonergic system regulating craving and satiety? This is nonsense. Or, rather, is their vulnerability mostly a result of long-standing, rapidly increasing social and economic chaos where, in many ways, psychologically and economically, cocaine offers a short-term but eventually disastrous solution? A few years ago Dr Herbert Kleber, in a talk at the 1989 annual meeting of the Committee on Problems of Drug Dependence, when addressing demand reduction strategies, referred to giving addicts 'a place in family and social structures where they may never have been before'. He considers this as 'habilitation' more than 'rehabilitation'. Maybe that 'habilitation' should be termed primary or complementary strategy, but it is certainly more than only an alternative.

Alternative strategies must eventually offer choices such as cocaine versus better housing, or cocaine versus jobs, or cocaine versus educational opportunities. To offer these choices means considerable economic investment in inner cities and in people for whom there has been little investment for many years, even though we spend considerable amounts of money to house some of them in prisons, and have spent much money abroad and at our borders to eradicate drugs.

Conclusions

A loss of community is a nationwide problem. It is most evident in America's inner cities. That is where the cocaine problem remains in the United States.

To manage or treat that social and social resource problem as a medical one by psychotherapy or pharmacotherapy, or to treat it as a problem of immoral or criminal behaviour, will not succeed. Cocaine is the focus now in America, but we have gone through similar cycles with other illicit and licit drugs without properly addressing the ultimate factors that regulate human drug use. In many ways, the scientific dimensions of cocaine (mechanisms of action, neurochemical matters and toxicity) are much easier to study and to understand than the relevant social dimensions. The social dimensions of cocaine use present little that has not been presented by other illicit drugs, but so far we have dealt with cocaine in the United States no better than with other drugs that have preceded it. When will we learn?

Acknowledgement

Research supported in part by grants DA00053 and DA01696 from the National Institute on Drug Abuse.

References

Alexander BK 1990 Alternatives to the war on drugs. J Drug Issues 20:1–27
Alexander BK, Holborn PL 1990 Introduction: a time for change. J Drug Issues 20:509–513
Brooke J 1991 Cali, the 'quiet' cocaine cartel, profits through accommodation. The New York Times. Sunday, July 14, 1991
Cahalan D 1991 An ounce of prevention: strategies for solving tobacco, alcohol, and drug problems. Jossey-Bass, San Francisco
Cheung YW, Erickson PG, Landau TC 1991 Experience of crack use: findings from a community-based sample in Toronto. J Drug Issues 21:121–140
Erickson PG 1990 A public health approach to demand reduction. J Drug Issues 20:563–575
Fagan J, Chin K 1991 Social processes of initiation into crack. J Drug Issues 21:313–343
Fiore MC, Novotny TE, Pierce JP et al 1990 Methods used to quit smoking in the United States. Do cessation programs help? JAMA (J Am Med Assoc) 263:2760–2765
Gawin FH 1991 Cocaine addiction: psychology and neurophysiology. Science (Wash DC) 251:1580–1586
Goldstein A, Kalant H 1990 Drug policy: striking the right balance. Science (Wash DC) 249:1513–1521
Jones RT 1987 Tobacco dependence. In: Meltzer HY (ed) Psychopharmacology: a generation of progress. Twenty-Fifth Anniversary Volume, American College of Neuropsychopharmacology. Raven Press, New York, 1589–1595
Kleber HD 1992 Treatment of cocaine abuse: pharmacotherapy. In: Cocaine: scientific and social dimensions. Wiley, Chichester (Ciba Found Symp 166) p 195–206
Kozlowski LT, Wilkinson DA, Skinner W, Kent C, Franklin T, Pope M 1989 Comparing tobacco cigarette dependence with other drug dependencies. Greater or equal 'difficulty quitting' and 'urges to use', but less 'pleasure' from cigarettes. JAMA (J Am Med Assoc) 261:898–901
Melkin D 1973 Methadone maintenance: a technological fix. George Braziller, New York

Morgan P 1991 Illicit drugs. J Public Health Policy (Spring):20–23
Musto DF 1991 Opium, cocaine and marijuana in American history. Sci Am 263(1):20–27 (p 40–47, US edn)
Nadelmann EA, Kleiman MAR, Earls FJ 1990 Should some illegal drugs be legalized? Issues in Science and Technology (Summer):43–49
National Institute on Drug Abuse 1989 Drug use, drinking, and smoking: national survey results from high school, college, and young adult populations, 1975–1988. DHHS Publication No. (ADM) 89-1638. US Government Printing Office, Washington, DC
O'Brien CP, McLellan AT, Alterman A, Childress AR 1992 Psychotherapy for cocaine dependence. In: Cocaine: scientific and social dimensions. Wiley, Chichester (Ciba Found Symp 166) p 207–223
Office of National Drug Control Policy, Executive Office of the President 1989 National drug control strategy. US Government Printing Office, Washington, DC
Treaster JB 1991 Cocaine manufacturing is no longer just a Colombian monopoly. The New York Times. Sunday, June 30, 1991
US Department of Health and Human Services 1988 The health consequences of smoking: nicotine addiction. A Report of the Surgeon General. DHHS (CDC) Publication No. 88-8406
Zimring FE, Hawkins G 1992 Ideology and policy: a look at the 'National Drug Control Strategy'. In: Zimring FE (ed) The search for rational drug control. Cambridge University Press, Cambridge, Chapter 1

DISCUSSION

Edwards: Reese Jones has been telling us about the broad societal response to cocaine in the USA. Let's try to get some idea of how other countries are responding. For a start, what is the difference between the Canadian approach to cocaine and that of the United States?

Kalant: I shall be going into some of the differences later, in my formal paper, but I would just mention two things here. First, the proportions of federal money that go into Canada's national Strategy on Drug Abuse are almost the inverse of those in the USA; in Canada, about 30% is spent on law enforcement and about 70% on demand reduction, through various programmes. Second, the courts have considerably more discretionary power in terms of sentencing than in the USA. Over 60% of sentences for cocaine possession in Canada consist of fines, or even conditional discharges.

Strang: In the UK, contrary to popular opinion, the approach by government is predominantly a control-driven approach, not so much because the 'control' component is very high, but because the treatment component is extremely low. As in Canada, though, there is considerable scope for discretion in the courts. What is evident from Reese Jones's paper is that this issue of whether one considers cocaine use as a moral disorder (and hence whether 'refraining from sin' is the approach that should be adopted) does not fit current thinking in the UK. In so far as cocaine use has been considered at all, it has been seen from the perspective of minimizing the harm resulting from HIV, of trying to reduce risk behaviour while the use of cocaine continues.

Alternative strategies

Edwards: Professor Uchtenhagen, what about the responses to cocaine in countries of continental Europe?

Uchtenhagen: The general picture is characterized by inconsistent positions and developments, although most European countries have ratified the single convention on narcotic drugs of 1961. Countries with rather liberal attitudes have introduced new legislation with stricter regulations. Sweden, for instance, has a new law including provisions for involuntary treatment; Italy has recently adopted legislation which makes drug consumption punishable; Spain has switched to a policy of the 'denormalization' of drug use (viewing it as undesirable) and strengthened law enforcement. On the other hand, other countries like Switzerland are debating new experiments in reducing repressive measures against drug users while reinforcing prevention campaigns; the new approaches concern the free availability of injection equipment, and sheltered living and working for drug users without making abstinence a prerequisite, providing opportunities for 'safe' injection in supervised shooting galleries, or introducing heroin and cocaine on prescription. Thus, repressive policies and harm-reduction policies follow each other like pendulum swings, because no country can really be satisfied with the effects of its policy.

Even within European countries you may find inconsistencies, based on differences in tradition and cultural background which make one or the other attitude preferable. A national drug policy, for example in Switzerland, is becoming increasingly difficult because of divergent cultural orientations in the different parts of the country.

Efforts are being made to gain more international consensus among European countries, favouring either a predominantly law-enforcement approach or a harm-reduction policy. One of the priority concerns is to develop a more rational basis for deciding which policy elements should be shared among European countries, as opposed to other elements of drug policy which should take local and regional needs and differences more into consideration. This process has just started, for example in a research project evaluating recent changes in drug policy by looking at their intended and unintended effects (a project of the European Cooperation in Scientific and Technical Research [COST], in which member States and non-member States of the European Community may participate).

Edwards: Dr Kaplan, is it true that Holland is moving towards a more repressive style of response to drugs?

Kaplan: That is true, in fact. In certain local regions in The Netherlands, especially bordering Germany, cities like Arnhem and Enschede are becoming very upset by having German heroin addicts coming and staying in their communities. In fact, a body called the 'drug tourism commission' has been set up by the Dutch government to review this process and to look very specifically at how more repressive measures can be used to make The Netherlands less attractive to foreign drug users. So Holland is responding almost completely pragmatically to the situation; it's almost a 'compact disc' of many different kinds of approach. One can find therapeutic communities, treatment, and a sense of tolerance, as well as repressive drug control measures. The problem of the national government is how to coordinate and provide platforms for all these views. The general political view, from parliament, is somewhat the opposite to the situation presented by politicians in the USA. The problem in The Netherlands is for the government to persuade politicians not to press for the legalization of drugs, because if they did so at this time, legalizing cannabis for example (for which a majority in the second chamber feels the time is right), this would only attract more 'drug tourism', whereas The Netherlands government wants to be a leading member of a larger political process that's going on internationally. They want to show restraint and to hold back for the time being.

There's an idea currently that discussions on the evolution of the cannabis policy should be linked with the discussion on the making of a cocaine policy (Cohen 1990). There is a feeling, going back to Canadian research on the cannabis–cocaine connection (Murray 1984), that this linkage needs to be understood, and that maybe, by allowing the natural development (within the practical constraints) of cannabis availability, one will decrease rather than increase cocaine use. Almost in the same way that relapsing cocaine addicts, in a situation where there is no substitute for cocaine, will return to it, what Canadian research has shown is that people who cease to use cocaine might smoke cannabis instead in a unique process of 'de-escalation' (Erickson & Murray 1989, p 151). So there is a move to open up the cannabis–cocaine dialogue, in The Netherlands.

Edwards: Let's now return to the picture which Reese Jones has been giving of the USA. His picture is of moralism rampant. Do others of you here who know America very well want in any way to revise or qualify his assessment? Is it possible, perhaps, that politicians have to make a lot of noise to get elected, but meanwhile very liberal processes are more quietly and covertly at work?

Woolverton: There certainly is a profoundly mixed message, in that official policy against drug use is so strong, and yet the marijuana smoking of a nominee for the Supreme Court has been deemed 'inconsequential'. After all, this is a crime for which a sixteen-year-old in the ghetto could be thrown in jail.

Jones: Remember that much of my information, although from newspaper sources, was from what are assumed by some Americans to be authoritative sources like *The New York Times*!

Gerstein: The USA, contrary to general opinion, is not one country. It is a large and complicated region of the North American continent, which includes States which vary, and Counties which vary. National policy is a thin fabric which looks smooth and uniform while afloat in the rhetorical atmosphere, but takes on the contour of every bump and hollow (and sinks entirely in places) once settled on the ground (or into the swamp) of local realities. I should add that it is significant that Reese quoted a specific national policy document (the September 1989 National Drug Control Strategy), and that virtually all his quotations were from the preface written by William Bennett (then Director of the Office of National Drug Control Policy). I would interpret that preface as a campaign speech, because of the marked contrast between the preface and the rest of the document. It is hazardous to interpret policy from the point of view of a campaign statement. This isn't to say that the preface represents an empty point of view, but that point of view is not the alpha and omega. It happens that 20% of the US population, if given the chance, would vote to put alcohol prohibition back into effect; but this is just one end of the spectrum of what the country thinks. These quotations are drawn, further, from the first of several national strategy documents, and there has clearly been an evolution of views in those documents. So, even as a portrayal of a point of view within the federal government of the USA, it is out of date.

Moore: If it is hard to give representations of the 'views' of any given country, it is even harder to give a picture of what US national policy is, whether one looks at declarations of purpose and justification, or at actual action at ground level. But there have been important changes in drug policy over the last 8–10 years that are worth considering. These are the areas in which I agree with Reese Jones.

It is true that for a long time, in the 1970s, the goal of drug policy was to minimize the adverse consequences of drug use for the users and their surrounding communities. Those utilitarian kinds of logic and calculation were the routine ways in which drug policy was discussed. Something that has been added to that since the arrival of the Reagan administration in 1980 is a notion that this might not be quite the right representation of what our goals should be, and perhaps not even the right way to talk about drug policy. What the Reagan administration added to this utilitarian conception was the further observation that drug use was a moral hazard to the individual—something bad for his soul as well as for his job prospects and his health. I don't see that as necessarily a harmful addition. It did tap into something that many people thought was a problem with drug use; they felt it to be a wilful choice to be irresponsible, and the wrong thing for a democratic citizen to do, and it was important to recognize that this was part of what was going on and should be resisted. So this moral perspective was added as an important goal of national drug policy.

In so far as that idea prevents discussion about how policy instruments do or do not achieve that objective, this was a dangerous change, in my view. I would prefer to have the policy conversation be a practical discussion, founded on widely agreed policy goals. I would like to have debate about whether the policies are effective at accomplishing given purposes, even if the purposes include the desire to minimize drug use and intoxication as such, and not just to eliminate the bad consequences.

To recapitulate, you can say that moralism comes into the discussion as an important goal to achieve. The argument runs as follows. It's the duty of an American citizen to be accountable for his or her actions and not be intoxicated, and not be dependent on drugs. Therefore, for those reasons, we shall try to reduce the use of abusable drugs. And you don't even have to tell me that it also makes you ill, or liable to get into road accidents. It's just wrong to put yourself in that state, so we are going to reduce drug use, at the level of either intoxication or dependence. That is a moral statement, but it doesn't mean that you have to decide that every effort has to be defended on behalf of the accomplishment of that goal, and that the only appropriate instruments are law enforcement and punishment. There may be many other things that can be done to help to accomplish the same goal.

The second thing that has been a problem in the USA has been obscuring the differences among drugs. This has made it difficult to have a rational discussion about the various drugs and the appropriate use of the law, and of enforcement mechanisms.

The third point, to which Reese Jones has rightly attracted our attention, is that in confronting what turned out to be an underlying cocaine epidemic at this particular moment in the history of the USA, we have reached for the use of the *authority* of the State to combat the problem, rather than the largesse of the State. That is, in a money-starved government, policy makers reach for all the instruments that use the government's authority to tell people how to behave, rather than use its power to raise taxes which would make money available that would allow us to persuade people to behave differently, through counselling, or educational programmes. All of that seems right to observe and to question. In my view, the worst effort to use State authority and power to accomplish these goals has been to make it a crime for pregnant women to use cocaine—a remarkable set of events happening now in the USA.

To all these extents I agree with Reese Jones. Where he went too far, in my view, was in delineating the attack that he claims has been made in the USA on civil liberties and freedoms, and not answering sufficiently the questions about what role laws and the criminal justice system could be made to serve in an overall drug policy. He implied that whenever, in the USA, these instruments are grasped, it must be because society has fallen into the grip of moralism and is on the brink of fascism, because no rational person could ever choose to deploy these instruments as instruments of policy. I would dispute that view quite vigorously.

Edwards: When we have this picture before us of America charging over the cliff of absolutism (a very slight exaggeration of what Reese has been saying!), I want to remind myself that Marian Fischman tells us she is able to give cocaine to experimental subjects, which you probably couldn't do in a country moving towards a police State. Furthermore, she gives cocaine to people who are known to be cocaine users, who presumably are willing to come forward in trust to see her, and she is not required to inform the police, and is not deemed to be compounding a felony.

There is a strange paradox here. I get on the one hand a feeling of enormous openness and massive investment in compassionate attempts to help people. Then on the other hand I am told that in the background there are people who are shouting strange slogans and preaching absolutism. The rest of the world has spent many years trying to understand the USA. Can someone help me to understand?

Moore: You have described the USA perfectly; that's the way it is!

Jaffe: The question as you put it is one to which I cannot respond within the time frame of this conference. There are many issues; policy is changing (although not as rapidly as Reese Jones's paper would indicate). The integrity and indeed the very possibility of scientific enquiry into problems of drug abuse, including the testing of the effects of psychoactive drugs, was resolved over the considerable objection of some law-enforcement groups just about 20 years ago, when the Special Action Office was given authority to develop policies with respect to the entire 'demand' side of the drug abuse problem. This policy, however, was built on a tradition of research that began when the government's own research programme was started in Lexington, Kentucky in the 1930s. How long this freedom of inquiry and experimentation will be able to survive, if the current swing toward moralism continues in the USA, is unclear. I don't see any vigorous movement to attack the concept of research directly, but there are attacks on drug abuse research of all kinds as either irrelevant or immoral. Putting someone with research experience—Dr Kleber—in a position of high authority and visibility in the White House office of the 'Drug Czar' provides a certain buffering of those who argue against the relevance of drug abuse research; but for how long this support will continue in the high level policy groups concerned with drug abuse problems is difficult to say. There are indeed inconsistencies in some respects in our drug policies, but then nowhere is it written that policy has to be consistent! There are inconsistencies, and that is probably part of our American history as well; it began that way and will continue.

Almond: There may or may not be moralism in American society, and I expect there is moralism, but you can't infer it from the legislation. That is to say, you cannot conclude, from the fact that there is anti-drugs legislation, that it is there simply in order to foster the moral improvement of the *individual*, so long as you can point to various ways in which the behaviour in question affects the *community*. And there can be little doubt that there are community effects involved here, which it is legitimate for governments to try to control.

Anthony: I would consider what Reese Jones has provided in his paper as a mosaic of recent experience in America. Perhaps individual pieces of the mosaic have been tilted a little bit in order for him to make certain points. Nevertheless, the mosaic should be regarded as a representation of experiences shared by many of us.

I would like to add that in our democracy (in spirit it still is a democracy) the leaders have failed to take full advantage of an unprecedented opportunity to put societal policy onto a more rational basis in relation to the individual psychoactive drugs, including cocaine. This opportunity is provided by the dramatic prevalence of marijuana use in the period from 1960 to 1980, to the extent that it became an exception for a high school graduate or college student, or someone of that age, to *not* use marijuana, and to *not* violate the controlled substances legislation. We could have used that base of experience with drugs and with drug law violations to transform the attitude of the nation toward one that attends more closely to the relative influences of the drug itself, the conditions under which the drug is administered, the ultimate consequences of drug use for the society, and the control of drug-using behaviour by alternative reinforcers and by the consequences of drug use. The opportunity to create a more rational policy by taking advantage of the marijuana experience of a large proportion of our population has escaped our leaders, I believe.

Musto: In the declining phase of these drug 'epidemics', drugs begin to lose their individual identities: they all become just 'drugs'. It is in the rising phase of drug toleration—as in the 1960s and 1970s—when careful distinctions are made among drugs. With alcohol, too, in alcohol-tolerant times, there are many distinctions among the various forms of alcohol—beer, wine, whisky, and so on—and even more distinctions among the brands in each category. But when a temperance movement shifts the image of alcohol from that of a beverage to that of a poison, all forms become just 'alcohol'. As Stephen Leacock wrote in an earlier temperance movement: 'There were days when we called it Bourbon whiskey and Tom Gin, and when the very name breathed romance. That time is past. The poor stuff is now called alcohol.' (Leacock 1918.)

This new image does reduce demand for drugs and alcohol. It is an extremely powerful trend, but, at least in the case of alcohol, its ultimate rejection may lead to a prolonged backlash—as after prohibition in the United States—that inhibits open discussion of the very real problems associated with its use.

Kleber: The US government was criticized for saying, in 1989, that the 'crack' problem in the United States was getting worse, when the data were clear—it was indeed getting worse. The fact that casual use of cocaine was going down did not contradict the fact that crack use was greater. Ironically, these days, when I say that the crack problem is getting better, I am attacked for so stating! Yet both statements are accurate, and it's irrational to attack them.

Secondly, as to marijuana, I find it interesting that people say that when we took over at the Office of National Drug Control Policy, in 1989, we should have considered it separately. By 1989, marijuana use was at its lowest level since 1975 in the USA. Its use peaks at around the age of 19 and then sharply declines. Any policy that would have legalized this drug would only have done so for the over-21 population—it has never been suggested that it be legalized for those under 21; even NORML (the National Organization for the Reform of Marijuana Laws) testified that it was considered a dangerous drug for adolescents. Any increased availability from change in its legal status would have reversed the trend of the past 10 years, and increased the availability, in the same way that alcohol gets to teenagers, for the one segment of the population that is most likely to use it and to be harmed by it.

So in my view, changing the country's laws on marijuana would have been an irrational thing to do. (Nor did we at ONDCP say that marijuana use by a Supreme Court nominee was 'inconsequential'; our office said 'it was a case of youthful poor judgement', which carries a very different connotation.)

Musto: What if it had been cocaine?

Kleber: For use below the age of 21, we would have said the same thing! (Judge Ginsberg's nomination to the Supreme Court was pulled back not because of youthful marijuana use, but because he used it when he had left law school and was already a Harvard Faculty Member, a very different stage.)

On cannabis strategy, and the suggestion that cannabis use would decrease cocaine use, I have to disagree with Dr Kaplan. Indeed, since cannabis is often used with cocaine, one of the most frequent causes of relapse by cocaine addicts is if they smoke cannabis. It then serves as a conditioned cue for them to want cocaine.

Regarding the availability of treatment, in 1987 800 000 Americans were treated for drug abuse problems. In 1991/2, we expect the treatment system will be able to deal with two million Americans per year, assuming that the individual States keep pace with the increased federal spending on treatment. Every country has to develop its own strategy, according to the nature of its drug problem. By 1989, 74 million Americans had used an illegal drug at least once—one-third of our total population. Much of it was not regular use, but, even so, that kind of number of users clearly called for a 'denormalization' strategy. In the 1960s, 1970s and early 1980s, illicit drug use had become 'normalized' in the United States. It was 'all right' to use marijuana or cocaine at school, at parties, in the workplace. To decrease our drug problem, this had to change. Denormalization strategies work to change public perception—to convince the population of the harm drugs do, not just to the individual but to the community and society in general.

Incidentally, Reese Jones underestimated one figure: the proportion of major companies that have drug-free workplace policies is now close to two-thirds, rather than half.

Des Jarlais: One dynamic that is peculiar to the USA and is affecting a lot of drug policy is that traditionally we have blamed certain minority groups for our drug problems. We are now in a further period of increased tension between different ethnic groups, too often expressed in racial violence in our large cities. With the increased resentment by Whites that racial minorities are getting preferential treatment in employment, racial issues have characterized political campaigns. The continued stereotyping of certain drugs, particularly cocaine, as being a Black and a Hispanic problem, contributes to the inter-racial tensions. This view is emphasized by television news programmes, which typically show a Black crack house being raided by police. When drug users or dealers are shown, they are almost invariably Black or Hispanic.

This all makes it easy for a moralistic tone to be taken towards illicit drug use, because this can play upon racial prejudices that the minority groups are basically immoral. As a result, the minority group community leaders in turn take a very moralistic stance and say drug use *is* bad, but that it is the fault of the White power structure that there is a problem for the minority communities, because the Whites are letting the drugs into the country.

The moralistic attitudes and racial tensions tie in with attitudes on the use of pharmacotherapy to treat drug abuse. Methadone is now more under attack by minority groups than at any time in the past 10 years. If we did come up with a medication effective against cocaine, it is questionable whether it would be politically acceptable to many minority group leaders; it might be seen as another White man's drug given to young Black people to control their behaviour.

Kleber: In 1987, the White House conference for a drug-free America attacked methadone maintenance programmes primarily, I believe, not for the real problems that exist with some of the programmes, but because of ideological reasons. In 1989–1990, our National Strategy stated clearly that methadone is an important part of an overall drug abuse treatment system. This is now the official government view.

Des Jarlais: I agree that there are voices of reason in the debate, but minority community opinion is more against methadone than 10 years ago. There are also instances where a harm-reduction policy is being adopted. There have been three court trials of people who ran syringe exchanges; these resulted in not-guilty verdicts. But to go against the prevailing ideology that all drug use is bad, you need some other strong ideology, such as preventing AIDS, to counteract the current politically correct view that even casual drug use is immoral.

O'Brien: It seems to me that there are 'liberal' and 'conservative' trends in any country. Perhaps the sociologists and historians can see that America is in a more conservative phase now—not just in voting patterns, but with more applicants for business school than for medical school, more concern with practical issues than idealism. Perhaps drug use patterns are related to those kinds of secular trends, as much as to active efforts on the part of government leaders.

References

Cohen P 1990 Drugs as a social construct. Universiteit van Amsterdam Press, Amsterdam, p 15–31

Erickson PG, Murray GF 1989 The undeterred cocaine user: intention to quit and its relationship to perceived legal and health threats. Contemp Drug Problems 16:141–156
Leacock S 1918 Frenzied fiction. John Lane, New York, p 200
Murray GF 1984 The cannabis–cocaine connection: a comparative study of use and users. J Drug Issues (Fall):665–675

The economics of drug use and abuse

Alan Maynard

Centre for Health Economics, University of York, Heslington, York, YO1 5DD, UK

Abstract. The markets for drugs such as cocaine are characterized by much ignorance about the nature of trading relationships, in particular the volumes and prices exhibited by overlapping national and international networks of buyers and sellers (i.e. markets), and by severe regulation by the State. The regulation of illegal markets is expensive; for example, in 1988 in the UK, over 5000 Customs officers and 1800 CID and uniformed policemen were involved in enforcing the law at a cost of about £140 million. The size of the markets can be only 'guesstimated': in 1989 just over 520 kg of cocaine was seized. If this is assumed to be 10% of the market, the total size of the cocaine market was somewhere in excess of 5000 kg. The 'cost-effectiveness' of both Customs and the police in enforcing the law may have declined in the late 1980s. What economic arguments are there for sustaining illegality and an expensive enforcement effort? Some arguments for State regulation are explored; for example, the drug user harms 'innocent' third parties, the drug user is less productive and reduces national income, the drug user will impose costs on the National Health Service, the drug user's behaviour is offensive, and the drug user should be protected from his own stupidity. Where do these arguments leave the case for maintaining public policy towards illicit drugs? Would it be cost effective to move towards the liberalization of these markets?

1992 Cocaine: scientific and social dimensions. Wiley, Chichester (Ciba Foundation Symposium 166) p 242–260

A market is a network of buyers and sellers. The market for cocaine, like that for other illegal drugs such as heroin and cannabis, is characterized by public ignorance about trading relationships; for example, data about volumes, purity and prices are not generally available and vary considerably according to the level of the market (import, wholesale and retail).

This paucity of data about the characteristics of traded illicit drugs is a product of the State's regulation of the market place. Governments put considerable effort into enforcing national laws and, through international networks, they seek to control the production, distribution and sale of drugs.

The objectives of this chapter are to examine the nature and effects of this regulation and to evaluate the economic arguments for the present form of regulation of these markets. Stigler (1971) has argued that regulation is supplied by the State and its enforcement agencies, and is demanded by the regulated (in this case, drug suppliers) because it gives them certain advantages. Is this general argument applicable to the market for illicit drugs?

Economics of drug use and abuse

The nature and impact of regulation

All markets, public and private, are regulated; that is to say, buyers and sellers act in response to their own internal rules and those imposed by outside agencies. These rules, by affecting the volume and quality of goods traded, and their prices, generate signals which influence behaviour by suppliers and demanders.

The economics of regulation

The quantity demanded by a buyer is usually assumed to be inversely related to its price (the demand curve). The quantity supplied by a seller is assumed to be positively related to its price (the supply curve). Markets (networks of buyers and sellers) are said to clear when the supply of a commodity equals the demand for it. The precise slope (the relationship between a small change in price and a small change in the quantity supplied or demanded is the demand or supply 'elasticity') of both supply and demand curves can be estimated empirically.

In Fig. 1, increased enforcement of the law aimed at sellers might shift the supply curve from S_1 to S_2. At the initial price (£10), suppliers will reduce their supply from 20 kg to 10 kg. Here demand exceeds supply, and the price will be bid up to £15, where 15 kg will be supplied.

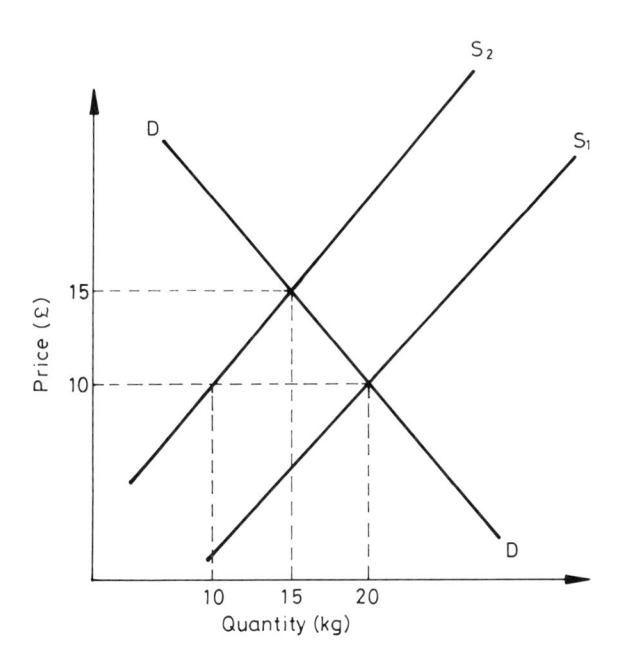

FIG. 1. The effect of increased law enforcement (directed at sellers) on the supply curve (S) and on the price of a commodity, given demand (D) elasticity.

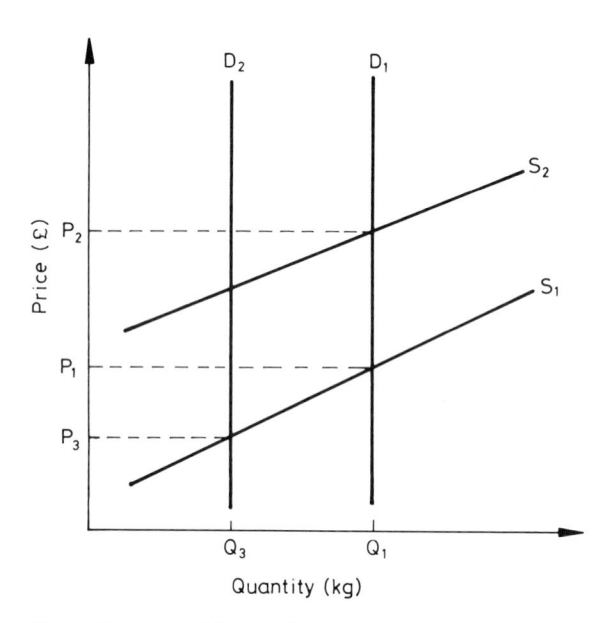

FIG. 2. The effect of increased law enforcement on supply (S) and price (P) when the demand curve is inelastic: prices rise (P1 to P2) but the volume traded (Q1) is unaffected. The effect of demand-side policies in the absence of supply-side law enforcement is also shown (prices are reduced to P3 and the quantity traded also falls, from Q1 to Q3).

However, if the demand curve is inelastic (Fig. 2), increased law enforcement will shift the supply curve (S_1 to S_2) and produces price increases (P_1 to P_2) with no effect on the volume traded. If demand-side policies (such as health education programmes, or enforcement aimed at users) are used (and supply-side enforcement policies are absent—that is, the relevant supply curve is S, and this does not shift), their effect is to shift the demand curve from D_1 to D_2, reducing both prices (P_1 to P_3) and the volume traded (Q_1 to Q_3).

The balance of supply-side (enforcement) and demand-side (health promotion) policies would be determined, if the efficient use of resources is the objective of government, by the cost-effectiveness of competing drug policies. Then the relevant question to be answered is whether such policies enhance the length and quality of beneficiaries' lives more or less than an equal expenditure on heart transplants or other relevant alternatives. All such choices should be informed by data about costs and benefits at the margin—that is, if activity increases by a small amount, how do costs and benefits change?

Of course, it is possible that the demand curve is not a linear relationship. In Fig. 3, which combines Blair & Vogel's speculation (1973) that demand is elastic at low prices and inelastic at high prices, with White & Luksetich's speculation (1983) that demand is inelastic at low prices and elastic at high prices,

Economics of drug use and abuse

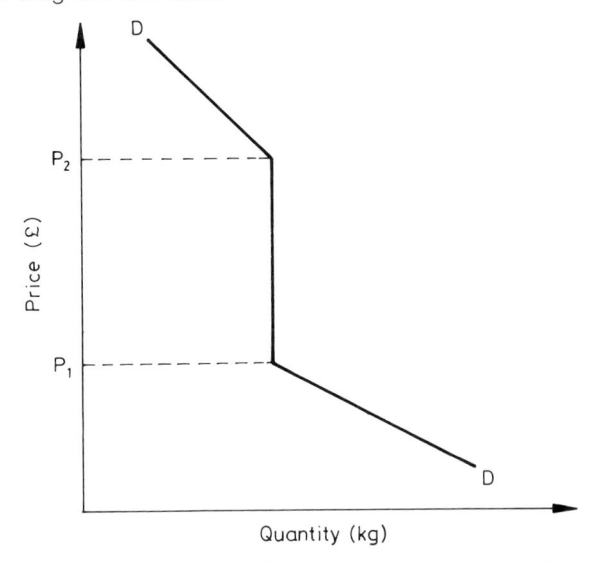

FIG. 3. Relation between price (P) and quantity traded (Q) on the assumption that the demand curve (D) is not a linear relationship (see text).

the hypothesis is that at low prices, non-addicts may curtail their drug use, and addicts may maintain their habits at a minimum level, if enforcement increases; and at high prices, the severe price pressure produced by enforcement may even reduce the use of addicts. In the P_1–P_2 range, where demand is inelastic, supply-side policies will have no effect on price or quantity.

Individual markets for drugs are clearly interdependent: successful enforcement which reduces supply in one market may spill over into another market and raise demand, prices and the volumes traded. The extent to which products are substitutes or complements can be estimated if data are available (the cross-elasticity of demand).

Other spillover effects also arise from enforcement. If enforcement is successful and prices are increased, addicts, to maintain their consumption, may have to raise more finance to fund their habits. For instance, in the United States, Silverman & Spruill (1977) estimated that a 10% increase in the price of heroin reduced consumption by 2.5% and that a 50% price increase in heroin would, after some months, increase the value of property crime by about 14%. Obviously, if enforcement is targeted at particular jurisdictions and raises prices there, criminal spillover effects may be greater in neighbouring jurisdictions, if drug enforcement puts more police into neighbourhoods and makes the risks of detection there, after crimes, greater.

The extent to which estimates of the effects of enforcement policies can be made is constrained by the paucity of suitable data. Little is known about the price elasticity of cocaine, or the price–crime spillover effects for this drug.

The degree to which public policy is formulated on the basis of ignorance is impressive.

The characteristics of the market

In the markets for drugs such as heroin, cannabis and cocaine, the State has ruled that the exchange of these substances is illegal. Despite this, the volume of trade in all three substances may have expanded considerably in Britain in the 1979-1989 period. Some estimates are presented in Tables 1 and 2. In 1979, 21.6 kg of cocaine were seized by Customs and by 1989 their seizure rate was over 400 kg.

Seizures by the police fluctuated considerably, rising from 2.4 kg of cocaine in 1979 to over 110 kg in 1989. Typically the police have higher rates of seizure than HM Customs, but the size of their seizures is much less. This is because Customs' activity is targeted at importers in particular and police make seizures from retailers generally. If the efficiency of enforcement agencies is judged in terms of seizure volumes, there is always the possibility of 'competition' between the two agencies to seize 'big hauls'. Such competition may inhibit cooperation, but has not led in the UK to the alleged accidental shoot-outs between competing enforcement agencies reported from the USA!

The purity of the drug seizures made by Customs and the police differs considerably. For instance, in 1989 the purity of cocaine seized by Customs at the import level of the market was 89%. Police seizures at the wholesale and retail market levels were 56 and 52% respectively. As a consequence of these differences in purity, any aggregation of the data in Tables 1 and 2 must be undertaken with care.

TABLE 1 Quantities of controlled drugs seized (1979-1989) in the UK by Customs (kg)

Year	Heroin	Cannabis	Cocaine
1979	43.6	11 586	21.6
1980	36.2	25 500	36.0
1981	85.8	24 210	15.7
1982	185.1	16 546	12.1
1983	215.9	18 892	74.0
1984	312.6	26 256	35.4
1985	334.2	20 905	78.7
1986	179.2	22 382	99.2
1987	190.0	16 293	362.4
1988	211.4	42 308	263.6
1989	338.3	50 903	408.8

Sources: Derived from Customs and Home Office returns and reported in Wagstaff & Maynard (1988).

Economics of drug use and abuse

TABLE 2 Quantities of controlled drugs seized (1979–1989) in the UK by the police (kg)

Year	Heroin	Cannabis	Cocaine
1979	1.6	547.4	2.4
1980	1.8	788.6	4.2
1981	7.6	547.4	5.4
1982	10.3	829.9	6.6
1983	20.3	628.5	6.0
1984	49.0	2814.5	30.1
1985	32.2	1259.6	6.7
1986	43.7	2754.3	3.4
1987	45.6	643.1	44.4
1988	24.3	3167.9	59.6
1989	16.2	3971.1	113.35

Source: Derived from Customs and Home Office returns and reported in Wagstaff & Maynard (1988).

The price of cocaine, as a consequence, varies between the different levels of the market. In 1989, the import selling price was about £29 000 for a kilogram of pure cocaine. The same amount and quality sold at the retail level would cost £154 000.

The total size and value (i.e. total expenditure) of the cocaine (and crack) markets is unknown. The rising trend in seizures may be the product of greater enforcement effects and/or an increase in the size of the market for this substance. The absence of data about market size for cannabis makes any estimate of its market size impossible. A 'guesstimate' of the value of the heroin market, between £162 million and £266 million in 1988, suggests that the market's size may have declined (it was £308 to £501 million in 1985).

Many of the deficits in knowledge about these markets could be reduced by more careful collection of data. However, such heresy (e.g. Wagstaff & Maynard 1988, chapter 7) has not led to much advance in the processes of 'confusing' policy choices by facts! As a consequence, on the basis of poor intelligence, the UK government created a 'crack' squad in 1989 to meet a non-existent crisis. Within a year this squad was disbanded and the resources were deployed, one hopes more productively elsewhere.

The nature of the enforcement

It is not easy to quantify the extent and cost of enforcement mechanisms in illicit drug markets. In 1988 HM Customs employed 1340 FTE (fulltime equivalent) staff who worked on drug enforcement (Table 3). The cost of this activity was over £38 million. Customs employed a further 4897 staff on general prevention duties (at a cost of £58 million). These officers spend some time on

TABLE 3 Drug enforcement efforts in the UK: manpower and expenditure 1988

| | FTE staff employed on drugs work ||
	Number	Expenditure (£1000s)
Customs[a]	1340	38 344
Police	2330	99 213

[a] A further 4897 FTE staff (at a cost of £58 million) were working on prevention (see text).
Source: Tables 2.2 and 3.6 of Claxton et al (1990).

drug enforcement, but HM Customs find it impossible to estimate the extent of preventive staff time spent on drug law enforcement activities.

The attribution of police manpower to drug activity is difficult, as with HM Customs, because it is not clear how much of the time of officers in Regional Crime Squads, police force Drug Squads, and the CID and uniformed branches is allocated to drug enforcement work. Some 'guesstimates' are presented in Table 3: 2330 FTE police staff at a cost in excess of £99 million were involved in drug enforcement in 1988.

The regulation of drug markets: a resumé

While it is possible to hypothesize about the ways in which drug markets work and how enforcement by police and Customs may affect the prices and volumes of traded commodities, it is difficult to test these predictions systematically because of poor data. The UK data available from police and Customs seizures is limited and useful, but it provides no indication of the total size of the cocaine market in terms of volume and expenditure. The volume of seizures increased in the 1980s but the costs of this enforcement were considerable: nearly £140 million in 1988.

How should the illicit drugs market be regulated?

The conventional economic approach

The conventional economic approach to drug abuse (see e.g. Culyer 1973) consists of an appraisal of a set of arguments which can be used to sustain the case for government intervention in the market for illicit drugs.

Third-party harm. If the drug user behaves in a way which harms other members of society, by violence or robbing people to finance his or her habits, there is a prima facie case for government regulation. It is known that drug use and crime are associated, but it is clearly possible that the volume of crime

Economics of drug use and abuse   249

is a product of the illicit nature of the trade and of the enforcement activities which raise drug prices and increase deviant behaviour.

Consequently, the relevant questions which need to be explored are: (a) what is the extent to which the volume of crime is associated with the level of prices of illicit products? And (b) what is the most cost-effective way of reducing the criminal behaviour of drug users?

Clearly, one policy option is the legalization of the drug trade. Would this reduce the third-party effects more effectively and at a lower cost than £140 million? This is an empirical question which can only be answered by careful evaluation of the precise nature and volume of all the third-party effects and an appraisal of alternative ways of mitigating them at least cost.

Reduction in national income. It could be argued that drug users, because of their limited participation in the labour force, reduce the size of the national income below its maximum possible level. In a country with two million unemployed, this argument is of little merit. Clearly, the adoption of the 'drug habit' may lead to productive workers leaving the labour force. They will be replaced by the unemployed with little long-term effect on the nation's output.

People who choose to fall off mountains, fall off their yachts, and hang-glide may also damage themselves and affect the value of the nation's output. They too can be replaced, but why are they considered so differently from drug users?

Costs imposed by the drug user on the National Health Service. It might be argued that where the £28 billion cost of the National Health Service in the UK imposes severe taxation burdens on individuals, the correct policy response is to prohibit drug use, to minimize the burden that users place on the NHS. This is a weak argument which, if developed, would require us to ban many foods (because of their cholesterol, salt and other 'harmful' contents), tobacco, alcohol, driving, walking . . . i.e. to make life so safe it would be unbearable!

Informational harm. Another argument that might be used to sustain the regulation of the drug trade is that the mere knowledge that I use drugs harms you. There are many things about me that may irritate you: I may be Black, homosexual, and a member of Militant Tendency (i.e. a Trotskyite). How do you differentiate these qualities from my drug-taking, and why make only the latter illegal? Such issues can only be decided by value judgements derived from the democratic process and based upon information about the cost-effectiveness of competing decisions.

Merit wants. If I judge your behaviour to be stupid, I may seek to change it. Should I be permitted to impose my values on you and organize your life for you? 'Merit wants' are activities deemed 'appropriate' by someone with 'superior' value judgements. Again, this is an issue which will be determined by political processes which reflect social values, and the case for making drugs a special case is clearly value laden.

Protecting children. The welfare of children is judged by their parents and if children are exposed to physical harm by drug use, then it may be efficient to protect them and avoid the inter-generational transmission of harmful habits. However, this may require not prohibition but the separation of users from children, as is done in the alcohol market.

Overview. Many of the arguments for viewing drug use as a 'special case' meriting special government regulation seem untenable. The mitigation of physical harm and the harm of children is unlikely to be achieved cost-effectively by prohibition: there are cheaper ways of mitigating these problems. As with the prohibition of alcohol in the United States, such regulation may create a system of social security for criminal elements such as the Mafia.

Some alternative arguments

Users are addicted. The conventional economic case ignores the impact of 'addiction'. Conventional economic theorists are utilitarian and believe that individuals are the best judges of their own welfare. However, if individuals are 'addicted', they may not be the best judges of their own welfare, and government regulation of the market for drugs may be necessary. But what is addiction? Is it continued drug use when the benefit is zero, or what? Whatever it is, does it exist? Does it exist any more (measured how?) in the illicit drugs market than it does elsewhere—in the alcohol or caffeine markets, for instance? If conventional (neoclassical) theory is to be rejected, more precision in the use (and abuse!) of the term 'addiction' is essential. Without such precision in definition, supported by good science, the neoclassical case remains a relevant basis for informing choices and doubting the efficiency of existing policies.

The benefits of regulation. Another possible reason for prohibiting trade in illicit drugs is that it benefits the regulators and the regulated. The suppliers of cocaine in Colombia and at the street level in consumer countries would sustain significant income losses if their trade was legalized and prices fell to reflect the cost of production. Governments would have less cause to invest in police and Customs enforcement and to buy votes by appealing to the law-and-order lobby. The suppliers of enforcement services would be redundant, and they and their relatives would vote to avoid liberalization if it threatened their income and employment.

Such behaviours are seen clearly in other markets where regulation is important (e.g. the pharmaceutical market) and reflects self-interest created by particular government policies. Such self-interest is inevitable, but is not a sensible reason for continuing inefficient policies such as prohibition.

How should the illicit drugs market be regulated?

Unless cocaine and other illicit substances have unique and significant addictive properties which create significant social costs, the case for prohibition either reflects what Theodore Roosevelt called the 'felt necessity of the time' and is based on the self-interest of the regulated and regulators, or is absent. This does not mean that all regulation should be abolished. All markets, public and private, are regulated. The issue for public debate is which policy is the most cost-effective method of reducing the 'harms' created by drug use. Unfortunately, many of these harms are poorly identified, let alone valued. The existing legislation which governs the production and consumption of alcohol provides a useful starting point for revising the regulation of the drug market.

References

Blair RD, Vogel RJ 1973 Heroin addiction and urban crime. Public Finance Quarterly 1(4):457–467
Claxton K, Wagstaff A, Maynard A 1990 Economic aspects of illicit drug markets and drug enforcement policies in the United Kingdom between 1984 and 1989. Interim unpublished report for the Home Office. Centre for Health Economics, University of York
Culyer AJ 1973 Should social policy concern itself with drug abuse? Public Finance Quarterly 1(4):449–456
Silverman LP, Spruill NL 1977 Urban crime and the price of heroin. J Urban Economics 4:80–103
Stigler G 1971 Theory of economic regulation. Bell J Econ 2(1):3–21
Wagstaff A, Maynard A 1988 Economic aspects of the illicit drug market and drug enforcement policies in the United Kingdom. Home Office Research Study 95. HMSO, London
White MD, Luksetich WA 1983 Heroin price elasticity and enforcement strategies. Economic Inquiry 21:557–564

DISCUSSION

Almond: I was interested in your reference to conventional or neoclassical economists. I wonder if this matches the definition of classical liberal, nowadays described as libertarian? A pamphlet from the Libertarian Alliance exactly reverses your argument in relation to legalizing drugs (Gabb 1990). It supports your conclusion, not on the empirical ground that individuals are the best judges of their own welfare, but rather on the *principle* that they should not be prevented from inflicting serious harm on themselves.

Secondly, you referred to the unemployment figures in relation to drug users, where it could be said that drug users who drop out of employment leave vacancies for others, so the costs to society are the same; but the argument about unemployment and social cost could be applied to the drug-enforcement personnel; their *non*-employment would increase unemployment, with the consequent social cost.

Maynard: If money was not spent on the enforcement agencies, it would be spent on something else; thus you create jobs for other people, so the net impact may be zero. If there is unemployment, ex-drug users may not be able to drop back into a job and the effects on Gross National Product may be minimal. Consequently, the social cost of drug use in respect of GNP may be small.

Kalant: I am reminded of Churchill's dictum that democracy is a terrible system except that all the others are worse! We have to look not only at the economics of the present control system, but at what predictions can be made about changes with alternative systems. Let us accept, for example, that expenditures on enforcement activities are disproportionately high now, in return for the benefits obtained, and the costs to the health care system of the use of illicit drugs are not seen as very large in relation to the total costs of health care. But suppose you were to legalize drugs and increase the freedom of their availability, and suppose that this changed the levels of use drastically, how would your economic analysis then change? I suggest that we should be on just as shaky ground in predicting that any alternative system would be better as we are with our present system in which drugs are not legalized.

Maynard: The basis for making predictions of that nature is very difficult. I would argue that we should be looking at 'the margins'. That is, we don't suddenly say that we want to make all drugs legal; we should begin to change the rigour with which we enforce the law, as various countries have done. Then, if we switched the resources from enforcement to other interventions, what observable effects could we actually measure? And that begins to inform us about margins. I would argue that any changes in policy should not be sudden; they must be incremental. I think there are an array of ways in which you could pull those policy levers; over any decade or in any country, you can see the emphasis on alternative aspects changing over time.

Edwards: You suggest, persuasively, that we should proceed incrementally, and make no hasty moves, but perhaps make a little adjustment here or there. Who could disagree? The other message that I hear is that economists are issuing predictions, for example that if you increase the price of heroin by 50% you will increase property crime by 14%. If you are telling us that you can make that kind of prediction with any degree of confidence, I would fear that your science might be over-reaching itself.

If you put up the price of heroin, fewer people may be recruited; people who are at the beginning of their heroin careers, and who are not heavily dependent and who still have other life options open to them, may quit because of the

Economics of drug use and abuse

price increase. Heroin users who are more heavily involved with the drug may be encouraged by the economic determinant to look for treatment. There are so many variables potentially involved that to start modelling, or offering guidance to policy on the basis of this type of data, seems to me risky.

Maynard: It depends on the level of question you want to ask. We are *not* advising the Home Office about whether they should try to raise the prices of drugs, because there are all sorts of imponderables about the effects of changing prices in illicit drug markets on other types and facets of behaviour. If I raise the price of alcohol, this will reduce your consumption of alcohol, but you won't then rob someone to buy alcohol, usually; whereas with the drug markets, because of the nature of the illegality, and also the substances, there are many covert relationships. I was trying to explain that at the theoretical level we can begin to look at those relationships, but the extent to which we have knowledge of them empirically is very slight.

If we move on to the issue of what we can say about competing policies, the economist's approach is to devise crude performance indicators whereby we can judge the success of enforcement policies by the police, and by Customs and Excise, in an explicit way. We can then try to measure what is actually happening on these performance indicators, and this is information which the Home Office can use, or not use, to decide whether it will put more money into Customs, or into the police force.

The third level is the issue of trying to emphasize, as I was doing in the diagrams of supply and demand (Figs. 1–3), that you can attack the problem of drug use from either side—supply or demand. If those involved in providing treatment want more money, for example, they must be able to show that the treatments, whatever they may be, are cost-effective and are better ways of spending money than on the police, or on Customs and Excise.

Moore: An important task of a law enforcement operation against drugs is to try to increase the effective price of drugs. To deal with the potential offsetting consequence of that, which can be either increased crime, or increased disability for the users, society should invest in a set of treatment programmes. In that important respect, law enforcement and treatment activities are *complementary* instruments of drug policy. They are not substitutes for one another. So the more you spend on enforcement, the more you will need to spend on treatment, and vice versa.

Strang: I am struck how the arguments differ for different drugs. In much of the debate it is presumed that we look at control strategy across all drugs. Yet Dr Moore has identified the need to have treatment available, to pick up the difficulties that a control strategy squeezes out of society; but that argument doesn't exist at all for some drugs. Nobody argues that we need marijuana-prescribing programmes for the people who get squeezed out as a result of cannabis control, or LSD-prescribing alongside LSD control. It is curious that we see these prescribing responses as appropriate for some drugs and not for others, if we think that they are actually governed by the same rules.

Moore: No; we arrange to have treatment for drug users taking drugs where the consequences for the individual, and for society, of increasing the price and inconvenience to the user turn out to be substantial. In that case, society wants to provide a soft landing for drug users, whom we are basically trying to frustrate and discourage by making it inconvenient and dangerous for them to use drugs. It is only where those consequences of continued use are significant that it is worth providing the treatment.

Jaffe: I am wondering whether an economist could produce a clear-cut set of criteria to decide when the efforts to control the supplies of drugs actually fail to contribute to reducing the extent of the problem. What would be the necessary and sufficient evidence? For example, if the costs of drugs were falling and the supply was increasing (at least as perceived by consumers), would an economist conclude that the effort to control the supply was necessarily ineffectual, or would he require additional data?

Maynard: You need to consider a range of data on drug use if you want to measure intervention performance, because the data are so poor, and there's no agreement about what you are trying to achieve. If your aim is to produce reductions in the volume of drugs, all you may get is drug price changes and crime rate changes, so you should be trying to look at indicators in those areas, and in related spheres, to see which way they evolve. They may move in ways which are contradictory, or they may move together. Our experience with the Home Office is that when you adopt this approach, the indicators move together, over certain subperiods, and therefore it is useful to the policy makers to see what is happening.

Moore: Jerry Jaffe is right about the method that could be used to estimate the impact on supply. We have developed an analytic approach to try to show whether a reduction in the supply of drugs has ever occurred (Moore 1990). This is an important question to ask, quite apart from the question of whether we were able to produce the reduction by law-enforcement efforts, or whether local guerilla wars or crop diseases produced the result. It turns out that if the observed prices of drugs in local markets are declining and estimates of the quantity consumed are increasing, then there has been an *unambiguous* increase in the supply of drugs. If, on the other hand, prices are increased, in local conditions, and the estimate of the quantity consumed is down, there has been a clear reduction in the supply of drugs. Using that framework, if we look across the last 20 years of American history, we find three periods in which we achieved reductions in supply, and one long period in which we had a significant failure in the supply reduction of illicit drugs.

The three periods in which the USA had supply reductions were (1) with heroin in the early 1970s; (2) heroin again in the late 1970s; and, unexpectedly, (3) a supply reduction success with respect to marijuana, over the decade of the 1980s.

The one disastrous failure to reduce supply that we have had in the USA has been with cocaine, again during the eighties. Recently, however, it looks as if we are beginning to see an unambiguous reduction in the supply of cocaine again to the United States. So there is a method available for estimating whether supply reductions have occurred.

On the impact of law enforcement on price, we found that when we make a drug illegal, we tend to push the price up, for a simple reason: life becomes very difficult for the drug dealers. It becomes difficult for two different reasons. Their most obvious problem is the threat represented by the law-enforcement agencies. The probably larger and more important threat to the dealers, however, is the one represented by the *other* bad guys—some of them dealers, and some robbers and extortionists. If you are a drug dealer, your biggest problem is not the law-enforcement agents threatening to arrest you, but other criminals who threaten to steal your supplies and to kill you. When we analyse the net effect of both things together, we find a dramatic elevation in price from what it would be in a legal market—even a taxed legal market. The difference between the legal and illegal prices for cocaine in the USA now is about 15 times, and the difference between the legal price of morphine and the illicit price of heroin, in the USA, is about 60 times. So when we are wondering whether we can produce dramatic changes in prices through combinations of making things illegal and enforcing those laws, the answer is that you can push the price up very high by forcing those who want to sell that product to do so in a market in which they are protected neither from their colleagues, nor from the State.

Maynard: You raise the question of what one's target is in trying to raise prices. This depends on the price elasticities of drugs. That's a very interesting area, and I look forward to reading what you have been talking about!

Uchtenhagen: In your cost-effectiveness analysis, Professor Maynard, you use the amount of drugs seized as one of your main measures of enforcement effectiveness. Can you tell me what effect an increase in expenditure on law enforcement would have on the proportion of seizures, in terms of total drug seizures? That is, if you doubled the expenditure on law enforcement, by how much would the seizures be increased?

Maynard: It depends whether one is thinking in terms of the pure volume of drug seizures, or the total seized as a percentage of the market transactions. We don't know the total amount of drugs being traded, unfortunately. It is clear that more expenditure on interventions is associated with increasing the seizures, but that may be because there is more drug to be seized. I am not sure what consequences you want to draw from this information. We may spend more on interventions next year, and our seizures rates may go up; that may be partly the effect of the enforcement agencies capturing more drugs, but it may also be that there is more there to capture, so it's easier for them to do it. So this is an ambiguous measure.

Uchtenhagen: Another message we hear is that it is not the *amount* of drugs seized that is the measure of the effectiveness of law enforcement in this field, but its *preventive* value. That is to say, if you reduced your drug seizure activity, the amounts being smuggled into your country would increase considerably. Do you have any methods of quantifying this effect?

Maynard: We should like to get information about how drug users feel their risks of being apprehended are changing, as preventive activity increases, but we haven't any information of that kind.

Strang: You don't seem to be taking into consideration the idea of an equivalent of a thermodynamic energy hump needed to bring about a change in attitude and behaviour. In other words, it is disproportionately difficult to bring about a small change in the *status quo*, even though, when you make that change in *status quo*, you get a stable state whereby a new set of balances is established.

Secondly, it seems to me that you are side-stepping the questions in just the same way that treatment agencies do: they say that they don't know the total population size, so they can't tell whether they are improving their ability to 'capture' clients. But we should be able to do better than this. For example, if we are 'capturing' more people, we would expect to be seeing people entering treatment at an earlier stage.

Similarly, why can't economists look at the impact of drug seizures? Consider some black market of unknown size: the police make a huge seizure, and I see the price double. I know that the seizure was a substantial part of the market. If the price goes up only a trivial amount, this particular seizure was only a drop in the ocean. Surely there is some more sophisticated way to say, not at a national level but at an individual seizure level, that particular seizures represent a certain percentage of the total market.

Maynard: What *would* happen at the local level, after a big drugs seizure? Would you see prices rise? The problem in the UK is our lack of good data about prices; the data we have show considerable variation from locality to locality. They are not adjusted in terms of the purity of the products being seizured. We have been trying to persuade the Home Office to acquire more systematic data, by actually buying drugs. The big problem in making predictions is that the data are extremely poor.

Kleber: A new natural experiment is about to take place in Iowa, which should be studied by economists: I am trying to get the federal government to consider funding this. A law has been passed in that State where they will fine anyone under 18 years $100 if they are caught in possession of a cigarette. It will be interesting to see what that does to the under-18 cigarette market.

Moore: This is to use the law as a demand-side strategy more than as a supply-side strategy.

Kleber: Yes. What I didn't hear in your analysis, Dr Maynard, relates to the existence of a legal market. Cocaine costs $4 per gram to produce legally and import into the US for medical purposes. Cocaine sells for $60–$100, depending on where you are in the country, on the illegal market. The problem in setting a price for cocaine, if you were to legalize it, is that you would want to do two opposite things. You want to diminish the number of people using it, which means you want to keep the price as high as possible; you also want to drive out the bad guys (the illicit suppliers), because they will wreck your strategy, and so you have to set the price low enough. The economists to whom I have talked say that this means the price of cocaine would have to be set (if it costs $4 a gram legally) at about $10–$15 per gram. At that low level, however, you have gone against your aim of trying not to cause more costs to society. The price of a dose of cocaine would be about $0.50 (fifty cents), well within the reach of 12-year-olds. The number of cocaine users would, I predict, rise sharply, as would both the direct and indirect costs resulting from the drug use. (The direct costs of health problems, and indirect costs such as motor vehicle accidents, cocaine-impaired infants, domestic violence, etc.)

Maynard: You say that a price of only about $10–$15 per gram would lead to a big increase in the costs to society. This gets back to the whole problem of what these costs are. When I look at the American attempts to assess the cost to society of the drug addiction problem, or of alcohol or tobacco, I am struck by how fundamentally flawed they are in the way in which the calculations are done. It looks more like a public relations exercise than a systematic analysis. I am worried by that. But supposing we do let the price go down, we may get an increase in drug utilization; that's an empirical question. The point you are emphasizing is that we may get increases in drug-related costs. Certainly we may; the interesting question is, if we begin to change drug policies slightly and slowly, can we get information which is relevant to identifying those costs to society? I came to this symposium wondering whether cocaine is more dangerous or less dangerous than alcohol; I am still not sure!

Kleber: I also felt that there was an assumption in your analysis that there is only one player in the equation. One of our problems with expanding treatment, for example, is that there are several players. We found that as we increase spending on treatment at the federal level, less is often spent for this at State and local levels. It becomes harder to get marginal or discretionary State dollars spent on this. To get the same amount of total increase in treatment availability, the federal government may need to put in $300 now as against $200 a few years ago. States and localities are drawing back. So there are different players in the game, and as you put more money into one kind of strategy, you affect other people who take out money.

Maynard: You say I assume there is only one player, and State and federal relationships may cancel each other out. That is a problem which one has to look at in each case; it will depend on the federal and political constitution of the country.

O'Brien: I'm confused by the recent history of the supply and demand situation for cocaine; there have been many reactions by the market place that don't fit into models such as those to which Alan Maynard and Mark Moore refer. First there was a radical change in the merchandizing of cocaine, from cocaine hydrochloride to alkaloidal cocaine in the form of small chips which can be sold for as little as $2-$3. That decline in price was going on at the same time as we were reading in the newspapers about seizures of huge quantities of cocaine. We have also had, in recent years, the perception of declining price combined with *increased* availability, in the face of a decline in use, which is unusual; use tends normally to parallel availability. And then we had another reaction, which as a clinician I think is related to these supply-side efforts. I am referring to an increase in the price of marijuana, because it's easier to seize, and a shift from foreign to domestic marijuana production. So we have had many changes in behaviour in the USA that possibly could be represented by some model, but I suspect that if we did that, future events would be different again. This throws doubt on the validity of models in an area where the subjects of study react and change the rules so much. The current situation seems to be different from anything we could have predicted from the past.

Des Jarlais: I find economic modelling and thinking to be very useful for some aspects of drug policy, but we should remember that economists are not so successful in predicting the economy or the stock market, and they certainly put more effort into that than they have ever put into predicting illegal drug markets.

Nevertheless, economic theory is useful when one thinks about the nature of the illicit marketing operations, and whether they are monopolistic or competitive. Monopolistic markets have clear implications for greater police corruption and for poorer quality of the product sold to the consumer. Profit maximization in a monopoly market comes with high profit margins, not maximum product sold. When drug organizations compete against each other, they tend to offer a better deal for the consumer, but also will have side effects of violent crime as a way of trying to reduce the competition.

A second place where economic theory is useful is in considering the relationship between the price of drugs and the mode of drug administration. As you drive up the price of drugs, you see shifts to more economically efficient methods of administering them, particularly to intravenous injection, which is the most efficient method in terms of getting a certain amount of drug from your pocket into your brain. It is far more efficient than sniffing, and much more so than smoking. You also see displacement, where, both in the USA and in Thailand, when effective laws were passed against the use of opium, a substantial number of those smoking opium went over to injecting heroin. The consequences of law enforcement driving the price up are complex; you don't only change the number of users; you alter the way in which drugs are used, towards greater economic efficiency.

Maynard: The merchandizing of cocaine certainly changes through time, as Dr O'Brien points out. There have been shifts in the marijuana market. But he is questioning whether it is sensible to try to model at all, in these areas. The answer really is to see whether economic modelling gives you any useful insights into the market. Clearly, trying to model the demand for automobiles is very different, because the shape changes, the colours change. Sellers change the way in which they market a whole variety of commodities, but you have plenty of people trying their best to predict how the markets will change. There is a set of techniques with economics; they may work in some cases and not in others. You have to be open about the approach and accept that sometimes the predictions will be wrong; as Don Des Jarlais said, quite rightly, most of my colleagues want to try to predict how the economy and the stock market will go, yet you never find a very rich economist! There is a need to evaluate economic data and to evaluate modelling, and also to evaluate the value of economists working in the area. There is a set of techniques that economists can offer which can give some insights into how the market works. If we could persuade drug regulatory agencies to collect better data, we could perhaps improve the clarity of those insights into the market. But basically, economics is a crude game; it's rather like medicine! Sometimes we make mistakes.

Edwards: The difference is that I may kill a patient; you may injure an entire country!

Kalant: In analysing the conventional economic arguments, you referred to the point at which these economic arguments impinge on value judgements. But in discussing what happens in the alternative models, you didn't touch on the extent to which the options open to you are dependent on the values of the society—the predominant moods, or the kinds of political shift to left or right that have occurred in different societies at different times. How does an economist deal with those variables?

Maynard: It is clearly so that the options available are determined by values. The economists come with a tool kit, with a particular set of values, and they have to be open about what those values are. The options that any society chooses to adopt in relation to regulating its drug market will be the product of the felt necessity of the time, and this changes. As jobbing economists, we try to provide useful information to decision makers. If they choose not to use that information, because it violates their values, that is their choice; as economists we are trying to offer the best information we have. How society uses it will change over time. One hopes that if we get better data, the way in which social values are fixed and how they change may actually be influenced.

Kaplan: Can one turn to the rats for any illumination? Bill Woolverton mentioned behavioural economics earlier. Are there any data, from any discipline, which show an optimal curve in terms of what degree of drug availability leads to what level of drug self-administration? Is the curve the same for all drugs, or is it different? Do the drugs differ in terms of, for instance, the amount of work that an animal will perform to obtain them?

Woolverton: Yes; research has made it clear that animals will work more to obtain some drugs than others. Cocaine seems to head the list.

Kaplan: And does that have to do with the schedule of availability of cocaine? What do we know about that?

Moore: The less hard you have to work, the more of it you use.

Kaplan: It would be interesting to know the limits within which this relation operates.

Jaffe: Even when you find an optimal dose for each drug, the amount of work an animal will perform to get that optimal dose differs. For some drugs, animals will work very hard; for others, as you raise the cost in terms of work, they simply decide not to work. So there are inherent differences between the psychoactive drugs.

References

Gabb S 1990 What to do about AIDS. Libertarian Alliance Pamphlet No. 12, London (Obtainable from: Libertarian Alliance, 1 Russell Chambers, The Piazza, Covent Garden, London WC2E 8AA)

Moore MH 1990 Supply reduction strategies and drug law enforcement. In: Tonry MH, Wilson JQ (eds) Drugs and crime. University of Chicago Press, Chicago, IL (Crime & Justice: An Annual Review of Research Ser vol 13)

Formulating policies on the non-medical use of cocaine

Harold Kalant

Department of Pharmacology, University of Toronto, Toronto, Canada M5S 1A8 and Primary Mechanisms Research, Addiction Research Foundation of Ontario, Toronto, Canada M5S 2S1

Abstract. The formulation of policy on cocaine, as on any other social issue, involves explicit or implicit cost-benefit analyses with many factors. Cocaine use carries many medical, psychiatric and social risks, and its inherent pharmacological risk of dependence is greater than for other drugs. The reported frequency of these problems has increased exponentially over the past fifteen years. However, current levels of use are decreasing in the general population, though still increasing among certain subpopulations in which it is accompanied by violent crime. On the other hand, the attempt to control use mainly or exclusively by reducing the supply has been of low efficacy and extremely expensive, in both human and monetary terms, for the consuming countries and economically and politically devastating for the producing countries. Yet past experience with other drugs suggests that legalization of cocaine would increase its use substantially. Moreover, legalization runs counter to public sentiment, even in those countries where the law is applied leniently against users and small-scale traffickers. The most practical policy appears to be to maintain prohibition as a sign of social disapproval, but to rely much more heavily on non-coercive measures to reduce demand by strengthening public consensus against all drug use.

1992 Cocaine: scientific and social dimensions. Wiley, Chichester (Ciba Foundation Symposium 166) p 261-276

Policies on a great number of matters are formulated at all levels of a society; the present paper deals only with the formulation of policies at the level of national governments. The process by which governments and international bodies formulate policies on cocaine is not fundamentally different from that which they use to formulate policies on taxation, nuclear weapons, schooling, health care, the sale of alcohol and tobacco, or any of the numerous other social issues with which they must deal. In brief, this process involves either explicit or implicit cost-benefit assessments of the various policy options available, and attempts to select that option which maximizes the benefits and minimizes the costs, *according to the perceptions, information and value systems* of those who make the assessment. In theory this sounds simple and logical, but in practice it is extraordinarily difficult because some of the costs and benefits are readily quantifiable and can be expressed in standard units, monetary or other, whereas other costs and benefits are emotional, or ideologically based, and thus extremely difficult to weigh objectively against the first type (Kalant & Kalant 1971).

The real differences between pragmatic and ideologically based policies are to be found not in the process, but in the relative importance assigned to essentially imponderable factors that go into the cost–benefit analysis. Thus, pragmatic policies concentrate on the minimization of identifiable costs that can be measured with some degree of accuracy, such as the health problems attributable to the use of cocaine or the law enforcement costs related to the attempts to suppress its use, and do not attempt to weigh these against moral or ethical aspects of drug use or its suppression. In contrast, policy proposals based on ideological considerations such as the right of personal choice or the defence of the moral ideal of a drug-free society imply that these abstract values outweigh any practical costs that might be incurred by the implementation of such policies.

Somewhat surprisingly, however, very little has been written about positive *benefits* to be obtained from the application of one or another policy, whereas a great deal has been written about the costs. The benefits of one policy are usually described in terms of elimination or prevention of the costs that would have been incurred by adoption of another. Very few advocates of legalization of cocaine and other illicit drugs argue that drug use is good *per se*, though some have eloquently defended the libertarian principle of non-interference with the right of individual choice. The great majority of those taking part in the policy debate consider drug use, or certainly heavy use, as undesirable, even if possibly inescapable. The main goal of policy decisions would thus be to reduce *total* harm to a minimum. This paper attempts to outline the reasoning that leads to a recommendation of pragmatic policies directed to this goal.

Costs of cocaine action and its consequences

Pharmacological considerations

Other contributions to this symposium deal in depth with the actions of cocaine. In the present context, only three points need to be summarized. The *first* is that cocaine, by inhibiting the re-uptake of catecholamines at noradrenergic and dopaminergic nerve terminals, enhances the effects of these neurotransmitters at postsynaptic receptor sites, and this action underlies both the rewarding effects of cocaine and most of the toxic effects of over-dosage. The *second* is that studies of drug self-administration by various species of laboratory animal, ranging from rodents to primates, have consistently shown that central stimulants, including cocaine and amphetamines, have very strong intrinsic pharmacological rewarding or reinforcing properties (Johanson & Fischman 1989). The *third* is that both types of effect are dose dependent; the greater the amounts of drug taken by the user in search of the rewarding effects, the greater is the risk of pharmacologically predictable adverse effects (Trinkoff et al 1990).

The nature of these adverse consequences is also predictable. They are produced either by an excess of local anaesthetic action (e.g. respiratory depression) or by over-activity of catecholaminergic pathways that results in a broad range of effects on different organ systems (Mueller et al 1990). A recent survey of such cocaine-related problems in one American hospital (Brody et al 1990) found that cardiopulmonary symptoms were reported in 56% of cases, neurological symptoms in 39%, and psychiatric symptoms in 36%; multiple complaints were present in 58%. It is unnecessary to review here the specifics of these adverse effects; they are described in many recent papers (e.g. recent reports of cardiovascular problems by Rezkalla et al 1990; cognitive and neurological problems by Tumeh et al 1990, Manschreck et al 1990 and Spivey & Euerle 1990; and psychiatric problems by Gawin & Ellinwood 1988). It is sufficient to note that toxic effects of cocaine are now common in hospital emergency services, and can be expected to increase in direct proportion to the level of use. In addition, cocaine dependence or addiction, at first thought not to occur, is now recognized as a relatively frequent and difficult problem (Gawin 1991).

'Crack' versus cocaine

As with any alkaloid, cocaine free base is much more volatile than its salts, and can therefore be vaporized in the smoke of a cigarette. Thus, the free base can be inhaled as the vapour, from which it enters the pulmonary capillaries and produces a very rapid onset of action which is prized by its users. This is entirely analogous to the use of amphetamine free base in the inhalers that first appeared on the market as hay fever and cold remedies, but that had to be removed soon after because of widespread misuse (Kalant 1973). 'Crack' is a crude form of cocaine free base, made by a simple and inexpensive process that has made the free base available in small portions at low cost to juvenile users who could not afford the more purified salt form (National Institute on Drug Abuse [NIDA] 1991). Consequently, it has greatly expanded the use of cocaine by juveniles in economically underprivileged groups in large American and Canadian cities. For example, in the general population of Toronto the rate of use of cocaine in 1989 was only 2%, and that of crack was under 1%, but among street youth in the same year 64% had used cocaine, nearly two-thirds of whom used it as crack. Of the 6% who were daily users, almost all used it as crack (Smart et al 1990). The actions after absorption are identical to those of the cocaine salts, as are the adverse effects, but the increase in use because of the lower minimum cost has also led to an increase in the frequency of adverse effects attributable to smoked crack (NIDA 1991).

Costs of attempted suppression of cocaine use

In contrast to the direct and predictable pharmacological adverse effects, the social and behavioural problems are not necessarily or predictably linked to the level of cocaine use in the population. Many are determined by the control policies adopted by a given society. At present, non-medical use of cocaine is prohibited in most countries. The absence of legal sources of supply for such use has been met by the creation of large-scale illicit traffic, which in turn has led to large-scale efforts by national and international authorities to suppress it. These efforts involve very large costs, both human and monetary. In the United States alone, the annual costs of police, coast guard and customs efforts to intercept supplies coming from abroad, and of judiciary and penal services required for prosecuting and incarcerating offenders, have been estimated at over ten billion dollars (Nadelmann 1989).

Costs associated with both the drug and its legal status

Other social problems are due in part to the illicit status of cocaine, and in part to the effects of the drug itself. Illicit drug traffic tends to attract young males with a propensity for risk-taking and often with antecedent histories of antisocial behaviour (Smart et al 1991). Vested interests in local illicit traffic are defended by violence if necessary. At the same time, the tendency for the drug to produce irritability, paranoid thinking and aggressiveness increases the risk that other causes of friction will give rise to violence among users. As a result, the subpopulations of heavy users of cocaine in North American cities also have high rates of violent crime (e.g. Budd 1989, Lindenbaum et al 1989).

In addition, the lucrative illicit trade has created grave problems for the cocaine-producing countries such as Colombia and Peru. Giant enterprises that produce and purify the drug, and transport and sell it to illicit wholesalers in North America and elsewhere, have created a parallel economy and power structure that rival or exceed those of the legitimate governments, and that disrupt the latter by corruption, violence and fear (Massing 1988).

Extent of the perceived problem

Cocaine first became widely used for medical purposes toward the end of the 19th century, and soon became popular for non-medical purposes, not only in North America, where controls varied widely from State to State (this volume: Musto 1992), but also in Europe, where it was controlled by medical and pharmacy regulations very early in its history (Maier 1926, Kalant 1987). In most countries, the problems associated with uncontrolled non-medical use led, in the first quarter of this century, to the imposition of strict legal controls, and the use of cocaine virtually disappeared for the next fifty years. When

Formulating policies on cocaine use

cocaine reappeared as a 'new' drug in the 1970s, the voluminous earlier literature on its adverse effects had been all but forgotten, and the knowledge had to be rediscovered by unhappy experience (Kalant 1987).

As a result of this costly lapse of public and professional knowledge, cocaine experienced an initial glamorization by the media and its use spread rapidly in North America. The National Household Survey, for example, indicated that among Americans aged 18–25 years, the percentage reporting use of cocaine within the preceding month increased from 3.1 in 1974 to 9.3 in 1979 (NIDA 1991). Together with increasing extent of use, there was a comparable increase in the frequency of associated problems, especially after crack use became widespread in the Black urban ghettos. In Los Angeles County alone, cocaine-related deaths increased exponentially from one in 1974 to 1160 in 1988, virtually all in young Black males (Budd 1989).

Since the mid 1980s, however, North American surveys have shown a consistent and significant downward trend in the use of all illicit drugs, including cocaine, in the general population. The latest annual University of Michigan survey of final-year high school students showed a decrease of the proportion using cocaine within the preceding month, from 6.7% in 1985 to 1.9% in 1990 (Johnston 1991). The biennial survey of high school students in Ontario showed a decrease in prior-year use from 5.1% in 1979 to 2.7% in 1989 (Smart & Adlaf 1989), and such use by Ontario adults had remained stable, at about 2% of the adult population, since 1984 (Adlaf & Smart 1989).

It is clear, therefore, that the decreasing extent of cocaine and other drug use among the general population, and the increasing use and associated problems among certain specific subpopulations, represent two different phenomena that presumably reflect different influences and perhaps call for different social responses.

Policy options

In recent years, growing attention has been given to what has been called the Great Legalization Debate (Saunders 1990), a narrow and sharply polarized consideration of two seemingly opposite alternatives: complete legalization and government-controlled sale of all psychoactive drugs, including opiates and cocaine, versus even stricter efforts to eradicate illicit drug production and traffic and to punish the traffickers (the 'War on Drugs' advocated by the governments of the United States, the United Kingdom, Colombia and others).

Those who advocate legalization argue that it would abolish most of the social costs at one stroke, eliminate the illicit traffic, remove the grave consequences of the criminalization of users, provide a new source of licit revenue to government or private enterprise, and offer an opportunity to regulate the quality and safety of the drugs. All this, it is argued, would involve little or no increase in the use of the substance in question (Nadelmann 1989, Chesher 1990, Homel et al 1990). Those who advocate an intensified War on Drugs argue that the drug epidemic is so great a calamity that the maximum possible effort should be mounted against it, as in a war for national survival (Nahas et al 1986, Barco 1990). In this view, the implicit assumption seems to be that the social and individual damages caused by the attempts to suppress the drug traffic, as well as the financial costs noted above, are analogous to the deaths and upheavals suffered in an actual war against an attacking power—the unfortunate but inevitable price that must be paid in order to win a victory over a greater evil.

In fact, as pointed out elsewhere, no exclusive dichotomy actually exists (Goldstein & Kalant 1990). A wide range of potential policy options is available, including harsher penalties (the War on Drugs), provision of illicit drugs to addicts by medical prescription, licensing of specific approved outlets, legal sale by regulated commercial enterprise or government monopoly, and different degrees of so-called 'decriminalization' ranging from discretionary non-enforcement of current laws to conversion of total to partial prohibition, or complete removal of criminal sanctions (J. Rolfe, cited by Farrell & Strang 1990).

As noted at the outset, the choice cannot be a completely logical one, because some of the considerations set out above cannot be quantified for purposes of comparison with each other. However, past and current experience can help to assess the validity of some of the premises.

Principles derived from past experience

A number of the arguments used to support one or another policy option can in fact be tested against empirical experience. Several points are important enough to warrant restatement here.

Does availability affect consumption?

There is a great deal of evidence that it does (other things being equal), for both licit and illicit drugs. The higher rate of opiate abuse among physicians, nurses and pharmacists than among the general population; the decrease in alcohol consumption, drunkenness, and cirrhosis death rate in Britain when pub opening hours were shortened in 1914–1918 (Smart 1974); the effect of cigarette-vending machines on smoking by minors; the increase in alcohol purchases in Ontario liquor stores that changed from clerk service to self-service; and the very high rate of opiate dependence among American troops in the Viet Nam war compared to the Pacific phase of World War II, all illustrate the simple and obvious fact that easier availability leads to increased use (Goldstein & Kalant 1990). The suggestion that easier availability would not increase cocaine use in Australia (Homel et al 1990) may perhaps reflect the fact that the respondents in that study were answering a hypothetical question rather than reacting to a real change in the availability of the drug.

Does price affect consumption?

Again, there is abundant evidence that it does. The inverse relation between unit price of alcohol in constant dollars and the per capita consumption in Ontario, as well as the death rate from alcoholic liver cirrhosis, confirms that not only social drinkers but also alcoholics are affected by the price (Popham et al 1975). The price elasticity of alcohol consumption by the two groups was even demonstrated experimentally (Babor et al 1978). The rapid expansion of cocaine use when the less expensive form of crack became available may be an analogous phenomenon (Musto 1990), although the simultaneous influence of smoking (a rapid, easy, highly effective and therefore highly reinforcing form of drug delivery) makes it difficult to assess the exact role of price. The argument that legal sale of cocaine, at prices low enough to eliminate illicit traffic, would not increase consumption greatly, appears to be wishful thinking. If increased consumption results in increased incidence of medical and social harm, the economic costs directly attributable to drug use can far outweigh the economic benefits arising from legal sale and taxation, as illustrated by Canadian experience with alcohol (Goldstein & Kalant 1990).

Does legal prohibition affect consumption?

Though less conclusively than for the preceding questions, the evidence supports the view that legal sanctions *do* affect consumption. For example, during the period of *de facto* alcohol prohibition in the USA (1916–1932), both the per capita consumption of alcohol and the death rate from liver cirrhosis dropped sharply (Klatskin 1961). It is often stated that the law will not deter the illicit use of drugs, because the users are already on the margin of the law and are accustomed to disregarding it. This may well be true, but it is irrelevant. The primary function of the law is to establish norms of behaviour for the *general population*, not for specific marginal or criminal subgroups. For the latter, the deterrent is not the law, but the firm application of punishment for infractions of it. In the usual operation of the democratic system, legislation in the field of drug use (as in other matters that are seen as moral issues) generally follows public opinion. The law is thus a codification of the values and standards of the society as a whole, and serves to remind the population of the limits of acceptable behaviour. The most effective laws are those in closest harmony with the ethical and moral standards of the population.

However, other factors modify the deterrent value of the law. It is therefore of interest to compare the manners in which apparently similar laws actually function in three different countries with dissimilar public value systems in relation to drug use: The Netherlands, Norway and Canada.

In *The Netherlands*, trafficking in illicit drugs is officially a crime, but for many years there has been *de facto* legalization of open sale of small quantities (less than 30 g) of marijuana or hashish, and the police have latitude in deciding whether or not to prosecute small-scale dealers in 'hard' drugs (cocaine, heroin or phencyclidine) who sell mainly to support their own drug use. Larger-scale trafficking, however, is still punished by prison terms that are, by Dutch sentencing standards, quite heavy. The Dutch people do not tend to see drug use as either a moral or political issue, and the emphasis of Dutch policy is on harm reduction and the reintegration of drug users into society. During the 1970s the tolerant attitude of the public and the authorities led to a period of 'unlimited tolerance' even for the use of hard drugs, but it was soon perceived as an overly idealistic failure and was replaced by a harder approach in which the authorities, rather than the users, set the limits of acceptable drug practices (Leuw 1991).

Norway has almost the opposite approach. Until the 1950s, cocaine and opiate dependence were seen as medical problems and were handled by legal prescription of drugs under the Opium Act of 1928. Since the mid 1950s, growing public concern about the use of new drugs, especially by teenagers, caused both use and possession to be designated as offences under the criminal code. There has been a steady increase in the severity of prescribed sentences; those for major trafficking are now the heaviest in the Norwegian penal code. There has also been a steady increase in police activity, seizures, and prosecutions. The general public is said to support this stern approach strongly (Hauge 1991).

Canada falls somewhere between these two extremes (Single et al 1991). The proportions of federal money spent on anti-drug measures are roughly 70% for demand reduction and 30% for supply reduction, almost the inverse of the pattern in the United States. The criminal code is strict, but the police and the courts have considerable discretionary power, and convictions for simple possession of cannabis or cocaine are usually handled by conditional discharges or fines, rather than prison sentences. The heavy sentences tend to be reserved for traffickers rather than users.

Despite these differences in tone and practice in the three countries, the statistics of drug use in the recent past have shown the same trends in all three. In The Netherlands there was a large increase in the number of cocaine and opiate addicts between 1974 and 1980, but the number has stabilized since then and their average age has increased, indicating that there are fewer young recruits (Leuw 1991). In Norway, surveys among 15- to 20-year-olds in Oslo indicated a rapid increase in the use of all illicit drugs from 1968 to 1974, and then a gradual decrease until the present (Hauge 1991). Drug use during the preceding year by Ontario students peaked in 1979–1981, and has fallen steadily since then; this pattern applies not only to cocaine but to virtually all drugs, including alcohol and tobacco (Smart & Adlaf 1989). This trend is essentially identical to that reported among high school seniors in the United States, where the 'War on Drugs' has broad public support. Similarly, among adult Canadians who had ever used cocaine there has been a striking increase recently in the percentage who did *not* use it in the preceding year (Adlaf & Smart 1989).

How are we to interpret this remarkable similarity of drug trends, despite wide differences in official policy? An easy conclusion might be that the law, and the manner in which it is interpreted and applied, make very little difference to levels of drug use, and therefore that drugs might just as well be legalized, thus avoiding all the problems created by their illegality. However, this may be a simplistic interpretation. World-wide use of alcohol has shown a periodic rise and fall, with a periodicity of about 60 years, that appears to depend not so much on legal status, economic situation, or international issues as on a slow building of public consensus in one or other direction (Skog 1986). It seems likely that the time scale for such swings is now much shorter as a result of modern communications and greatly increased travel.

We may very well be witnessing the same phenomenon with respect to other drug use, including that of cocaine. The rapid spread, among youth of all Western countries in the 1970s, of an ethos that equated drug use with freedom and self-realization, now appears to be followed by a growing perception of the hazards and costs of such use (Bachman et al 1988). This perhaps accounts for the relative lack of effect of the partial decriminalization of cannabis in a number of American States on the levels of cannabis use in those States (Single 1989). Despite the differences in their degrees of lenience or severity toward drug users, The Netherlands, Norway and Canada share a public disapproval of hard drug use and a predominant sentiment, even among the age groups most affected, against legalization even of cannabis, let alone of cocaine. In these three countries, which differ in the general harshness of their criminal codes, drug trafficking remains among the most severely punished offences. Thus, in all three countries the law does reflect a public consensus, and may very well be helping to reinforce the swing away from drug use in the general population.

An interesting contrast, however, is offered in the case of cannabis, which, as noted above, is regarded much less seriously by the Dutch authorities and public than by those of the other countries. Its open sale in 'coffee houses', without risk of prosecution, appears to indicate both greater availability and less strong consensus against its use, despite the fact that outright legalization of cannabis is not favoured by the majority of the public. This may explain why the level of cannabis use has not fallen since 1980, as it has in Norway, Sweden, the USA and Canada (Driessen et al 1989), but has apparently risen.

Suggestions for a pragmatic basis of policy

From the foregoing considerations, there emerge several principles for a pragmatic, rather than a dogmatic, basis of policy concerning cocaine and other drugs (Goldstein & Kalant 1990). What a government proposes in this area must be consistent with the type of society that the majority of the population desires. The following suggestions appear to be in keeping with the wishes of most democratic societies.

(1) Given the admittedly low rate of success and the high human and monetary costs of efforts to prevent illicit drugs from reaching the market, pragmatism would suggest a major reduction in these efforts, and a greater concentration on all types of demand reduction, including preventive education, increased availability of treatment for users, and greater attention to the socioeconomic circumstances that appear to foster drug use among some specific subgroups within countries.

(2) Recognition of the role of the law as a codification of the prevailing values of a society, and the fact that even the most lenient of societies retain anti-drug laws, suggest that we should retain legal proscription of cocaine and other currently illicit drugs as an expression of disapproval of their use. At the same time, giving specific educational programmes and wider discretionary powers to the police and judiciary could reduce the unintended hardships that strict application of the law can produce.

(3) The startling success of anti-smoking campaigns demonstrates that public consensus is perhaps the most powerful controlling influence of all. Health-oriented campaigns to increase the anti-drug consensus, with respect not only to cocaine but to the non-medical use of all drugs, both licit and illicit, may well be the most effective strategy for reducing cocaine consumption and its consequences, while avoiding the extravagant costs of reliance on repressive measures.

A note of caution is indicated, however. The building of consensus should not be confused with the mounting of moral crusades. It is too easy for moral crusades to turn into tyranny by the majority, and the history of the 20th century demonstrates the grave dangers that this can pose.

Acknowledgements

I am greatly indebted to Dr O. J. Kalant for valuable discussions of this topic, and to Dr Peter Reuter for permission to cite papers presented at the Rand Corporation Conference on National Drug Policy. The views expressed above are those of the author and do not necessarily represent the policy of the Addiction Research Foundation of Ontario.

References

Adlaf EM, Smart RG 1989 The Ontario adult alcohol & other drug use survey 1977–1989. Addiction Research Foundation, Toronto

Babor TF, Mendelson JH, Greenberg I, Kuehnle J 1978 Experimental analysis of the 'Happy Hour': effects of purchase price on alcohol consumption. Psychopharmacology 58:35–41

Bachman JG, Johnston LD, O'Malley PM, Humphrey RH 1988 Explaining the recent decline in marijuana use: differentiating the effects of perceived risks, disapproval, and general lifestyle factors. J Health Soc Behav 29:92–112

Barco V (Ex-President of Colombia) 1990 Cited in 'News and Views'. Drug Alcohol Rev 9:377

Brody SL, Slovis CM, Wrenn KD 1990 Cocaine-related medical problems: consecutive series of 233 patients. Am J Med 88:325-331
Budd RD 1989 Cocaine abuse and violent death. Am J Drug Alcohol Abuse 15:375-382
Chesher GB 1990 Controlled availability as an alternative. Drug Alcohol Rev 9:369-371
Driessen FMHM, Van Dam G, Olsson B 1989 De ontwikkeling van het cannabisgebruik in Nederland, enkele Europese landen en de VS sinds 1969. Tijdschr Alcohol Drugs 15:2-14
Farrell M, Strang J 1990 Confusion between the drug legalization and the drug prescribing debate. Drug Alcohol Rev 9:364-368
Gawin FH 1991 Cocaine addiction: psychology and neurophysiology. Science (Wash DC) 251:1580-1586
Gawin FH, Ellinwood EH Jr 1988 Cocaine and other stimulants—actions, abuse and treatment. N Engl J Med 318:1173-1182
Goldstein A, Kalant H 1990 Drug policy: striking the right balance. Science (Wash DC) 249:1513-1521
Hauge R 1991 Drug problems and drug policies in Norway. Paper presented at Conference on National Drug Policy, Rand Corporation, Washington, DC, May 1991
Homel P, Flaherty B, Reilly C, Hall W, Carless J 1990 The drug market position of cocaine among young adults in Sydney. Br J Addiction 85:891-897
Johanson C-E, Fischman MW 1989 The pharmacology of cocaine related to its abuse. Pharmacol Rev 41:3-52
Johnston LD 1991 Use of crack and other illicit drugs has declined significantly among young Americans. University of Michigan news release 23 January 1991. U of M News and Information Services, Ann Arbor, MI
Kalant H, Kalant OJ 1971 Drugs, society and personal choice. Addiction Research Foundation, Toronto
Kalant OJ 1973 The amphetamines: toxicity and addiction. University of Toronto Press, Toronto
Kalant OJ 1987 Maier's Cocaine addiction (Der Kokainismus). Addiction Research Foundation, Toronto
Klatskin G 1961 Alcohol and its relation to liver damage. Gastroenterology 41:443-450
Leuw E 1991 Drugs and drug policy in the Netherlands. Paper presented at Conference on National Drug Policy, Rand Corporation, Washington, DC, May 1991
Lindenbaum GM, Carroll SF, Daskal I, Kapusnick R 1989 Patterns of alcohol and drug abuse in an urban trauma center: the increasing role of cocaine abuse. J Trauma 29:1654-1659
Maier HW 1926 Der Kokainismus. Georg Thieme, Berlin. For English translation, see Kalant 1987
Manschreck TC, Schneyer ML, Weisstein CC, Laughery J, Rosenthal J, Celada T, Berner J 1990 Freebase cocaine and memory. Compr Psychiatry 31:369-375
Massing M 1988 The war on cocaine. NY Rev Books 35(20):61-67, Dec 22
Mueller PD, Benowitz NL, Olson KR 1990 Cocaine. Emerg Med Clin North Am 8:481-493
Musto DF 1990 Illicit price of cocaine in two eras: 1908-1914 and 1982-1989. Conn Med 54:321-326
Musto DF 1992 Cocaine's history, especially the American experience. In: Cocaine: scientific and social dimensions. Wiley, Chichester (Ciba Found Symp 166) p 7-19
Nadelmann EA 1989 Drug prohibition in the United States: costs, consequences, and alternatives. Science (Wash DC) 245:939-947
Nahas GG, Frick HC, Gleaton T, Schuchard K, Moulton O 1986 A drug policy for our times. Bull Narc 38 (1&2):3-14

National Institute on Drug Abuse [NIDA] 1991 Drug abuse and drug abuse research. Third triennial report to Congress from the Secretary, DHHS. DHHS Publications, Washington, DC

Popham RE, Schmidt W, de Lint J 1975 The prevention of alcoholism: epidemiological studies of the effects of government control measures. Br J Addict 70:125-144

Rezkalla SH, Hale S, Kloner RA 1990 Cocaine-induced heart diseases. Am Heart J 120(6, pt 1):1403-1408

Saunders JB 1990 The great legalization debate. Drug Alcohol Rev 9:3-5

Single EW 1989 The impact of marijuana decriminalization: an update. Public Health Policy 10:456-466

Single E, Erickson P, Skirrow J 1991 Drugs and public policy in Canada. Paper presented at Conference on National Drug Policy, Rand Corporation, Washington, DC, May 1991

Skog O-J 1986 The long waves of alcohol consumption: a social network perspective on cultural change. Soc Networks 8:1-32

Smart RG 1974 The effect of licencing restrictions during 1914-1918 on drunkenness and liver cirrhosis deaths in Britain. Br J Addict 69:109-121

Smart RG, Adlaf EM 1989 The Ontario student drug use survey: trends between 1977-1989. Addiction Research Foundation, Toronto

Smart RG, Adlaf EM, Porterfield KM, Canale MD 1990 Drugs, youth and the street. Addiction Research Foundation, Toronto

Smart RG, Adlaf EM, Walsh GW 1991 Adolescent drug sellers: trends, characteristics and profiles. Addiction Research Foundation, Toronto

Spivey WH, Euerle B 1990 Neurologic complications of cocaine abuse. Ann Emerg Med 19:1422-1428

Trinkoff AM, Ritter C, Anthony JC 1990 The prevalence and self-reported consequences of cocaine use: an exploratory and descriptive analysis. Drug Alcohol Depend 26:217-225

Tumeh SS, Nagel JS, English RJ, Moore M, Holman BL 1990 Cerebral abnormalities in cocaine abusers: demonstration by SPECT perfusion. Radiology 176:821-824

DISCUSSION

Kleber: We should clarify a point you made about crack. You said that crack is sold 'at low cost'. Crack is *not* cheap; it is only sold cheaply. One gram of cocaine hydrochloride sells for $100; when converted into crack, it yields about $150 worth of crack. This is an expensive way to buy cocaine, in fact. It is equivalent to buying drinks at a bar for $3 each when a bottle of the same whisky would sell for $12 at a store and yield 15-20 drinks.

Secondly, are your demand:supply figures for Canada comparable to the US figures? That is, are your demand reduction efforts, as far as treatment is concerned, all supported by federal efforts? In the US, the federal contribution to treatment is only about 25%, and the rest is State and local expenditure.

Kalant: In Canada, the costs of demand reduction are met at both provincial and federal levels, on the basis of the constitutional division of powers and responsibilities. My percentages (p 268) for demand and supply reduction (70% and 30%) referred only to federal funding.

Formulating policies on cocaine use

Des Jarlais: So if provincial funds were added to federal sources, this would increase the proportion spent on demand reduction still further.

Kalant: Yes, because operation of the health care system, as well as education, is a provincial responsibility.

Negrete: In Canada, criminal law enforcement is a responsibility of the federal government, whereas health services are run by the provinces; so the drug control costs are mostly a federal (national) expenditure, and the service (treatment) budget is mainly a provincial one. Inclusion of non-federal spending in the calculation would make the disparity on demand reduction expenditure between Canada and the USA even greater.

Kleber: In the USA, we estimate that the 70% of our drug-related expenditure which goes to supply control is roughly spent half on law enforcement inside our borders and half outside, on international and border efforts. Is Canada able to keep its supply control budget low by taking advantage of the efforts of countries such as the USA in Thailand and in the Andes?

Kalant: In all fairness we would have to say yes, but the difference between US and Canadian patterns also reflects a difference in the view of what it is worth spending money on.

Jaffe: There seem to be some approaches to decreasing drug use that aren't clearly either demand reduction or law enforcement (supply reduction). A whole technology is evolving in the United States for testing people to determine whether they have used drugs, and the sanctions are never (or rarely) criminal. Typically, the sanctions are that you can't get a job, or an appointment to a particular public office, if you are shown to be a drug user. On which side of the supply/demand equation does this belong? That is what interests me.

Kleber: Jerry Jaffe is referring to our 'user accountability' measures that could lead, for example, to loss of a driver's licence if you're convicted of a drug-related offence. This appears to me to be clearly a demand reduction effort, not a supply reduction effort. You haven't affected the availability of the drug. Since we may never be able to make drugs physically unavailable, the task of demand reduction efforts is to make them psychologically unavailable. That's more than just education and treatment.

Edwards: Your paper, Dr Kalant, was an interpretation of great rationality and humanity; there's a sense of balance in it. As I see it, you have broadly concluded that in many countries the prevalence of the use of illicit drugs (and indeed the prevalence of alcohol consumption) is falling, and your interpretation is that this fall is more due to change in societal appraisal of the dangers than to enforcement efforts. But I wonder whether this view is a conjecture, a postulate for further testing, or a confident assertion? You referred to public policy and the operation of drug control legislation in Norway, The Netherlands and Canada. But I am uncertain whether a sufficiently systematic analysis has been done over time, for a large enough number of countries, for these conclusions to be drawn.

For instance, in the UK, the number of notified addicts (largely heroin) rose in 1990 by a greater percentage than in any year since we had records. It went up by 20%, and there are alarm bells ringing. Again, it would worry me if we left out of our reckoning the situation in the developing countries, including South America. Also, do you think we can at present adequately understand the multivariate nature of the field, when there are changes going on at the same time in societal appraisal, in drug supply, and in law?

Kalant: I hoped I had made it clear that I was offering a postulate, not a firm recommendation! The actual databases are not very solid; many of the important quantitative components are just not documented reliably. I didn't discuss third world countries because, for most of them, reliable figures are not available. Even in those developed countries which have the means to gather the information, often it hasn't been properly gathered. I am proposing my schema as a model based on a comparison of trends in a limited number of countries with different policies, and attempting to say why, despite these different drug control policies, they are all showing the same trend. I am also suggesting what data we need to gather to document this well enough to be able to say with confidence whether it is a correct interpretation or not.

Moore: I have one comment on this question of the role of the law in drug policy, which is inevitably at the heart of the discussion. Often, when we think of 'the law', we contrast it with 'education', on the one hand, or with people accumulating experience and changing their views, on the other. The implicit assumption is that there is a 'natural' process by which society learns voluntarily and collectively about the hazards of cocaine use; and then there is some 'foreign' process involving the passage of a law, which has to be in tune with the society in which it will operate. What Harold Kalant has quite properly emphasized is that this distinction breaks down. The act of passing new laws is an instrument of education and is itself a way in which the society comes to understand and believe certain things. Once a law is in place, it often becomes something that is used to educate people about where the norms of the society are, in terms of what behaviour is appropriate. So instead of seeing 'the law' as standing outside the society, we should think about it as an instrument that society uses to debate with itself about what is appropriate, and to change its views and provide guidance about what constitutes appropriate behaviour. Indeed, legal scholars used to talk about the *promulgation* of the laws as an important part of the act of passing them. That is an educational process, and an important one.

Kalant: I agree completely with that, but I would just repeat that in democratic societies the laws don't happen until the society has already changed its attitude. A political party which advocates a particular policy has to be elected, and therefore it has to have won enough public acceptance for that policy; and public views also have to have gained enough acceptance by the party that is proposing a law which will codify and express those views.

Economics of drug use and abuse

Edwards: But, as you say, such considerations pertain only in democratic countries.

Gerstein: I have two comments on this analysis. One concerns value judgements. Among the things that need to be measured are the distribution and intensity of the values held by members of the society, because these values—these images of the desirable—are what determine the indices on which costs and benefits are measured. People value things differently (and quite legitimately so). Moreover, it is always difficult to balance values against each other. Concerns about crime, public health and moral fibre translate into different kinds of costs and different kinds of benefits.

Second, there may be a problem of language. When we talk about the 'moral crusade' against drugs, we are actually not thinking of drugs in the sense of a 'sin', but in the sense of criminal behaviour. Most of the time we view the drug problem largely in a criminal rather than a theological light. This is why the war on drugs becomes a police war, rather than something largely waged through the pulpit.

Kalant: On values, I was not so much disagreeing with your views, but indicating a different and additional point at which value judgements enter the process. On your second point, it would be wrong to interpret the word 'moral' literally, as being equated with religions. When I use the term 'moral crusade' I am thinking not of a religious crusade as such, but of a crusade based on a common assumption of what is 'good' and 'right', against what is 'wrong' and 'evil'.

Negrete: As in China or Cuba?

Kalant: Or in Nazi Germany; this wasn't a religious movement but a moral crusade based on some concept of Aryan superiority. I use the word 'moral' in that sense.

Gerstein: I must admit that the phrase 'drug-free America' leaves a certain disquieting echo of '*judenrein Deutschland*'; nevertheless, I am deeply reluctant to compare any American moralists to Nazis (except the American Nazi Party itself).

Almond: It would be interesting to hear comment on the cases of Spain and Italy, where I understand that cannabis was legalized, and legalization was followed by an increase in the use of hard drugs, and then an increase in the incidence of AIDS, and so in both countries they have gone back to the original situation. Is that correct?

Kleber: Italy has the highest death rate and highest overdose rate from heroin in western Europe. As a result, it recriminalized the possession of heroin for personal use in 1990.

Strang: I don't think the link from cannabis use to heroin use can be made—certainly not just by considering Italy. The change in the law in Italy had to do with the removal of penalties for the personal possession of all drugs, including heroin. It wasn't through the intermediate step of cannabis legislation.

Almond: There is, though, the Spanish case, where the transition was indeed from cannabis, through hard drugs, to HIV/AIDS, leading to a serious AIDS problem in the city of Madrid.

Drug use and abuse: the ethical issues

Brenda Almond

Social Values Research Centre, University of Hull, Hull HU6 7RX, UK

Abstract. Drug abuse is both a personal and a public issue, raising questions about individual rights and the boundaries of law, as well as about national sovereignty and international control. Ethical issues that arise under these headings may be related to certain broad ethical positions. The implications of adopting utilitarian assumptions may be contrasted with basing ethics on a theory of individual rights, closely related to a theory of human nature. Neither position justifies a libertarian presumption against control, for, first, an individual decision to expose one's mind and personality to the control of drugs cannot be ethically justified and, second, there are no ethical reasons, nor any compelling arguments from social and political theory, for decriminalizing non-medical drug use.

1992 Cocaine: scientific and social dimensions. Wiley, Chichester (Ciba Foundation Symposium 166) p 277-293

'Man', said Aristotle, 'is a rational animal'. As a defining characteristic, this is more important than that man is a maker and user of tools, a social creature, a hunter-gatherer or featherless biped. If rationality is the significant hallmark of a human being, however, it is paradoxical that people sometimes defend, in the name of autonomy, a right to destroy or damage that rationality through drugs that affect both mind and personality.

It is fashionable to follow Aristotle these days, particularly in ethics, where there is current a view that he approached the matter the right way round. That is to say, he began by asking what it is that is distinctive of a human being, and went on to ask what is necessary for a human being so characterized to flourish—to find happiness or fulfilment in a fully human way. He also saw, as did Plato, that the answer to this question cannot be separated from a second question: what sort of society will provide the best conditions for this flourishing? He recognized, that is to say, that ethical, social and political questions are closely interwoven, and that law is the element that mediates between them.

This interconnection is particularly striking where the specific issue of drug abuse is concerned. (I shall use this term although it is not entirely satisfactory in that it appears to guarantee the wrongness of the behaviour under discussion. For purposes of this chapter, however, it may be regarded as a neutral description of habitual drug use outside legitimate medical areas.) The issue of drugs, then, raises ethical questions, closely followed by legal and political ones, at the personal level, at the social level, and also at the broader political level of international relations between States.

At the personal level, an initial presumption in favour of hedonistic enjoyment and a right to freedom of choice is balanced by a number of less favourable considerations, in particular an established link with factors such as psychiatric illness, general incapacity and possible early death. As far as society is concerned, drug abuse is often associated with a variety of health and social problems: drug addicts may live in poor conditions, including diet and shelter (often *no* shelter other than city streets), while both women and young males who are addicts may resort to prostitution to pay for their habit. Increasingly today it is inextricably linked with the problem of AIDS (acquired immune deficiency syndrome)—studies in Edinburgh, for example, showed recently that 50% of intravenously injecting drug users tested positive for HIV (the human immunodeficiency virus), and that 50% of those diagnosed as HIV-positive were intravenous drug users (Robertson 1990). There is also a link with crime—in the case of crack, pointlessly *violent* crime—to pay for a habit which can escalate uncontrollably in cost. (A recent newspaper article in the UK reported one drug addict as saying that, whereas it had been hard for her and her boyfriend to take more than £50 worth of heroin a day each, they had spent £1500 in four days on cocaine 'rocks' [Warwick 1991]). As long as the 'crack' lifestyle is incompatible with holding down a job, the link with crime is likely to be there, whether or not access to the drug is legal or illegal. In general, then, drug abuse carries heavy economic and social costs without corresponding social benefits. For this reason, it is a legitimate concern of governments and, because of conflicts of interest between producer and consumer countries, it is a concern at the international as well as the national level.

The ethical questions that arise at these three levels may be summarized as: firstly, at the personal level, the question for the individual of what moral attitude to take to drug use and abuse; secondly, at the community level, the question of where the boundary is to be drawn between law and individual autonomy; and thirdly at the international level, the question of where the limits of national autonomy lie and how far intervention by States in the internal affairs of other sovereign States can be justified.

At all these levels, conclusions are likely to be shaped and influenced by the broad ethical position adopted as an underlying premise. One of the most influential of these is utilitarianism. This is the theory that policies should be appraised in the light of their practical consequences, and that courses of action should be chosen so as to maximize benefits and minimize costs. In contrast to this view, which focuses on the consequences and outcomes of action, ethics may be grounded on a theory of individual rights, based on a conception of human nature and the conditions necessary for human flourishing. This may lead to a more principle-based morality, in which broad moral values such as honesty, compassion, justice, consideration for others and respect for freedom have an independent justification. In what follows, I shall consider briefly the moral issues that arise for individual, society and the wider international community before returning to the question of which broad ethical position provides the soundest basis for decisions at these differing levels.

The personal equation

Few people would want to sell themselves into slavery, even to a good owner. An addictive drug is not a good owner, but it does represent enslavement, as many addicts are prepared to testify. So there is an immediate choice in individual terms between long-term freedom and short-term pleasure. This is not an unknown dilemma either in philosophy or life.

The philosopher Joseph Butler, in his capacity as Bishop of the Church of England, urged his congregation at least to choose to follow 'cool' self-love, rather than the impetuous short-term variety which, he argued, more often than not leads us disastrously astray. On the contrary, he insisted: 'Conscience and self-love, if we understand our true happiness, always lead us the same way. Duty and interest are perfectly coincident.' (Gladstone 1896.)

So, on the personal level, there is a case for at least a calculated selfishness— for preferring more solid and long-term pleasures, including in particular the pleasures of health, to immediate ones. For there are also, of course, physically harmful side effects of drug consumption. In addition, there are psychological hazards, such as an altered attitude to risk-taking, which can have consequences for physical health. That is to say, there are various health risks, of which AIDS is a prominent example, which can be avoided with care, but care and a consequent commitment to taking precautions are likely to be abandoned under the influence of drugs.

There is also a well-established moral argument, associated with Kant, based not on self-interest, but on the principle of universalizability, which is relevant here. Indeed, Kant took as examples for applying this principle duties to the self, including a duty not to commit suicide and a duty not to neglect the cultivation of any talents one might have. A person contemplating suicide, or personal neglect, Kant maintained, should ask the question, 'Could I will that the principle I am acting on here should become a universal law?' Whether or not one accepts the ethical system in which this principle is embedded, Kant's question does draw attention to the fact that to choose self-neglect or suicide is indeed to make a morally unjustifiable exception of oneself, for it is not possible to will such a policy for everyone else. If consistency is a necessary requirement for an ethical position, then, it is not to be found here. A life on drugs is a life parasitic on an otherwise functioning society.

But supposing there were *no* harmful side effects, no danger to health, would this change the balance of the equation? Two well-known examples are relevant to this question, one from literature, one from philosophy. In Huxley's *Brave New World* (1932) the drug Soma was widely and harmlessly available. And yet the reader of this book does not identify with or envy those characters in the story who maintain an even tenor of psychologically experienced happiness. The identification is with those who struggle, those who have, despite grief, the experience of choice. Similarly, in the philosophical literature, there is discussion of what is sometimes called The Experience Machine. In a fanciful hypothesis it is proposed that a scientist has invented a computer which may be programmed with the appearance of the fulfilment of all a person's lifetime goals and desires. Once connected to this machine, a person, whilst never again leaving the laboratory, will experience the illusion of a full and satisfying life, exactly suited to his or her own specification. If happiness is all-important, it seems this should be what any human being should want. And yet, clearly, the average person, approached by the scientist for this experiment, would recoil in horror, preferring freedom and its hazards, to the certainty of this insubstantial pleasure.

What is one to conclude from this? Only that most of us have—like Aristotle—a conception of what is best, and, where the mind is unclouded and the issues are understood, a desire to pursue it. The pursuit of this may bring happiness, but happiness as a goal in itself is, as Butler also argued, a nothing. In addition, of course, the individual may also have duties and obligations which should have priority in his or her personal life, and drug addiction will be incompatible with their fulfilment. I have preferred here to address the harder argument of the personal issue for someone whose morality is more limited than this—even a morality limited to the promotion of personal self-interest.

The social argument

Whatever choice the individual makes, the question for society is whether to permit the degree of freedom of action that the mention of choice implies. It is a matter, in other words, of the boundary between law and individual autonomy.

The classic defence of individual liberty was presented by John Stuart Mill in his *'On Liberty'*. In this essay, first published in 1859, he argued that interference by the State in the life of the individual should be limited to the minimum necessary to prevent harm to others. As he wrote, 'the only part of the conduct of anyone, for which he is amenable to society, is that which concerns others. . . . Over himself, over his own mind and body, the individual is sovereign.' (Mill 1982.) This principle represents a line of division between the public and the private realm, and it began a debate which continues to the present day. The Wolfenden Report, in 1957, for example, making recommendations concerning the laws relating to homosexuality and prostitution in the United Kingdom, followed Mill in insisting again that it is not the function of the law to intervene in the private lives of citizens, or to seek to enforce any particular pattern of behaviour.

There are a number of reasons, however, why Mill should not be too quickly enrolled as a drug libertarian. Firstly, as I have already pointed out, because of the problem of addiction, the only real choice in relation to drugs is the early choice to become involved. Thereafter, the kind of choice in which Mill himself was interested, and which he valued highly, is eliminated. An essential aspect of Mill's view of politics and society was that it is only in the exercise of choice that a human being uses his or her unique and peculiar mental and moral powers. Hence he saw no problem in ruling out as an option that of selling oneself into slavery. No such contract, he believed, could be valid.

Secondly, he excepted, in any case, from the scope of his liberty principle 'children and young persons below the age which the law may fix as that of manhood or womanhood.' (Mill 1982.) In relation to the current drug scene, and particularly cocaine use, which peaks between the ages of 18 and 21, this is an extremely important qualification.

Thirdly, Mill gave a striking example of justifying interference even outside these restricted areas. If someone was approaching a bridge, he argued, which was in a dangerous condition, then an onlooker would be justified in physically restraining him from going onto the bridge if there was no time to warn him of the danger. At least as a metaphor, this provides a justification for paternalistic interference by an onlooker in an emergency.

On the other hand, in considering the practical application of the liberty principle, Mill gave a rather different answer. Taking as an example excessive alcohol consumption, he argued that society was *not* entitled to interfere directly as far as the individual's drinking habits were concerned. However, if as a result of that alcohol consumption, the individual was failing to perform his social duties—in relation, for example, to maintaining his dependants—then society *would* be entitled to interfere, but only to secure the fulfilment of those responsibilities. This may seem a somewhat disingenuous argument, however, in the case of substances which are known to cripple the ability of users to hold a job and so to fulfil their social obligation, even that of self-support.

Some contemporary libertarians would, however, follow Mill in this respect, arguing that drugs are harmless apart from their criminal connections and that there is a right of access to such substances. As one libertarian has put it, 'Everything considered bad about heroin is an effect of trying to ban it.' (Gabb 1990.) According to this view, the effect of law in this area is to encourage police corruption and provide a tax-free gift to drug traffickers. However, more thoughtful libertarians, including even some 'free market' economists, recognize the relevance of what are known as 'neighbourhood effects'—a consideration actually implicit in Mill's alcohol example. Milton Friedman uses such an argument to justify compulsory education, Nozick to justify a police force

(Friedman 1962, Nozick 1974). The effect of substance abuse is to produce a change in the social context within which an otherwise uninvolved individual must operate. Hence the non-user's freedom is affected by the existence of users. At a minimum, walking home late at night becomes a hazard, but also taxes and social payments must be raised to pay for those who cannot support themselves or their dependants.

Mill's harm principle, then, is not, after all, violated by a community's attempt to control the conditions of its own existence. Just as an individual in the 19th century could not alone choose a healthy environment—clean air, sanitation, pure water—so an individual in the 20th century cannot choose a harmonious and safe social environment except by corporate action, enforced by common laws. Is this to sacrifice freedom, then? To quote Lord Devlin on this, 'If we are not entitled to call our society "free" unless we pursue freedom to an extremity that would make society intolerable for most of us, then let us stop short of the extreme and be content with some other name.' (Devlin 1978.)

At the social level, then, there can also be a social view—a public morality—on which action in the public sphere may be based; and society is entitled to use the weapon of the law to enforce the conduct essential for the kind of harmonious and fruitful social order it has chosen. Much depends, too, on how strongly the threat is construed. For in the case of a serious onslaught on a country's way of life by an army of drug distributors and sellers, a principle of collective self-defence becomes operative, which will justify that society in taking measures to prevent its own disintegration.

The international dimension

This brings us finally to the issue of relations between States. I shall say little on this subject, since it is an area where political expediency is likely to take precedence over ethical argument. The root issue, however, is one of a conflict of interests between producer and consumer countries. Because the division between these coincides to a considerable extent with the division between the developing and developed world, it also prompts reflection on the relation between rich and poor, North and South, with an attendant risk that pressure from the rich consumer countries to curb supplies may be viewed as a form of neo-colonialism.

But the effects of small-scale entrepreneurship in Bolivia may be linked, by a fairly solid causal chain, to the death of strangers in New York. It is not hard, therefore, to claim both a duty and a right of self-defence. Of course, attacking demand in the consumer countries through education and through control of trafficking at street level must be a substantial part of the reaction of countries in the developed world committed to minimizing drug abuse. But it is generally acknowledged that this cannot be effective on its own without also attempts to reduce the supply at source. Whatever the ethical justification for direct interference might be, however, this can only be achieved with the consent of the producer countries—a consent most likely to be gained by well-conceived programmes offering crop substitution, rural development programmes, and help towards the creation of an industrial infrastructure.

Conclusions

I have argued here, firstly, that an individual decision to expose one's mind and personality to the control of drugs cannot be ethically justified. Secondly, at the social level, I have suggested that there are no pressing *ethical* reasons for decriminalizing non-medical drug use, nor are there any compelling arguments from the point of view of social and political philosophy. Much turns here, however, on the *facts* of the matter, particularly if a utilitarian moral philosophy is adopted. And on the broader community level, it seems we operate in the realm not of science but of speculation. Appeal may be made to certain limited experiments involving free access to certain soft drugs, particularly cannabis, such as have taken place in Amsterdam and Madrid; or to historical experiences, such as the free use of opium and cocaine in Britain in the last century.

But these examples tell us nothing of the social impact for major population centres of mass-market hard-selling methods used to promote highly addictive substances, particularly those in chemically concentrated form. Nor do they tell us how, today, to prevent escalation in drug-taking, how to protect the young, or how to control the AIDS risk accompanying intravenous drug use. I conclude that even for the utilitarian, concerned to maximize social benefits, a liberal approach must be highly problematic. For those prepared to form their moral judgements on a less pragmatic basis, whether that of individual rights or a fuller conception of human nature, including its spiritual, intellectual and cultural dimensions, there can be no moral case to answer. To argue otherwise in the name of ethics is to take on a heavy responsibility.

References

Butler J Fifteen Sermons. In: Gladstone WE (ed) 1896 The works of Joseph Butler. Clarendon Press, Oxford (First published 1726)
Devlin P 1978 The enforcement of morals. Oxford University Press, Oxford
Friedman M 1962 Capitalism and freedom. Chicago University Press, Chicago
Gabb S 1990 What to do about AIDS. Libertarian Alliance Pamphlet No. 12, London (Obtainable from: Libertarian Alliance, 1 Russell Chambers, The Piazza, Covent Garden, London WC2E 8AA)
Huxley A 1932 Brave new world. Chatto & Windus, London
Mills JS 1982 On liberty. Penguin, Harmondsworth (First published 1859)
Nozick R 1974 Anarchy, state and utopia. Blackwell, Oxford
Robertson R 1990 The Edinburgh epidemic: a case study. In: Strang J, Stimson G (eds) AIDS and drug misuse: the challenge for policy and practice in the 1990s. Routledge, London
Warwick P 1991 A life cracked. The Guardian, London, June 29, p 13

DISCUSSION

Anthony: Your cost-benefit analysis has interesting possibilities. I suggest that the analysis, as you have applied it to cocaine use, could also be applied to the consumption of alcohol, or to the habit of shaking salt on our eggs in the morning at breakfast, or perhaps even to sexual activities after the reproductive years. That is, on the high moral ground of your cost-benefit analysis, perhaps it should be argued that we all should stop drinking alcohol, stop shaking salt on our eggs, and stop having sex if there is no clearly demonstrable advantage to survival of the species.

I am also wondering if you are considering the *functions* of drug use in humans at all? You have spoken mainly in terms of *pleasure,* but I wonder if that is the controlling influence on drug use in humans, and whether there are functions that drug use serves.

Finally, I believe that, depending on the societal context, human beings sometimes have been quite willing to 'enslave' themselves. The British historian, R.W. Southern, in his *The Making of the Middle Ages* (1953), wrote about men who were willing not only to put themselves into serfdom to other men, but also to put their offspring into perpetual serfdom, in order to gain good during their lives. So the presumption that people acting rationally would not enslave themselves might be called into question, at least in the context of that particular experience in the Middle Ages.

Almond: I was not arguing that people don't enslave themselves; they obviously do enslave themselves, and are willing to do that. The question is whether this is something that one should support from a rational ethical perspective, and there I think the answer is that one should not.

Anthony: Southern's argument was that this was quite rational within the context of the society of the Middle Ages.

Moore: You can say that that society was an immoral society, and that it was an advance of human morality to establish a society on a different basis.

Almond: Yes, that is a possible response. However, Dr Anthony's first point concerned the comparison of drugs with other substances. I am certainly not suggesting that the facts of a situation are irrelevant to one's conclusions, nor do I think that cost-benefit analyses have no part to play; but I believe that a very different cost-benefit analysis results, depending on the example you take. I would particularly mention alcohol. Although alcohol gets such a bad press, human beings have lived in a symbiotic relationship with alcohol from the dawn of time. It has many positive aspects, and its adverse effects are pretty controllable. With the other examples that you mention, the balance is obviously tipped in favour of leaving decisions to individuals as to what risks they care to run.

Musto: The point has been made that very few claims are advanced for a benefit from the use of these drugs. This is not the case in the American experience. There have been periods in which the drugs (including alcohol) are seen as very valuable, when used correctly and in moderate amounts. Then we come to times like the present in which no use of certain drugs is permitted. So US society goes through phases of seeing drugs as very useful and then seeing them as of no value whatsoever. I have heard many wonderful things said about cannabis, LSD, cocaine and heroin. Drugs have had their promoters, from Aldous Huxley to Timothy Leary, although their recommendations are often qualified by the advice to use drugs in 'moderation'.

Moore: I think these swings in attitude give many people a feeling of unease. How could it be true that one view was held by society at one time, and another view at a later time? It can't be that the drug has changed pharmacologically! People are looking for an 'anchor' for how they ought to view various drugs. One part of that anchor seems to come from scientific evidence about their operations and effects on people, another from epidemiological evidence about what a drug seems to do when it is used in the society. However, there is already an element of uncertainty at that point, because once we see it operating in the society, we no longer see the 'pure' effect of the drug; we see the effect of the drug in a particular legal regime being used by particular people.

So we come to the complex question of what part of the drug's effects we should attribute to the drug itself and what part to other aspects. Given America's weakness as a society for looking for simple explanations and ignoring complicated ones, we tend to attribute more to the drug than we should and therefore to 'demonize' it.

One 'anchor' is therefore to try to determine what the effects of the drugs are, and much of this conference has focused on that. The other way to find an anchor is to try to develop our moral intuitions about whether the effects of drugs should be reckoned as beneficial for people, and whether we should try to see what the possibilities of attractive drug use are, or whether we should decide to suppress those aspects of drugs and try to heighten our picture of all the possible bad consequences of drug use, and then adopt a moral stance toward the good versus the bad effects of the drugs on individuals. What is frustrating is that both grounds shift constantly—both our scientific knowledge about what the effects are, and our moral stance as to whether we see drugs as things that give pleasure and enhance human capabilities, or as things that enslave us. Therefore, it feels to people who like to believe that there are permanent truths, and who like to act on that basis, that it is impossible to act rationally in this area, because you can't work out what the proper ends of policy should be, nor the underlying facts about the effects of drugs. That gives us a very anxious feeling—or at least it does me.

Benowitz: I question the concept of enslavement as being a consequence of drug use in general. Historically, the early phase of the cocaine epidemic consisted of cocaine use by middle-class youth, taking relatively low doses, primarily by sniffing; and most of the use was casual. There was a relatively low addiction rate, and thus no enslavement or great incapacity was engendered. Cocaine became a major health and societal problem when cocaine use (especially intravenous cocaine and crack) became associated with violence on the streets and crime. Only then did the concept of enslavement apply. So I question whether 'enslavement' can be the basis for ethical decisions about cocaine.

Almond: This is again where questions of fact are relevant. If there are drugs which are unarguably non-addictive and harmless, then we must have a different attitude to those drugs—unless, of course, we think that making these fine distinctions is something that will make it socially impossible to control substances acknowledged to be more dangerous.

Jones: I am not sure there is any human behaviour to which some subset of people *don't* seem to become at least temporarily enslaved. I know people who seem to be enslaved by their work. They seem to be out of control in going about their daily work and forget their friends, family and health. Even people seeking good health appear to become enslaved by some things. I have known of people who have suffered multiple stress fractures and still go on jogging! They seem unable to stop.

We haven't mentioned any of the beneficial effects of cocaine, other than in the historical context. Yet only 25 years ago, thoughtful people in the USA argued that there was a positive, utilitarian reason to use cocaine in moderation. Now, this view can be mentioned only with a great deal of guilt. Attitudes change.

Kalant: The point has been raised again that the majority of users of any psychoactive drug, even of heroin or cocaine, do not become addicted. If they can experience sensations which are of interest to them, which give them a view of their own existence and a sense of well-being that is different from what they would have had without using the drugs, is that view not ethically defensible?

Related to that is the question of whether it is theoretically possible, in the view of an ethicist, for any concept of society to exist with full individual freedom. The mere fact of living in a society means automatically some sacrifice of an individual's freedom, because you can't co-exist with another person and both have complete freedom where you impinge on each other. Where do you define the shifting point of optimization?

Almond: My position is largely a matter of supporting the idea that society is entitled to exercise certain constraints on the individual; as far as I know, there isn't any viewpoint, short of anarchy, that would challenge that. I would not like to press a general argument that anything to which one may become addicted is *ipso facto* wrong, however. I was particularly focusing on forms of addiction which affect the mind and the personality.

Kleber: I found your analysis compelling. In terms of some of the specific comments that have arisen in criticism of it, it is interesting that people say that cocaine use earlier on was not 'enslaving', but Charlie Kaplan has told us that a significant percentage of the early cocaine abusers did end up addicted.

They end up in trouble with the drug, either because they have changed the route of administration or because they change the amount that they take.

One of the reasons that certain drugs are permitted by certain societies, over time, in some contexts, and others are not, is this question of relativity. Caffeine has been tolerated by society with relatively few attempts to suppress it, because it is viewed as having useful effects and relatively few users get into trouble from it or have difficulty stopping it if they do. We have made periodic attempts at the prohibition of alcohol, but we have had 2000–3000 years during which alcohol has largely been accepted, for the reason that the majority of people who use it do so moderately and do not get into trouble. Those issues should not be lost sight of when we talk about the policies that society should follow.

Fibiger: Do we know what percentage of alcohol users get into trouble, and how this number compares with the percentage of cocaine users who get into trouble?

Anthony: We have crude measures for the conditional cumulative probability of becoming dependent on alcohol (or for becoming a problem drinker), compared to becoming a daily user of cocaine. (These are estimates for individuals who drink and for individuals who have used cocaine.) Both values are well under 25%, over the life course of adults surviving through the ages of greatest risk. For cocaine, during the period from about 1974 to 1985, the most likely values were substantially less than 25% (Helzer et al 1991, Anthony & Helzer 1991, Anthony & Trinkoff 1989). From those admittedly flawed data, I would guess that a greater proportion of individuals become casualties from their consumption of alcohol than became casualties from their consumption of cocaine, during the most recent cocaine epidemic in the USA.

Fibiger: If that's the case, what is the rationale for having different laws regulating cocaine and alcohol use?

Anthony: The explanation is not because the human species has a substantially longer relationship with alcohol than with opium or cannabis, or perhaps even with coca leaves, because human experience with each of these substances goes back to before written history.

Edwards: I am worried by figures being quoted for the prevalence of harm from any drug, as if this were a natural law rather than something culturally, socially and economically determined. There are villages in Pakistan where the prevalence of opium dependence reached 80%, while, in other villages, opium was virtually unknown. In the hill tribe area of northern Thailand, you find some people (usually in the lower layer of the socioeconomic farming stratum) widely using opium: others, who had their own land and were doing quite nicely, didn't seem to have much use for it. Thus I would hate to see these figures being given universal generality.

Anthony: I agree. Our experience is based on our epidemiological studies of adults in the US population, and I was summarizing the experience for the period from about 1974 to 1985. John Helzer and an international collaborative research group have published relevant figures on alcoholism for a number of countries, including Taiwan, Korea, Canada, Puerto Rico, and the USA (Helzer et al 1990). This work shows a broad range of estimates across those different countries. So the value is certainly not a constant; it is variable. Nonetheless, to answer Dr Fibiger's question, we have to try to hold all else constant while looking for differences between alcohol and cocaine. This is why I tried to compare the recent American experience with cocaine to that obtained with alcoholic beverages.

Kleber: To my mind it would be in any case more accurate to say that the average user of alcohol can continue to use it moderately over a long period of time, say 10–30 years. In the USA we think we have 110 million people who drink, and we have 12–18 million alcoholics and problem drinkers (15%). The cocaine user is more likely to stop after a period of time; if they continue, eventually a higher percentage of cocaine users, certainly a higher percentage than the 15% for alcohol, will get into serious trouble. This is why I do not believe we shall see societies such as the United States permit free access to cocaine. Once you go beyond the raw product, the chewed coca leaf, and into more sophisticated delivery systems, such as smoking or injection, the drug becomes much too addicting. There seems little likelihood of society permitting heroin or cocaine, because the epidemiological evidence is ultimately compelling that these are much more addicting drugs than alcohol to the bulk of people who use them.

Kalant: Just as we stand to learn a lot by comparing different societies in different stages of development and with different social values, we have to remember in evaluating control systems within our own society that comparing alcohol and cocaine can be deceptive. What we should really compare is alcohol as it is—licit—with cocaine as it might be if it too were legal, rather than compare one drug which has heavy restrictions put on it with another which doesn't. In assessing the inherent risks, we have to try to equalize the situation.

Des Jarlais: I also was impressed with Brenda Almond's paper. The question is, as she says, subject to the facts of the situation, for both legal and illegal drugs. Within her analysis, it is hard to understand why we do not make nicotine use illegal! We should also remember that we don't have simple, unified consensus societies where the laws necessarily reflect popular opinion on all issues. These complex societies also contain a lot of conflict. They do change over time. So we need to define an ethical position that will take into account social change and attempt to minimize the adverse effects of people using psychoactive drugs, both legal and illegal. How do we go from an ethical analysis that says that people should not use drugs, to an analysis that includes some people using drugs, and historical changes over time? What ethical positions would help dampen out some of the adverse effects of drug use? Those are the problems to be addressed in the ethics of drug use.

Negrete: I was once asked to look at approaches to prevention. I compared different models of demand reduction and came to the conclusion that the most powerful and effective form of preventive influence on the behaviour of prospective or actual drug users was a moral and ethical one, a common orientation that a particular social group had taken at a given moment in history—not an individual decision, but a collective decision. This is what happened with opium smoking in China, or with marijuana and cocaine use in Cuba. Certainly that is what happened with alcohol drinking in Iran, when the Ayatollah Khomeini returned, starting a powerful social movement based on certain moral principles.

The problem is that collective morality movements are short-lived; they keep shifting, as has happened in Cuba, and is happening in China too; it started with tobacco but they will soon be smoking other things, perhaps heroin. Even in Iran some of the revolutionary guards are already drinking alcohol again. The point is that collective moral attitudes are seldom established as truths forever. We are trying to find a permanent code of socially desirable behaviour, but it doesn't exist.

Strang: I am interested in the question of behaviour *within* drug use. Brenda Almond said that 50% of drug users in Edinburgh who inject intravenously are positive for HIV infection, but these are not necessarily using illegal drugs; most of them in 1990/91 are injecting buprenorphine and temazepam. So it is not a simple question of legality or illegality. What we also need to address is the moral arguments about the current harm-minimization movement (at the level of public and individual policy towards drug users), which is aimed at reducing the damaging nature of the continued use of various drugs— especially injectable drugs. This is an active issue; should one be giving health care to make sure that those who continue to do what we don't want them to do, do it in a 'better' way? This is becoming a large international movement.

Almond: Certainly, whatever rules you make, some people are going to break them. I do agree, then, that you must take account of the facts, and if the law operates so as to *prevent* harm minimization, for example by attempting to close down needle exchanges which facilitate safer drug use through clean syringes, then one has to think again and accommodate one's ideals to the realities of the situation.

O'Brien: I am very impressed with individual differences among drug users, and with our progress in identifying biological mechanisms that may enable us, in the future, to identify people who are likely to become enslaved to drugs. Conversely, there will be people whom we may be able to identify who will be almost guaranteed not to become enslaved. Where does the moral argument take us then, if we have people who could be assured of using a drug like cocaine with just the pleasant aspects of it, and without becoming addicted? Would we be able to prohibit it just from those who were susceptible, and could we give a licence to those whom we can show are genetically determined *not* to become enslaved?

Almond: As far as this argument is concerned—that some people would be all right, at least with some drugs, and should therefore be left to go their own way—again much would turn on the facts of the matter. But even if the facts were favourable, I suspect the argument from example might feature again here. This is the argument that it might be too dangerous for the susceptible majority to allow a minority who are not susceptible to exercise their freedom. This is a possibility.

Kaplan: I think it's extremely important that Brenda Almond has laid out the moral terrain. We should be aware that reason is multiple; there's pure reason, and practical reason. Now, in Frankfurt, there is something called 'aesthetic reason', and also 'cynical reason'. So there are many different kinds of reasoning, and they are tied to particular social, cultural and historical variations.

Almond: The question of which rationality and which morality to adopt is a good question, and it has surfaced a great deal here, implying a background assumption of the relativism of morals. It was with this prevalent assumption in mind that I began my paper with the Greeks, because they were well aware of the relativity of morals, but they thought nevertheless that if you looked at the concept of a human being, you could find principles which would override the differences that depend on place and locality.

Negrete: It seems to be emerging that the cocaine abuse problem is starting to resolve itself, certainly in that part of the world in which it has reached its most active expression, namely North America. Perhaps in Europe the cocaine problem may increase a bit further and then follow the downward trend that started a few years ago in the USA.

That is not the picture in South America. The cocaine problem there is acquiring a magnitude that is truly amazing and is involving more and more people; it is not just the corruption, or the new-found source of labour, or the illegal economic development that is occurring around this drug, but the use of it in a way never known until now.

Coca chewing has been a stable practice for many centuries. It is not part of the current problem in South America; coca chewing will probably continue and outlive what is happening now. But the use of cocaine in its new highly toxic version (coca paste smoking) is perhaps paralleled only by the use of heroin in Southeast Asia when young people started to shun opium smoking. It is something that is likely to expand enormously, not just because the urban population that is mostly involved is growing, and likewise the unemployed and the young who have no sense of purpose, social role or possibility; but also because the drug is there, readily available. This makes the situation very different from that in North America, where cocaine will disappear when people stop buying it. So the picture in South America is different from what has been described for the northern hemisphere. Indeed, it is probably the most threatening drug situation anywhere today.

The ethical issues

O'Brien: While I accept the epidemiological trends showing that the cocaine epidemic is waning in the United States, at the level of the treatment programme where I work in Philadelphia, there is no evidence of a let-up. We are still inundated with requests for treatment, with people desperate for help, coming in psychotic or depressed. I am sure we shall eventually see some of the changes, but we don't see them yet.

Secondly, and related to that, is that there are clearly vulnerable populations. We have touched on the populations of people who are less educated and those who are younger, and certainly people who are poor. Another important population is the mentally ill. In our chronic schizophrenic population in Philadelphia, of those receiving injectable neuroleptics, one-third have cocaine metabolites in their urine. This is very surprising, because these people developed schizophrenia generally before cocaine was available. I don't know whether they are taking the cocaine to combat their schizophrenia-induced anhedonia (lack of pleasure), or, as was suggested earlier, to counteract some of the anhedonia or slowness induced by the neuroleptic drugs. But taking cocaine is antitherapeutic, because cocaine itself can induce psychosis. The drug is so available and so cheap that these people, with their pension money (because they are not organized enough to commit crime for money) are able to finance a certain amount of cocaine use which at the very least is not healthy. This points to another population which those countries that haven't yet been touched by the cocaine epidemic may have to pay attention to.

Balster: I would agree that there is a need to be concerned abut the initial exposure of people to dangerous abused drugs such as cocaine, but I take away from this symposium a renewed belief in the importance of what public health experts would call secondary and tertiary prevention—namely, trying to do what one can to intervene in the escalation to more serious cocaine use, and then to develop adequate treatments for those who need it. What we require is a greater proportion of available money and energy to be spent on demand reduction and on the development of treatments for drug abuse.

Moore: Relating this discussion to earlier comments on what is the right fraction of our effort to put into treatment versus law enforcement and supply reduction, if we do believe that there are epidemic features of drug use, which rises and then falls, it's possible that the right proportion of investment will also change over time. At the beginning of a drug epidemic, before a large number of people are exposed and are advancing down these probabilistic pathways towards disastrous use, it would be important to get primary prevention instruments in place, the principal ones being the mobilization of society, the use of laws to educate people, the effort to control supply, and an effort to get the message across to remind people that these drugs are not entirely harmless. This would be the right approach to take at the beginning phase of an epidemic. Then, as those measures began taking effect, we should move to secondary and tertiary prevention to deal with the casualties that we didn't prevent because our primary prevention instruments came into place too slowly. It is of course important whether you believe that that's the picture that we face—that there are drug epidemics that rise and fall, rather than *endemic* high levels of use that we are constantly dealing with all the time. If you believe in epidemics, you need a way of adapting the instruments to each particular moment that you are facing in the drug epidemic. If that is true, and if our analysis of the epidemic is correct, then everything that people have been saying, which is that our portfolio of policy instruments should be shifting dramatically in the direction of treatment, and special efforts should be made to reach especially vulnerable populations (such as the poor), would be the right way to begin thinking about policy at this stage. This is the important lesson that I take away from the conference. Previously, I did believe that drugs came in epidemics, but I feel more confident about that now than I did before.

Strang: There is something attractive about the idea of having a different profile of response at different stages. But that is a rational analysis. My fear is that there is something about the early stage of society's response to a drug 'epidemic', its strong moral tone, that interferes with our ability to change the profile subsequently. I certainly can see that in the UK.

Moore: You are right; but the challenge for leadership that we face now in dealing with cocaine is precisely that challenge. At the opening of the epidemic, the challenge was to sound the alarm; the challenge at the later stage is to repress the alarm and get a more differentiated response.

Kalant: What has also come out of our discussion is that we cannot talk of 'an' epidemic of cocaine use; we have to talk of several cocaine epidemics, because what has happened in the general population in the USA is very different from what has happened in the Black and Hispanic populations in certain larger urban centres there. And developments in South America are very different from what is happening in Western Europe. So we need much more careful observation, analogous to clinical histories, or natural histories of disease; but they must be natural histories of subpopulations, rather than an exclusive emphasis on statistical data on very large populations that are actually made up of a number of distinct subpopulations.

References

Anthony JC, Trinkoff AM 1989 United States epidemiologic data on drug use and abuse: how are they relevant to testing abuse liability of drugs? In: Fischman MW, Mello NK (eds) Testing for abuse liability of drugs in humans. (National Institute on Drug Abuse Research Monograph 92) US Government Printing Office, Washington, DC, p 241–266

Anthony JC, Helzer JE 1991 Syndromes of drug abuse and dependence. In: Robins LN, Regier DA (eds) Psychiatric disorders in America. The Free Press, New York, p 116–154

Helzer JE, Canino GJ, Yeh EK et al 1990 Alcoholism—North America and Asia. Arch Gen Psychiatry 47:313-319
Helzer JE, Burnam A, McEvoy LT 1991 Alcohol abuse and dependence. In: Robins LN, Regier DA (eds) Psychiatric disorders in America. The Free Press, New York, p 81-115
Southern RW 1953 The making of the middle ages. Yale University Press, London (see especially Chapter 2)

Summing-up

Griffith Edwards

Addiction Research Unit, National Addiction Centre, Institute of Psychiatry, London SE5 8AF, UK

Listening to all that has been going on in this symposium I am persuaded that although our debate has evidently been about the immediate problem of cocaine, it has also and at a deeper level been about cocaine as exemplar of society's general use of, worries about, and responses to, mind-acting drugs. At the immediate cocaine level, the Ciba Foundation has succeeded in bringing together people who have provided an unusually comprehensive series of review statements, and the discussion has usefully clarified both the state of today's knowledge and the gaps in what is known. Most of the relevant research comes from the USA, and I suspect that we are all left with a sense of admiration for the elegance and ingenuity which has been a feature of this research, coupled with dumbfounded awe at the American capacity for get-up-and-go, and the ability to find the funding to make the research happen.

Turning from the drug itself to cocaine as exemplar of the questions which relate to drugs in society, a number of themes can be identified as having run through our debate. Let me try to list some of them, although the ordering does not imply weighting or priority. The general challenge of trying to make a connection between the understandings given by different types of science has been with us, or latent, in our discussions all the time: you can either regard the issue of interdisciplinarity as boring, a cliché, or as an absolutely fundamental challenge which will not go away, although it is all too seldom effectively addressed. Linked to that theme has been an element in the debate which, rather than centring on collaboration between disciplines in the common task of explaining drug use and dependence, has on the contrary circled rather delicately around rivalry, hegemony, and who gets the dollars. It is notable that a significant proportion of the American research budget for cocaine has been directed at biological and biomedical questions, and in comparison only vestigial support has been given to history. Some of us might perhaps be attracted to the revolutionary notion of the world turned upside down, with multimillion dollar support given to a historical research initiative on drugs, or with the money put toward work on the dynamics of drug epidemics, with just a little funding around the margins for molecular biology. Absurd, most people will say. But why? This meeting at least approached that kind of question.

Summing up

The theme of a 'drug epidemic' is certainly a fundamentally important concept which has cross-cut several of our debates, and the disturbing point which David Musto makes about society's capacity to experience memory blackout for past drug epidemics could be widely generalized beyond cocaine. Could one perhaps conclude that across the whole field of drug problems, drug research, the treatment of drug users and drug prevention policies, we too often get locked into short-term anxieties and dealing with immediate problems? Should we instead be more ready to admit that while research of many kinds can usefully add to this or that part of the immediate sum of knowledge, the larger issue is how we are to deal with drug problems which affect many individuals over a life course, and work for a better understanding of the dynamics of drug epidemics which ebb and flow over decades or even centuries?

Lastly, perhaps I may as Chairman be allowed to thank you all for your courtesy and goodwill which have made our time together so pleasurable, and thank the Ciba Foundation and its staff for their organization of this meeting.

Index of contributors

Non-participating co-authors are indicated by asterisks. Entries in bold type indicate papers; other entries refer to discussion contributions

Indexes compiled by John Rivers

Almond, B., 36, 144, 186, 237, 251, 275, 276, **277**, 284, 286, 289, 290
*Alterman, A., **207**
Anthony, J. C., **20**, 34, 35, 36, 37, 39, 55, 56, 76, 145, 163, 177, 192, 201, 237, 284, 287

Balster, R. L., 54, 89, 92, 112, 115, 162, 205, 290
Benowitz, N. L., 37, 52, 74, 91, 92, 122, 125, 143, 144, 146, 147, 174, 217, 285
*Bieleman, B., **57**
*Brown, E. E., **96**

*Childress, A. R., **207**

Des Jarlais, D. C., 35, 79, 119, 146, 164, 178, 181, 188, 189, 204, 217, 239, 240, 258, 273, 288

Edwards, G., **1**, 18, 35, 39, 74, 75, 80, 93, 123, 144, 146, 147, 186, 189, 193, 201, 205, 216, 222, 232, 233, 234, 236, 252, 259, 273, 275, 287, **294**

Fibiger, H. C., 36, 90, 92, **96**, 111, 112, 113, 114, 115, 117, 118, 119, 162, 178, 179, 205, 287
Fischman, M. W., 51, 52, 74, 116, 117, 122, 145, **165**, 173, 174, 175, 176, 177, 178, 179, 201
*Foltin, R. W., **165**

Gerstein, D. R., 19, 55, 56, 203, 217, 234, 275

Jaffe, J. H., 33, 93, 94, 117, 118, 120, 121, 122, 144, 202, 203, 204, 218, 220, 237, 254, 260, 273
Jones, R. T., 50, 52, 74, 75, 78, 93, 94, 120, 121, 122, 177, 188, 201, 222, **224**, 234, 286

Kalant, H., 16, 71, 38, 52, 53, 77, 79, 90, 113, 114, 121, 145, 161, 162, 163, 174, 175, 176, 192, 205, 221, 232, 252, 259, **261**, 272, 273, 274, 275, 286, 288, 292
Kaplan, C. D., 53, **57**, 73, 75, 78, 79, 80, 119, 163, 233, 259, 260, 290
Kleber, H. D., 14, 15, 34, 35, 52, 55, 75, 79, 91, 92, 93, 112, 113, 116, 117, 120, 146, 147, 186, 188, 189, 193, **195**, 201, 202, 203, 205, 219, 222, 223, 238, 239, 240, 256, 257, 272, 273, 275, 286, 288
Kuhar, M. J., 17, **81**, 90, 91, 92, 114, 117, 118, 162, 193

*McLellan, A. T., **207**
Maynard, A., 56, 144, 188, **242**, 252, 253, 254, 255, 256, 257, 259
Moore, M. H., 35, 54, 73, 76, 186, 190, 203, 204, 205, 220, 235, 237, 253, 254, 256, 260, 274, 284, 285, 290, 292
Musto, D. F., **7**, 14, 15, 16, 17, 18, 39, 50, 123, 179, 191, 238, 239, 284

Negrete, J. C., 17, 36, **40**, 50, 51, 52, 53, 54, 77, 90, 113, 115, 118, 119, 120, 143, 146, 173, 174, 179, 187, 192, 200, 203, 218, 273, 275, 289, 290

296

Index of contributors

O'Brien, C. P., 37, 77, 92, 111, 121, 178, 192, 204, **207**, 216, 217, 218, 219, 221, 223, 240, 258, 289, 290

*Phillips, A. G., **96**

Strang, J., 51, 119, 120, 121, 147, 177, 192, 219, 232, 253, 256, 275, 289, 292

*TenHouten, W. D., **57**

Uchtenhagen, A., 15, 233, 255, 256

Woolverton, W. L., 90, 91, 92, 113, 115, **149**, 161, 162, 163, 164, 176, 177, 189, 234, 260

Subject index

Acquired immune deficiency syndrome (AIDS), HIV infection and, cocaine users, in, 181-194, 275, 276, 278, 279, 283
  areas for future research, 185-194
  intravenous injection and, 181, 182, 183
  sexual behaviour and, 183, 184, 185
  See also 'Crack'
Addiction See Cocaine dependence
African-Americans, cocaine dependence among, 77
AIDS See Acquired immune deficiency syndrome
Alcohol
  abuse
    adverse consequences, 287
    animal models, 176, 177
    psychotherapy for, 207, 216
    cocaine effects potentiated by, 11, 89
    price and consumption, 267
    public image of, 238
    role in priming for drug use, 38
  use
    cocaine use and, 56, 287, 288
    cost-benefit analysis, 284
    patterns of change in, 76
Amantadine, 198
Amphetamines, 87, 91, 99, 100, 102, 226
  toxicity, 147
Amsterdam, surveys, 58, 59, 69
  See also Netherlands
Anaesthesia, local, cocaine in, 9, 125, 127, 128, 129, 151
Anhedonia, 168, 196, 291
Anhydroecgonine methyl ester, 129
Antidepressants, tricyclic See Desipramine
Antipsychotic drugs, 115
Anxiety, cocaine abuse, in, 129
Apomorphine, 99
Aristotle, 277, 280
Arrhythmias, cardiac, 130, 133, 143
  β-blockers in, 144
Ascending methodologies, 75, 76

Athletics, cocaine use in, 7, 8
Attention deficit disorder, 79, 198
Autonomy
  individual, 277, 278, 279, 280, 281, 283, 286
  J. S. Mill and, 280-282
  social issues in, 280-282, 283, 286
  national and international, 278, 282

Basuca, 43, 51
Behavioural abnormalities, cocaine abuse and, 129, 145
Behavioural economics, 163
Benzylecgonine, 83, 127, 128
'Binge', 34, 37, 74, 77, 79, 166, 167, 181, 196
  animal equivalent, 175
Bromocriptine, 198
Buprenorphine, 113, 205, 289
Butler, Joseph, 279

Canada, cocaine problem in, 232, 263, 265, 268, 269
  demand reduction efforts, 268, 272, 273
  legal status, 268
Cannabis
  – cocaine connection, 234, 239
  legal restraints against, country variations, 269
  Spain and Italy, in, 275, 276
  UK seizures of, 246
Carbamazepine, 200, 202
Cardiovascular complications of cocaine abuse, 128, 129, 130, 132, 133, 143, 167, 168, 169, 170, 263
Catecholamines, elevated in cocaine abuse, 91, 92, 129, 130, 143, 262, 263
Central nervous system stimulation, cocaine causing, 128, 129, 130, 263
Chlorpromazine, 87, 97, 179
Chocolate cocaine tablets, 10, 11, 50

Subject index

Coca-Cola, 7, 10, 50
Coca leaf, 7, 8, 17, 41
  chewing, 2, 8, 40, 41, 43, 44, 50, 290
    cocaine dose absorbed, 50, 51
    cultural history of, 51, 53, 54
    mental impairment causing, 47
  growing, 40, 41, 42, 43
Coca paste (*pasta basica*), 5, 17, 119
  manufacture, 42, 43
  smoking, 45, 46, 290
    health problems in, 47, 52
    increasing use of, 52, 53
    onset, 51
    social patterns in, 45, 53
Coca wines, 7, 9, 10, 11, 50
Cocaethylene, 89, 201
Cocaine
  abuse *See Cocaine abuse*
  action *See Dopamine hypothesis*
  addiction to *See Cocaine dependence*
  alcohol potentiating, 11, 89
  alternative reinforcers, 26, 155-157, 158, 163, 164, 175, 190
  analogues, 83, 89, 127, 128
  behavioural responses to, 149, 150, 152, 154
  binding sites, 82, 83, 90
  blood levels, method of administration and, 116, 126
  brain levels, rate of change in, 116, 117, 120, 122
  caffeine potentiating, 11
  central nervous system stimulated by, 128, 129, 130
  chocolate, 10, 11
  clinical pharmacology, 126-128
  'crack' *See 'Crack'*
  craving for, 145, 154, 163, 167, 170, 196, 197, 211, 212, 214
  demand, control of, 268, 273, 282, 290
    health-orientated campaign, 270
    increase in effort, 270
  epidemic, 20, 21, 292, 295
    See also US cocaine problem
  half-life, 127, 128, 129
  hypertension caused by, 128, 129, 130, 131, 143, 201
  intoxication *See Cocaine abuse; Cocaine dependence*
  local anaesthetic, as, 9, 125, 127, 128, 129, 151
  locomotor stimulant effects, 102, 103
  metabolism, 127
  molecular mechanisms, 81-95, 190
  neonatal effects, 133-135, 144
  pregnancy and, 133, 134
  receptor for, 81, 82
    See also Dopamine transporter
  reinforcing properties, 7, 8, 9, 11, 12, 13, 17, 27, 45, 81, 82, 86, 87, 90, 96, 97, 118, 128, 149, 150, 262
    breaking point, 97, 99, 107
    cholinergic systems and, 92
    dopamine and, 114, 115
    environmental/behavioural determinants, 154-157, 158, 159, 163, 164
    genetic determinants, 150
    method of ingestion and, 168
    pharmacological determinants, 150, 151-153, 157, 158, 159
    reward and, 161, 162
    schedules of, 97, 100, 107, 154, 163, 164
  -related death, 125, 130-132, 146, 147, 265
    hyperthermia in, 129, 147
  reproduction and, 133-135
  self-administration *See Cocaine self-administration, animal; Cocaine self-administration, human*
  sensitization to, 152
    conditioned stimuli and, 103, 111, 112, 115
    enhanced dopaminergic response in, 102, 103
  serotonergic activity in, 22, 29, 31, 91, 92
  structure-activity studies, 82, 83, 87
  supply, control of, 204, 268, 290
    cost of, 264, 268
    international co-operation in, 282, 283
    reduction in effort, 270
  tolerance to, 128, 167, 168
  toxicity, 125-148
    assessment of, 135-141, 145, 146
    behavioural consequences, 145
    chlorpromazine and, 179
    cigarette smoking contrasted with, 140, 141, 144
    hospital treatment, 146, 147
    intravenous injection and, 177, 178
    mechanisms of, 129
    oral ingestion and, 126, 127
    unicausality, 135, 144

Cocaine abuse, 196, 199, 214
  acute, medical complications, 129, 131
  cardiovascular effects, 128, 129, 130, 132, 133
  chronic, 129
  dopamine system changes in, 92, 93
  euphoriant effects *See Euphoria*
  liability to, 165, 166, 176
  life-threatening complications, 129, 130
  neurophysiological adaptation in, 196
  noradrenaline uptake blockade and, 91
  outside compulsion to stop, 175, 273
  sensitization in, 102, 111
  treatment approaches, 86, 87, 195, 202, 203
    combined approach, 199, 215
    pharmacological *See Pharmacotherapy*
    psychological *See Psychotherapy*
    recovery in, 199
    relapse in, 199, 211, 212
    scientific vs political considerations in, 192, 193
    substitution, 119
    withdrawal symptoms in, 168, 196
  See also Cocaine use, non-medical; Cocaine users
Cocaine dependence, 10, 77, 79
  crime, as, 227, 228, 236
  treatment strategies, 119, 185, 187, 191, 207
    cost-effectiveness, 188
    goals of national strategy, 188, 189
    models for, 228, 229
    policies for, 229, 230, 238, 239, 290
    psychotherapy for *See Psychotherapy*
    public health approach, 228, 229
    science vs law and morality, 123
    social dimensions, 230, 231
Cocaine hydrochloride, 43, 52, 53, 126
  smoking, 121
  'snorting', 53, 54
Cocaine 'kids', 71
Cocaine-producing countries, problems of, 264, 282
Cocaine self-administration, animal, 4, 96, 97, 98, 100, 149–164
  alternative reinforcers in, 155–157, 158, 163, 164, 190
  behaviour in, 82, 86
    predictive of human behaviour, 150, 158, 165, 175, 176, 177, 178
  choice in, 154, 155, 156, 157
  dopamine levels in, 105, 106, 107, 113, 114
  elasticity of demand in, 263
  nucleus accumbens lesions in, 98, 99
  preference in, 155
  prefrontal cortex, to, 100
  punishment in, 154, 155, 158, 189
  sensitization to cocaine and, 164
  serotonin and, 107
  simple rate measures, 97, 100
  See also Cocaine self-administration, human
Cocaine self-administration, human, 165–180
  alternative reinforcers, 175
  choice in, 167, 168, 170
  desipramine maintenance, 170–172, 179, 197, 200, 201, 202
  dose levels in, 167, 168, 171
  drug abuse liability and, 165, 166, 176
  drug-taking behaviour, 166, 172, 179
    animal models predictive of, 150, 158, 165, 175, 176, 177, 178
  method of ingestion, preference in, 168, 170, 173, 174, 177
  subjective effects, 167, 168, 169, 170, 171
  tolerance to, 167, 168
  treatment medication, 169–172, 174, 175
  verbal reports, 165, 168, 172
  volunteers, 166
  withdrawal symptoms, 168
Cocaine use, non-medical
  adverse consequences, 125, 133, 263, 278, 279
  animal studies, 2, 3, 4, 96, 97, 98, 99, 149–164
  availability and consumption, 266, 267
  'binge' *See 'Binge'*
  cost-benefit analysis, 278, 279, 280, 284, 285
  costs of, 262–264, 269, 278
    measurement of, 144
  crime associated with, 264, 275, 278
  cultural context, 2, 3
  determinants of, 22, 26–28, 54
  epidemiology, 20–39, 54, 55, 56, 190
    See also US cocaine problem
  ethnological studies, 2, 60, 67, 74, 79, 189

Subject index

health impact, 28-32, 56
health policy issues and, 70, 71
heroin use and, 27, 28, 33, 34
historical context, 1, 2
illicit status, problems of, 264
laboratory studies, social and medical applications, 3, 186, 189, 190, 191
legal controls, 264, 270, 274
  consumption and, 267-269
mental and behavioural disturbances in, 22, 27, 28-31, 45
methods of ingestion
  chewing *See Coca leaf chewing*
  elimination and, 120
  intravenous injection, 18, 53, 70, 77, 96, 120, 122, 126, 127, 135, 168, 173, 174, 177, 178, 258
  peak concentration and, 121, 122
  smoking, 17, 18, 31, 45, 46, 70, 74, 77, 119, 120, 121, 122, 126, 135, 168, 173, 174
  'snorting', 53, 54, 70, 119, 120, 126, 127, 135, 174
moral and ethical aspects, 262, 267, 270, 275, 277-283
pattern of change in, 74-76, 77
patterns of, 78
perceived effects, 27, 28-32
perspectives on, 1-6
prevention, 187
price and consumption, 267
risks of, 263, 269, 278, 279
  assessment of, 147, 148
risk-taking, altered attitude to, 279
social aspects, 280-282
social contact variables, 60-63
US, in *See US cocaine problem*
withdrawal syndrome in, 168
Cocaine users
basis for categorization, 67
categories of, 59, 60, 77-80
  casual, 58-63, 66, 67, 68, 69, 70, 71, 77, 79, 228
  compulsive, 67, 68, 69, 70, 74, 75, 77, 78, 79, 166, 228, 250
  controlled, 60, 67, 68, 69, 70, 71, 73, 74, 77, 78, 79
  daily, 74, 75, 76, 77, 78, 79, 181, 228
  salient, 68, 69, 70, 71, 78
clinical populations, 58
community-based surveys, 58, 59, 69
patterns of change in, 74-76, 77

situational factors, 79
'snowball sampling' methodology, 63-65, 75, 80
See also Cocaine abuse; Cocaine dependence; Cocaine use, non-medical
Conditioned responses, 103, 111, 112, 115, 211, 212, 213, 218
'Crack' (cocaine free base) smoking, 12, 31, 35, 51, 52, 70, 119, 120, 121, 126, 168, 227, 238, 263, 265, 272
  link with crime, 278
  -related sexual behaviour, 183, 184, 185
  sexually transmitted diseases and, 183, 191
'Crack baby' syndrome, 134, 144
'Crash', 167, 196, 199, 214
Cortex, prefrontal
  cocaine reinforcement and, 102, 119
  cocaine effect on dopamine in, 102, 113, 114
  cocaine self-administration to, reward and, 100, 114, 119
  6-OHDA lesions and 102, 114

Death, cocaine-related, 125, 130-132, 146, 147, 265
'Decriminalization', 266, 283
Delirium, agitated, cocaine abuse, in, 129, 132
Delusion/hallucination, 31
'Denormalization' policy, 226, 229, 233, 239
Dependence *See Cocaine dependence*
Depression, 26, 27, 31, 34, 35, 36, 37, 168, 196
Desipramine, cocaine self-administration and, 170-172, 179, 197, 200, 201, 202
Dopamine
  CNS synapses, in, 159
  concentrations
    behaviour pattern and, 114
    cocaine dosage and, 112, 113, 114
    cocaine self-administration, in, 105, 106, 107
    rate of change in, 116, 117
Dopamine hypothesis of cocaine action, 86, 87, 97, 112, 113, 163

Dopamine receptors D_1, D_2
  agonists, 151, 153
  antagonists, 151, 152, 153
    cocaine reinforcement and, 97, 98, 103, 111
    cocaine reinforcement and, 119, 152, 153, 158
  See also Dopamine transporter
Dopamine transporter, 81, 82, 87, 90, 115, 205
  characterization, 83, 85
  chronic cocaine administration and, 92
  cocaine binding at, 82, 83
  cDNA cloned, 85, 87, 205
  receptor blockers, 86, 87
  re-uptake, cocaine inhibiting, 81, 83, 86, 90, 102, 151, 153, 158
Dopaminergic neurotransmission, cocaine reinforcement and, 151
Drug dependence, 227, 250
  WHO definition, 68
  See also Cocaine dependence
Drug education projects, 186
Drug epidemic, 295
  See also Cocaine epidemic
Drug markets
  economics of, 243-246, 252, 253, 254, 258, 259
    behavioural economics, 259, 260
    demand elasticity, 243, 244, 245, 253
    price elasticity, 254, 255, 256
    social values and, 259
    treatment programmes and, 253, 254, 290
  regulation of, 242, 243, 248-251
    addiction and, 250
    benefits of, 250
    control of supply, 254, 255
    law enforcement and, 242, 243, 244, 245, 246, 247, 248, 253, 255, 256, 290
    legalization, arguments for and against, 249, 250, 251, 252, 257
Drug policies, cost-effectiveness, 244
Drug-seeking behaviour See Cocaine craving
Drug treatment, alternative strategies, 224-241
See also Pharmacotherapy, Psychotherapy
Drug use and abuse, 225
  criminal activity in, 258
  criminal behaviour and, 249

ethical, social and political issues, 277-293
falling prevalence in some countries, 265, 268, 269, 273, 274
harm minimization in, 289
moral attitudes to, 288, 289, 290
punishment through law, 225, 226, 229
user accountability measures, 175, 273
See also Cocaine abuse; Cocaine use, non-medical; Cocaine users

Ecgonine, 83, 127, 128
Enslavement, addiction seen as, 279, 285, 286, 289
  willingness to experience, 284
Erythroxylum spp., 40, 52, 53
Ethical issues, 277-293
  social and political issues interconnected, 277
Ethnographic surveys, 2, 60, 67, 74, 79, 189
Euphoria, 9, 12, 68, 161, 172, 179, 196, 198, 214
Europe, Western, cocaine abuse in, 292
  legal controls, 264
  prevalence levels, 58
  responses to, 233, 234
Fluoxetine, 107, 198
Flupenthixol, 86, 97, 198
c-*fos* gene, cocaine activation of, 108
Freud, Sigmund (1856-1939), 8, 16, 39

GABA transporter, cloning of, 85
GBR 12909, 83, 90

Hall's wine, 11, 50
Haloperidol, response to intravenous cocaine and, 87, 97, 115, 116, 117, 118, 119, 179
Halsted, William Stewart (1852-1922), 9, 10
Happiness, short-term vs. freedom, long-term, 279, 280
Harm minimization approach, 232, 233, 240, 289
Harrison Act (1914) See US cocaine problem
Headache, cocaine abuse, in, 130

Heroin, 226, 227, 285
  legal status, Netherlands, in, 268
  price, consumption and, 245, 252, 253
  price-crime spillover, 245
  seizures, UK, 246
  stimulant properties, cocaine compared, 27, 28
  use and abuse
    AIDS and HIV infection and, 181, 187, 188, 204
    cocaine use and, 33, 34, 121
    combined treatment, 204
    Italy, in, 275
    methadone treatment, 93, 94, 203, 204
    psychotherapy for, 216
HIV infection *See Human immunodeficiency virus infection*
Holland, drug abuse in *See Netherlands*
Human immunodeficiency virus (HIV) infection, AIDS and cocaine users, in, 181–194, 275, 276, 278
  other drug use, in, 289
6-Hydroxydopamine (6-OHDA) lesions, 98, 99, 102, 114
5-Hydroxytryptamine (5-HT) *See Serotonin*
Hypertension, cocaine abuse, in, 128, 129, 130
Hyperthermia, cocaine abuse, in, 129, 147

Infertility, drug abuse and, 32
Italy, drug abuse in, 233, 275

Law enforcement, drug market and, 242, 243, 244, 245, 246, 247, 253, 264, 267–269
  educational value of laws, 274
  individual autonomy and, 278
  social considerations and, 280–282
  See also Legislation; US cocaine problem
Legalization, cocaine use, of, 262, 265, 266, 283
Legislation
  cocaine and, 225, 226, 227, 228, 229, 230, 232, 233
  marijuana and, 238, 239
Libertarianism, 251, 262, 280–282
Lithium, 197

LSD (lysergic acid diethylamide), 12, 138–139 (tables), 176, 226, 253, 285
Locomotor activity, 114
  conditioned, 103, 111

Mania, 31
Marijuana, 12, 139, 141, 145, 226, 227, 238, 253, 258
  legal status, 238, 239
  use, cocaine use and, 37, 38, 39
Mesolimbic system, 102
Mesolimbocortical pathway, dopamine and, 82, 86, 87
Methadone, 93, 94, 203, 204, 205, 240
Methylphenidate, 86, 198
Miami survey *See US cocaine problem*
Microdialysis, 100, 101, 102, 103, 107, 111, 113, 114
Mill, J. S., 280, 281
Mood disturbances, 22, 29
Mydriasis, cocaine abuse and, 129
Myocardial infarction, 132
Myocarditis, 143

Naloxone, 94
Naltrexone, 118
Netherlands, drug abuse in, 268, 269
  legal situation, 267, 268
  response to, 233, 234
  See also under Amsterdam, Rotterdam
Neuroleptics
  cocaine abuse treatment, in, 198
  cocaine self-administration and, 97, 98, 179, 180
  schizophrenia treatment, in, 291
  See also Flupenthixol, Haloperidol
Neuroleptic malignant syndrome, 132, 147
Neurotransmitter
  re-uptake, cocaine inhibiting, 81
  systems, cocaine action and, 91, 112, 115
  transporters, 81, 85
Nicotine
  animal models of abuse, 177
  intravenous, tobacco smoking compared, 122, 123
  self-administration, 174, 175
Nifedipine, 117
Noradrenaline (Norepinephrine)
  receptor antagonists, cocaine self-administration and, 97
  transporter, 85, 90
  uptake
    cocaine inhibiting, 91, 112, 151

Noradrenaline (Norepinephrine) *(cont.)*
  uptake *(cont.)*
    reinforcing action of cocaine and, 151, 152
  uptake blockade, cocaine toxicity and, 91
Norway, drug abuse in, 268, 269
Nucleus accumbens
  cocaine reinforcement, in, 102
  dopamine concentration increased by cocaine, 102, 105, 106, 107
    environmental stimuli and, 103
  dopamine transporter in, 84, 85, 90
  lesions of dopaminergic innervation, 98, 99

Obsessive-compulsive disorder, 22, 31
Opiate addiction, 59, 136, 196, 213, 229, 266, 268, 287
  law enforcement, 15, 258, 268
  research on, 93, 94

Panic attacks, 22, 31, 35, 36, 129
Paternalism, 281
Personal self-interest, 279, 280
Pharmacotherapy, 162, 197-205
  alcohol and, 201
  drug development for, 205
  efficacy, 201, 202
  evaluation, 168, 169
  side effects, 197, 198, 199, 200, 201, 215, 240
Phencyclidine, 139, 140
  legal status in Netherlands, 268
Pimozide, 97, 111
Place preference, 118
Policy formulation, 261
  cost-benefit assessment, 261, 262, 275
  value judgements in, 275
  See also under Drug abuse; US cocaine problem
Preference, cocaine self-administration, in, 155
Procaine, 90, 176, 177
Propranolol, 143
Prostitution, drug-related, 183, 184, 188, 278
Psychiatric disturbances, cocaine abuse, in, 22, 31, 32, 36, 37, 52, 77, 129, 263
Psychobehavioural variables, cocaine use, in, 59, 70

Psychotherapy, drug dependence, in, 197, 202, 207-223
  after-care, 220, 221
  counselling and, 213, 215
  cue densitization in, 212, 215, 218
  extinction, 213, 214, 215, 218
  implications for future policy, 220
  responses to, 214, 219, 220
  social and moral purposes in, 222
  subject selection for, 208, 216, 217, 218, 219
  'success' vs. relapse, 220, 221
  supportive-expressive, 213, 215
Punishment
  cocaine self-administration and, 154, 155
  drug abuse deterrent, 225, 226, 229

Random assignment clinical trials, 207
Rehabilitation
  day hospital, 207, 208-211
  in-patient, 208-211
Relapse after treatment, 199, 211, 212, 213, 220
  cocaine-related cues in, 212
Respiratory arrest, cocaine abuse, in, 129
Reward, cocaine-induced, 96, 97, 98, 100, 107, 118, 262
  dopamine systems and, 161, 162
  lesion studies, 98, 99, 100
  neural circuitry of, 107, 108
Richardson, Benjamin Ward, 1, 3, 191
Risk-taking, drugs affecting attitudes to, 279
Rotterdam, cocaine use in
  'casual' users, 58
  'snowball sampling' methodology in, 63-65
  See also Amsterdam, Netherlands
'Rush' phenomenon, 117, 118, 161, 174

SCH 23390, 97
Schizophrenia, paranoid, chronic drug abuse, in, 129
Seizures, 32, 52, 129, 130
Serotonergic activity, 22, 293
Serotonergic neurotransmitter system, 112
Serotonin (5-hydroxytryptamine, 5-HT) uptake, 91, 92
  cocaine inhibiting, 91, 112, 129, 151

Subject index

cocaine self-administration and, 107
reinforcing action of cocaine and, 151, 152, 158
re-uptake blockers, 198
Sertraline, 198
'Snowball sampling' methodology, 63–65, 75
Social contact variables of cocaine use, 60–63, 65, 67, 68, 69, 70, 73, 74
  involvement in network relationships, 59, 61, 62, 64, 65, 66, 67, 68, 71
  social network density, 62, 68
  scope of settings, 61, 62, 64, 65, 66, 67, 68, 69, 74
South America, cocaine production and use in, 40–56, 274, 290, 292
  AIDS and HIV infection and, 185
  epidemiology, 41–46, 52, 54, 55
  health problems, 47, 52, 54
  social, economic and ecological consequences, 47, 49, 54
  See also Coca leaf chewing; Coca paste smoking
Spain, drug abuse in, 233, 275, 276
Striatum
  dopamine concentrations, cocaine increasing, 101, 102
  dopamine transporter in, 84, 85, 90
Stroke, 32, 52, 130
Suicide attempts, 22, 29–31, 34, 35, 36, 37
Sulpiride, 97

Temazepam, 289
Tobacco smoking vs. intravenous nicotine, 122
Transporter proteins, cloning of, 85
  See also Dopamine transporter
Tryptophan, 199
Tyrosine, 199

United Kingdom
  approach to cocaine problem, 232
  demand reduction efforts in, 272, 273
  drug market, 246–248
    law enforcement in, 242–248
    price, 247
    seizures, 246, 247, 256
United States, cocaine problem
  African-Americans, in, 77
  AIDS and HIV infection and, 181–194
  American Association of Poison Centers Survey, 136, 137
  Anti-Drug Abuse Acts (1986, 1988), 12
  cocaine epidemic, 20, 21, 23–26, 265, 290, 291, 292
    alternative reinforcers, availability, 164
    changes in cocaine use, 57
    changes in perception of cocaine use, 57, 190, 191
    exposure opportunities, 24, 25, 38
    initiation and progression of use, factors in, 22, 26–28
    perceived consequences, 22, 27, 28, 29
  constitutional rights and, 225, 226, 227, 230, 236
    individual vs community rights, 237
  Drug Abuse Warning Network (DAWN) Report, 135, 136, 139, 140, 145, 146
  demographic trends, 21
    age-specific prevalence, 23, 24, 25, 37, 38
    population susceptibility, 24, 25, 37, 38, 291
    prevalence, duration and incidence, 23–26, 37, 38, 57
  funding for treatment and research, 93, 237, 257, 294
  government policy, 225, 229, 234, 235, 238
  Harrison Act (1914), 11, 13, 15, 17
  illicit market, 10, 11, 13, 16, 17
    street price, 10, 14, 15, 16, 17, 255
  law enforcement in, 225, 226, 227, 228, 229, 230, 232, 236
  legal status and availability, 8, 9, 10, 11, 12, 13, 15, 18, 19
  Miami Survey, 59, 69, 70
  moral perspectives in, 225, 226, 229, 235, 236, 237, 240
  National Household Survey data, 139, 146
  nineteenth century, 7–11, 17, 264
  public attitude to, tolerance/intolerance patterns, 12, 13, 15, 16, 18, 37, 190, 191, 192, 193, 284, 285, 286
  San Francisco Friendship Network Survey, 59, 60, 74, 75
  social and racial factors, 15, 16, 19, 23, 26, 27, 226, 230, 231, 239, 240
  treatment policy, 230, 239, 291
  twentieth century, 10–13, 14, 15, 16, 17, 18, 19, 207
  War on Drugs, 224, 226, 227, 265, 266, 268

Universalizability, 279
Utilitarianism, 235, 278, 283

Ventral tegmental area (VTA), 6-OHDA lesions, 100, 113
   dopamine in, 102

Vin Mariani, 7, 8, 10, 11, 17

War on Drugs, The, 224, 226, 227, 265, 266, 268